T0212121

Contemporary Issues in Gerontology

Promoting Positive Ageing

V. MINICHIELLO AND I. COULSON
EDITORS

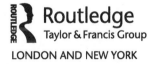
Routledge
Taylor & Francis Group

LONDON AND NEW YORK

First published 2005
by Routledge
2 Park Square, Milton Park, Abingdon, Oxon, OX14 4RN, UK
Simultaneously published in the USA and Canada
by Routledge
605 Third Avenue, New York, NY 10017
Simultaneously published in Australia and New Zealand
by Allen & Unwin
83 Alexander Street, Crows Nest, Sydney, NSW 2065, Australia

Routledge is an imprint of the Taylor & Francis Group, an informa business

© 2005 Victor Minichiello and Irene Coulson

Typeset in 10/12 pt Hiroshige by Midland Typesetters, Maryborough,
Vic., Australia

Notice:
Product or corporate names may be trademarks or registered trademarks, and
are used only for identification and explanation without intent to infringe.

British Library Cataloguing in Publication Data
A catalogue record for this book is available from the British Library
Library of Congress Cataloging in Publication Data
A catalog record for this book has been requested

Publisher's Note
The publisher has gone to great lengths to ensure the quality of this reprint
but points out that some imperfections in the original may be apparent.

ISBN 13: 978-0-415-36429-4 (hbk)

Foreword

Human ageing is a global phenomenon, linking north, south, east and west. Indeed, while the more developed countries aged substantially in the last century, it is the less developed ones that will see the greatest and most rapid increase in the number of people aged 60 years and over during the first half of this century. The global increase in this age group will be from 10 per cent of the total population in 1998 to 21 per cent in 2050 (from around 600 to almost 2000 million) and, in the less developed countries, the absolute numbers are expected to quadruple.

In the face of this demographic revolution, which presents major challenges to families and communities as well as governments, a strategy is required to ensure that the extra years added to life are quality years rather than being spent in poverty, ill-health, disability and isolation. To paraphrase the World Health Organisation: 'Years have been added to life—now we must ensure that life is added to those years'. Instead of the 'apocalyptic demography' and alarmist newspaper headlines that often greet new data on the scale of population ageing with negative images, what is required is a positive perspective that sees ageing as a lifelong process and older people as significant contributors to family, community and economic life; whose potential is not realised.

That is where this book scores handsomely. As its subtitle suggests, this collection is orientated towards positive ageing and this theme is pursued consistently from chapter to chapter. While its positive focus on active life expectancy is more than sufficient for me to commend this collection to students of gerontology everywhere, it also has an admirably practical dimension alongside its scientific core. Each chapter includes case studies and proposed activities, policy prescriptions and guidance for practitioners. This will make it invaluable as a textbook for practitioners—such as nurses and care workers who are training to work with older people. The chapters themselves are substantially literature reviews covering the key issues under each topic and these issues range widely across the gerontology field. Victor Minichiello and Irene Coulson have assembled a talented cast and, therefore, each contribution is of a very high quality.

The book begins with a powerful argument against ageism (labelled in the United Kingdom as the last unrecognised discrimination) as the basis for positive ageing. In Chapter 2 the centrality of health to positive or active ageing is demonstrated. The increasingly important topic of mental health is discussed in Chapter 3. While recognising the multiple determinants of well-being in old age the importance of social networks and social support are highlighted. Minichiello is one of the pioneers in the field of sexuality and ageing and Chapter 4 dispels some of the grossly ageist stereotypes on this topic, especially the myth of the asexual older person. This Chapter challenges the commonplace ageist assumptions behind how society views the sexuality of older people. Chapter 5 provides a valuable guide to the prevention of dementia, pointing to the key roles of self-actualisation or spiritual growth and healthy lifestyles. The need for a new policy paradigm on work and retirement is demonstrated in Chapter 6. Then Catherine Bridge and Hal Kendig, in their consideration of housing and the built environment in Chapter 7, argue for an environmental approach to supporting older people. Again there are plenty of practical interventions that aim to promote wellbeing. Chapter 8 is an extensive review of gerontological research on caregiving. Among many other topics Neena Chappell and Glenda Parmenter refer to the trend across the more developed countries to concentrate care resources on those in greatest need, a policy which undermines the preventative potential of supportive services. The following chapter on service delivery complements nicely this account of informal care. Chapter 10 concentrates on the promotion of positive ageing and looks at interventions and lifestyle choices not commonly found in gerontology textbooks, but used increasingly by older people themselves to achieve active ageing and a positive outlook. These include natural therapies, such as acupuncture and massage, spirituality, music and wellbeing. Health professionals are given clear guidance in these novel areas. The final chapter examines the role of technology in independent living and relates gerontechnology to a broad-based health promotion model. The central message here is the need to involve older people in shaping the technology that affects their lives.

As this foreword indicates, the scope of the book is wide while the analysis achieves depth as well. Having been, for the last five years, director of the largest social science research programme ever mounted in the United Kingdom, the Growing Older (GO) Programme on Extending Quality Life, I am struck by the similarities between that research and this volume, emphasising again the universal nature of ageing. Comparative material can be downloaded from the GO website (http://www.shef.ac.uk/uni/projects/gop/index.htm). I have no doubt that this textbook will be a much sought after reference for students and professionals in gerontology for years to come and, because of its laudable emphasis on promoting positive ageing, also has the potential to help to make active life expectancy a reality.

Professor Alan Walker
Department of Sociological Studies, University of Sheffield, United Kingdom

Contents

Figures and tables

Contributors

Samantha Ackling Doctoral student in the School of Health at the University of New England in Armidale, Australia, undertaking studies on sexual intimacy in later life.

Chris Bourne FACSHP Staff Specialist and Medical Unit Manager at the Sydney School of Health Centre, Sydney Hospital.

Catherine Bridge PhD Director of the Home Maintenance and Modification Clearing House in the School of Occupation and Leisure Studies at the University of Sydney, Australia.

Colette Browning PhD Associate Professor in the School of Public Health at La Trobe University in Melbourne, Australia.

Neena L. Chappell PhD Professor in the Department of Sociology and a Canada Research Chair in Social Gerontology in the Center on Aging at the University of Victoria in Victoria, Canada.

Irene Coulson PhD Professor and Dean of the Faculty of Nursing at the University of Prince Edward Island in Charlottetown, Canada.

James L. Fozard PhD President of the Florida Gerontological Research and Training Services, Florida, USA, and serves on the adjunct Faculty of Saint Leo University, Florida, USA.

Judy Harris PhD Lecturer in the School of Health at the University of New England in Armidale, Australia.

Terrence Hays PhD Lecturer in the School of Education at the University of New England in Armidale, Australia.

Rafat Hussain PhD Senior Lecturer in the School of Health at the University of New England in Armidale, Australia.

Andrew Joyce Former doctoral student in the School of Psychological Sciences at LaTrobe University in Melbourne, Australia, who recently completed his studies on social activity in older people.

Hal Kendig PhD Professor and Dean of the Faculty of Health Sciences at the University of Sydney, Australia.

Jeffrey Kottler PhD Professor and Head of the Department of Counseling at California State University in Fullerton, California, USA.

Rodrigo Mariño PhD Senior Lecturer in the School of Health at the University of New England in Armidale, Australia.

Cathryn McConaghy PhD Senior Lecturer in the School of Education at the University of New England in Armidale, Australia.

Jenny McParlane Associate Professor in Nursing in the School of Health and Associate Dean in the Faculty of Education, Health and Professional Studies at the University of New England in Armidale, Australia.

Victor Minichiello PhD Professor of Health and Dean of the Faculty of Education, Health and Professional Studies at the University of New England in Armidale, Australia.

Ina Olohan Lecturer in the School of Health at the University of New England in Armidale, Australia.

Glenda Parmenter Lecturer and Nurse Practitioner in the School of Health at the University of New England in Armidale, Australia.

David Plummer PhD Associate Professor in Community and Public Health in the School of Health at the University of New England in Armidale, Australia.

Linda Rosenman PhD Professor and Executive Dean of the Faculty of Social and Behavioural Sciences at the University of Queensland in Brisbane, Australia.

Alan Scott Doctoral student in the School of Professional Development and Leadership at the University of New England in Armidale, Australia, undertaking his studies on ageism and society.

Margaret Somerville PhD Associate Professor in the School of Professional Development and Leadership at the University of New England in Armidale, Australia.

Lyndall Spencer PhD Research Fellow in the Department of Medicine at the University of Queensland in Brisbane, Australia.

Vicki Strang PhD Professor in the Faculty of Nursing at the University of Alberta in Edmonton, Canada.

Yvonne Wells PhD Research Fellow in Lincoln Gerontology Centre in the Faculty of Health Sciences at La Trobe University in Melbourne, Australia.

Peter Wright PhD Senior Lecturer in the School of Education at Murdoch University in Western Australia.

Acknowledgments

The inspiration for writing this edited collection has come from talking with older persons about their lives and learning that there is nothing to fear from growing old. In fact, we have been enriched by the many positive stories and experiences that accompany the journey of people as they grow old, despite the many challenges they face.

The book attempts to value growing old and to support older people in their campaign to combat ageism in our society. We also hope that the younger reader will rethink his or her misconceptions about older people and respect the human right of older persons to experience the same rich opportunities for social, cultural and productive roles and not be subject to selective discrimination because they are 'older'.

This book reflects a collaboration between many people. First, we are indebted to the many older persons we spoke to, and particularly our senior postgraduate research students at the University of New England in Armidale, Australia. Second, we are grateful to Jeanette Tan and Gloria Davidson for assisting us with typesetting the manuscript, chasing reference details, and providing excellent support. Third, the contributors have been most patient with us. We want to thank them for participating in this project. And finally we want to acknowledge the support we have received from Emma Cant and Jeanmarie Morosin at Allen & Unwin.

Special acknowledgment for the assistance received by the authors for particular chapters is noted. Richard Rohrshiem and Glenn Harvey provided research assistance and compiled some of the data presented in Chapter 4.

Professor Victor Marshall provided copies of some of the material used in Chapter 11 and made comments on an earlier version of this chapter. Dr John C. Thomas also made many helpful comments on an earlier draft of this chapter.

Professor Victor Minichiello

Professor Irene Coulson

Preface: The context of promoting positive ageing

Victor Minichiello, Irene Coulson

The challenge

The past century saw astronauts landing on the moon, medicine mastering human organ transplant, people communicating across the globe using email, mobile phones, faxes and instant Internet connections—but, alas, finding no antidote to stop the ageing process, the so-called 'fountain of youth'. In our view, however, we should not be disappointed that such a remedy has not been found, because there is nothing inherently bad or abnormal in growing old.

We age from the moment we are born. But somehow western societies want to put a stop to the ageing process at about the time a person reaches the age of 21 or so. Why? So that they can retain and preserve the physical appearance and attractiveness associated with those so heavily featured by fashion, advertising and youth-preserving technologies and lifestyle industries. Perhaps our problem is not so much with ageing, but with our lust for youthfulness.

The new millennium has, however, brought what might appear to be longer life expectancy and better health for older citizens. 'Successful ageing' is no longer an oxymoron but a reality. We will leave the subsequent chapters to argue the impressive statistics associated with life expectancy these days and the health status of ageing populations in western societies, although it is important to make two points. One is that some groups do better than others. For example, minority groups such as Indigenous people experience risks in their lives that adversely influence life expectancy (Thomson 2003). The life expectancy for Indigenous Australians is much lower than for white Australians; similarly, the life expectancy for people living in Australia, the United States, Canada and the United Kingdom is far higher than for people living in Rwanda, Uganda or Sierre Leone, three countries amongst those with the lowest life expectancy rates. Second, Fries (1986) studied the life expectancy of humans in general and documented that average life expectancy can expect to remain at around 85 years, plus or minus seven years, depending on how well disease and other influencing lifestyle factors can be controlled. The theory put forward by Fries, however, is that human life is finite. What has been occurring over time is not the extension of life per se, but rather that the onset of disease has been delayed to produce what he refers to as a 'rectangular survival curve'. This curve is represented by a decline in infant mortality and in the number of deaths from accident and violence during the middle years of life, together with a decline in the number of deaths from acute and chronic diseases in the later years, thus allowing more people to reach the life span of the species. Zimbabwe, however, presents a stark reminder of how quickly improvements in life expectancy can be eroded, for over the past few decades it has dropped in that country from 67.5 years to about 33 years due to HIV/AIDS (Tirrito 2003).

The new millennium has also brought general improvement in the health status of older people. Take, for example, the results of the longest study of ageing in the world, the Study of Adult Development at Harvard University that includes three separate cohorts of people born in 1911, 1921 and 1930 (Vaillant 2002). It documents overall improvements in health over the span of the study, although the argument about differences between groups made above also holds true here. Some groups show much better health outcomes than others. This American study reveals findings duplicated in many other studies across western nations. Increasingly, people in developed nations are growing old without brain disease, are not depressed and maintain a modest well-being until the final months before they die. This picture reflects our own experiences with our grandparents. For example, both grandparents of one of the authors lived independently and grew old relatively illness free until a heart attack (a few minutes) or cancer (a few weeks) quickly terminated their lives. The authors still have their parents living independent and active lives and in good health.

Of course, we recognise that some older people do experience prolonged loss, poor health and dependency in later life. This too is a part of the reality of the ageing experience. Do we believe Robert Browning, who urges us to 'grow old along with me! The best is yet to be . . .', and accept this related view:

> Contrary to all expectations, I seem to grow happier as I grow older. I think that America has been sold on the theory that youth is marvellous but old age is terror. On the contrary, it's taken my sixty years to learn how to live reasonably well, to do my work and cope with my inadequacies.
>
> For me youth was a woeful time—sick parents, war, relative poverty, the miseries of learning a profession, a mistake of a marriage, self-doubts, booze and blundering around. Old age is knowing what I'm doing, the respect of others, a relatively sane financial base, a loving wife and the realisation that what I can't beat I can endure (quoted in Vaillant 2002, p. 14).

Or do we accept William Shakespeare's assertion that old age 'is second childishness and mere oblivion; Sans teeth, sans eyes, sans taste, sans everything'. We concur that both scenarios can be someone's reality and lived experience.

The new gerontology

Holstein and Minkler (2003) describe the 'new gerontology' movement that is replacing the study of disease and disability. The popular discourse found in the gerontology literature and at conferences these days is that which 'seeks to counteract and replace the old decline and loss paradigm' (Holstein & Minkler 2003, p. 787). What is emerging is a 'successful ageing' agenda that uses a preventative discourse model to provide insights that avoid or delay losses and physical and mental decrements. This book welcomes this shift in emphasis—let us be clear about this point. Like our colleagues Holstein and Minkler, who make their argument so convincingly, we believe that successful ageing as defined by Rowe and Kahn (1998) to include the avoidance of disease and disability, the maintenance of high physical and cognitive functional capacity, and active engagement in life, is much too limiting.

Good health is only one of the issues on a much larger social agenda that includes the attainment of happiness, wellness, fulfilment, respect and equality in later life. We cannot simply assume that every individual can take sole responsibility and control over their life and make autonomous and informed choices to achieve the above outcomes. To do so would assume that everything else is equal and that every person has the same means and resources made available to them by their society. Eating well, not smoking, having safe sex, exercising (all of the good health promotion messages we constantly hear) are important. But if we are to change how people think and experience ageing and later life, we need to consider the contexts and constraining factors that influence access to, for example, affordable housing, adequate income, clean environments and quality health care. Policies are required to support the equitable distribution of resources to poor and disadvantaged older persons and reverse the ageist attitudes formed over many decades, if not centuries. And we would need to recognise and address the fact that society privileges some groups over others. Holstein and Minkler (2003, p. 792) make a good point when they argue:

> [An] individualistic analysis doesn't ask if the 80-year-old skier had county club privileges and a winter home in Colorado, or the 80-year-old in the wheelchair had cleaned houses for a living while holding down a second job as a nurses' aide on the graveyard shift in a nursing home. Nor does this analysis inquire about the inner or family life of our 80-year-old in the wheelchair. These contextual features, at a minimum, shape the conditions of possibility for individuals and determine how they choose what to value. If the ideal is not practically feasible for all, or even most, people—even with the best intentions—then it serves to further privilege the already privileged, a danger that a feminist perspective identifies.

Positive ageing

This book shows that we are experiencing a notable departure from the narrow focus on disability in later life and a movement towards a broader approach using wellness and primary health care concepts. Primary health care is defined by the World Health Organization

(1998) as essential health care made universally accessible to individuals and families in the community by means acceptable to them, through their full participation and at a cost that the community can afford. In order to promote positive ageing, health care policies and practices need to take a life course perspective that focuses on health promotion, disease prevention and equitable access to resources. Positive ageing policies need to focus on improving the life experiences of older people as a group and create an environment that offers opportunities for continuing participation in society, and an understanding of how cultural factors, gender, economic status and geography, for example, influence life chances. Definitions of health for older people must also include health and wellness as being inseparable from identities and experiences accumulated throughout the life span (Kendig 1996b).

This book invites the reader to examine the challenges we face this century, in terms of an ageing population and the diversity of issues we need to re-evaluate, including housing, technology, ageism, sexual health and intimacy, the role of health promotion, work and retirement, social support, the cost of care, and alternative ways to empower and promote positive ageing. We describe the challenges of ageism in a society that still discriminates against older people merely because of their age. We predict that in the decades to come an unprecedented number of baby boomers and future generations of older citizens will and must exert social and political influence to change the current discourses about ageing.

How quality of life will be experienced in later life will become of paramount importance to all of us. Quality of life is defined as an individual's perception of their position in life in the context of their culture and value system, and in relation to how society allows its citizens to achieve their aspirations and goals, as well as address their concerns. It is a broad-ranging context, incorporating in a complex way a person's physical health, psychological state, social status in that society, social networks and relationships to salient features in the socio-political environment.

The chapters that follow shed light on how ageing can be better understood and affirmed and spoken about in more empowering and humane ways, and not, to use a sociological term, as the 'other'. This edited collection attempts to address the questions: How can later life be enjoyed with all its strengths and complexities in more meaningful ways? and: How can older people be liberated to change the ageist fears that are internalised by so many of us? Without a doubt the basic structures of our societies will need to be re-examined and redefined to meet the expectation by older people for a better and different life to what we currently know as 'old age'. Failure to fulfil this expectation will give rise to opposition and conflict.

1

The challenges of ageism

Victor Minichiello, Margaret Somerville, Cathryn McConaghy, Jenny McParlane, Alan Scott

No one can doubt that sexism and racism revolutionised the way people and institutions in our society had to rethink relations between dominant groups and women, black and Indigenous people. Women are now found, for example, in large numbers in medical schools and general practitioner (GP) practices, businesses and government. They hold key positions of power such as vice chancellors of universities, chief executive officers of large multi-national corporations, ministerial cabinet positions and so on. Legislation makes it illegal to discriminate on the basis of gender, race/ethnicity and sexual orientation (see Chapter 4). Forms of oppressions, such as domestic violence and segregation, have been given public exposure and both legal and political measures have been put in place to reduce the effects of such oppressions on the lives of social minority groups.

Without a doubt the 21st century will see a revolution in terms of the relationship between older people and other age groups and the way society views the status and position of older people. Why is this? Older people are devalued and discriminated against. They will not tolerate this treatment for much longer, especially given that they are growing in numbers and have the potential to be an influential activist group.

Ageism is a current reality in the lives of older people and we will come back to discussing the research that supports this statement later in the chapter. Ageism reflects a deep-seated uneasiness on the part of the young and middle aged and is frequently internalised by older people themselves. Ageism is a personal revulsion towards and distaste for growing old, disease and disability, and a fear of powerlessness, uselessness and death (Butler 1975). Bytheway reminds us that we find being 'old' in western society difficult or undesirable:

> So are we all sensitive to revealing our age? How self-conscious do we feel when asked outright how old we are? Do we shriek? Do we feel our energy ebbing? Do we feel uncomfortable as we stutter over the answer? Do we find ourselves elaborating it with comment about how we feel and what we do? (Bytheway 1995, p. 7).

This chapter discusses the concept of 'ageism', how it is manifested and its consequences. It documents how widespread ageism is in our society, including in the health and aged care sectors. Current discourses about older people and ageing are presented to highlight the assumptions that are underpinning such discourses. The role older people will play to reverse the impact of ageism on their lives is discussed.

What is ageism?

Before discussing ageism in more depth, let us briefly explain how ageism is created. Bytheway (1995) argues that ageism is the creation of values in society that have developed over centuries. Many of the ingrained ideas that western culture holds about ageing have come to us from ancient Greece and Rome. Amongst them was the idea that the state of youthfulness, being slim and having no defect, was most desirable, and that being 'old' was offensive. Euripides in the *Suppliants* (c.423 BC) tell us: 'Old age, that irresistible foe, how I loath your presence. I also hate those who desire to lengthen their span of life, seeking to turn the tide of death by foods and drinks, drugs and magic spells; people that death should take away when they cease to benefit the world, leaving the young their place.' Pythagoras, Hippocrates, Plato and Aristotle all found the idea of becoming old offensive, yet they were 80, 90, 82 and 62 respectively when they died. Gossip (1952, p. 593), commenting on Aristotle's views, makes the point that: 'Few pages in literature are more depressing than that in Aristotle, who, casting aside his customary calm, savagely depicts old men as "human nature fallen into ruin, selfish and unenthusiastic, knowing and mean".'

Cicero (1971), amongst his other writings, has left us the earliest substantive work we have on ageing, in the essay 'Concerning Old Age' (44 BC). In it, he condemns the fallacies, myths and stereotypes of ageing that were rife in Roman society and identifies the four stereotypes used to identify older people. These were: 'they find life wearisome', 'they move away from active work', 'they are deficient in sensual pleasures' and 'they are worried about the nearness of death'. It is now more than 20 centuries since Cicero penned his efforts to try to dispel these myths and stereotypes, yet today we still have to argue the same case. As Perdue and Gurtman point out:

> It is commonly accepted that the elderly in our society find themselves viewed in predominantly negative fashion, victims of a pervasive form of discrimination and disparagement sometimes referred to as 'ageism'. The attitudinal basis of ageism appears to be systematically negative evaluations of older persons, including (generally inaccurate) stereotypes of their character and capability. The aged are often described as more ill, tired, slow, forgetful, withdrawn, self pitying, defensive and unhappy (1990, p. 199).

Such deep-seated beliefs are widely reflected in the media, the health care system, the workplace, and in interpersonal relations. These beliefs place high emphasis on reproduction, production, consumption and youthfulness (see Chapter 4), and shape access to power and resources in ways that disadvantage older people. Consider, for example, how it is that in a youth-dominant culture the body is an important signifier to others and to the self of the 'passing of time, qualified by the socially constricted definitions associated with that image' (Briggs 1993, p. 52). The cosmetics and fashion industries constantly remind older people that their bodies are undesirable, unattractive, unwanted and devalued. When was the last time you saw a fashion event using an older woman or man as a model?

So what is ageism? Bytheway (1995, p. 14) states:

1. Ageism is a set of beliefs originating in the biological variation between people and relating to the ageing process.

2. It is in the actions of corporate bodies, what is said and done
    by their representatives, and the resulting views that are held by
    ordinary ageing people, that ageism is made manifest.

The term 'ageism' was coined in the early 1960s by Robert Butler
(1975), a psychiatrist living in the United States. Butler was involved
with the civil rights movement at the time and was offended by the
systematic stereotyping and discrimination of older people simply
because they were old. As the term gained greater acceptance it was
introduced, for example, in the *American Dictionary of the English
Language* in 1979 and became the subject of gerontological research
and debate.

The biomedicalised view of later life at the time—focusing on the
less healthy, the frail and the problems of ageing persons—helped to
further reinforce many of the common stereotypes held by both
younger and older people. In a study that examined the impact of an
educational intervention program on the attitudes and knowledge of
students aged 17–18 years, Scott et al (1998) found that students
held negative attitudes towards older people and that the intervention program did little to change their attitudes, largely because the
curriculum focused on the biological losses associated with ageing.
It is interesting to note that psychologists have also made negative
assumptions about later life. For example, Shield and Aronson
(2003, p. 67) critically comment that the inherent logic of self-esteem
studies is to test the hypothesis 'that a decline in self-esteem is
responsible for many of the overt symptoms of aging'. However, this
explanation, offered by an older person, provides an alternative view
as to why they may have low self-esteem:

> Who was ever in any doubt that the self-esteem of the elderly de-
> clines in this society which indicates in every possible way that it
> does not value the old in the slightest, finds them an expense and an
> embarrassment, laughs at their experience, evades their problems,
> isolates them in hospitals and Sunshine Cities, and generally ignores
> them except when soliciting their votes or ripping off their handbags
> and their Social Security checks? And which has a chilling capacity
> to look straight at them and never see them. The poor old senior
> citizen has two choices, assuming he is well enough off to have any
> choices at all. He can retire from that hostile climate, or he can shrink
> in his self-esteem and gradually become the person he is constantly
> reminded he is (*The Spectator Bird* 1976, p. 116).

Even sociological theories, such as the disengagement theory put forward by Cummings and Henry in the 1960s, in which they theorised a disengagement from life as a person ages, influenced policy and social planning in such a way that it reinforced the view of the dependency status of older persons. Barrow (1996) termed this 'compassionate stereotyping'. As another example, Estes (1979) shows that the social policies of the 20th century were formulated to 'help' older people by creating what she refers to as 'an ageing enterprise'. These ageing enterprises, as she points out, have not eradicated poverty, discrimination and social ills. Instead, their establishment 'paradoxically has created their own problems and inadvertently perpetuated some of the other problems' (1979, p. 2). Carol Estes' critique

> was one of the first to demonstrate how the programs and policies created an industry of helping organizations that had, and still have, a vested interest in understanding the elderly as needy and problematic. This stilted way of looking at the elderly has become its own industry. As programs and policies are created to fix the ills, and people are trained and hired to fill the positions to help clients get services, an environment of entitlement and depend-ency begins. Rather than solving the problems, the problems perpetuate. The people hired to fill the positions do not want to see their programs eliminated (Shield and Aronson 2003, p. 93).

These notions of need and dependency may explain why one of the frequently cited myths that young people have of older people is that they live in nursing homes, when the truth is that the vast majority live independently in the community as neighbours (see Chapter 8).

As the concept of ageism was subjected to academic and public scrutiny, social scientists challenged the 'disengagement discourse' of ageing, and the work of feminists and writers such as Simone de Beauvoir in France highlighted the social, economic and psy-chological roots of ageism. De Beauvoir (1970, p. 7) wrote these powerful words, which made a remarkable contribution to the establishment of a popular anti-ageist consciousness in Europe:

> When their economic status is decided upon, society appears to think that they belong to an entirely different species: for if all that is needed to feel that one has done one's duty by them is to grant

them a wretched pittance, then they have neither the same needs nor the same feelings as other [people].

So we now know what ageism is, even though we know it less well than sexism and racism. But what are the consequences of ageism? Bytheway (1995, p. 14) offers some insights:

(a) Ageism generates and reinforces a fear and denigration of the ageing process, and stereotyping presumptions regarding competence and the need for protection.
(b) In particular, ageism legitimates the use of chronological age to mark out classes of people who are systematically denied resources and opportunities that others enjoy, and who suffer the consequences of such denigration, ranging from well-meaning patronage to unambiguous vilification.

Evidence for ageism

Research shows that older people are viewed as a problem— a financial and health care burden at least. Interestingly, women had to overcome a similar situation. For example, Shield and Aronson (2003) show how women have been medicalised and pathologised by western biomedicine. Feminists have raised serious questions about how childbirth was treated by physicians and fought to re-establish the normalcy of such uniquely female physiological experiences as menarche, pregnancy, childbirth and menopause.

Viewed as a helpless problem group, older people (like women) are similarly subjected to all kinds of intervention, often couched in paternalistic terms and seen as well-intentioned. Whether past western societies viewed older people differently is debatable. Shield and Aronson (2003) argue that perhaps older persons were still seen as 'different' but because their numbers were so low in proportion to the rest of the population, they were tolerated by dominant groups. As they also note, 'when the numbers go higher, tolerance tends to recede. Do people feel threatened by the proximity of these "others"? When the numbers increase, so do comments about greedy geezers, old fogey drivers, and the like' (2003, p. 104). As in previous centuries, more festivity accompanies the birth of a child than the celebration of retirement or the beginning of the senior years!

Shield and Aronson (2002) provide a simple but common example to illustrate the point of the well-intentioned carer acting to protect the helpless older relative, something one of the authors experienced himself when his grandfather died and the family considered the risk of his grandmother living 'alone', making the decision to move her to be with a daughter. Demographic statistics about living arrangements reveal that many older widowed women live alone (frequently with pets, although this is not counted in the census). The majority of these women will not re-marry and for some this decision is a preference, an alternative to having lived with a spouse for most of their lives. Many express freedom in such new living arrangements and resist attempts by the family or health care providers who may view them as isolated, frail, lonely, vulnerable and in need of help. Many refuse such offers of help. As Shield and Aronson (2002, p. 76) argue:

> Is this a bad thing? Is this a catastrophe waiting to happen? Or is not intervening a sign of respect for their individuality, their autonomy? Maybe we need to tolerate our own uneasiness when people prefer to live in ways that we judge unsafe or unsound.

Research shows that such women are not without support and often create their own sense of community and coping strategies (see Chapter 8). For example, Hochschild's classic study, conducted back in 1973, found that such older women living alone often create their own community of support and level of cohesiveness and cooperation. For example, they would let each other know that 'they were all right by opening their curtains in the morning. Closed blinds alerted the others that something was awry and needed immediate attention' (Shield and Aronson 2003, p. 77).

Sociologists have long argued that older people have been given a 'spoiled identity'. What does this mean? Like other marginalised groups in society, we believe that older people are not quite human like us and, on this assumption, we tend to impute to them, to use Goffman's (1969) own words, 'a range of imperfections' and exercise various forms of discrimination. At the popular cultural level we can easily interpret that ageing is not viewed as desirable. Consider the following advertisements: the anti-ageing cream label of Estée Lauder, Christian Dior's 'age-defense renewal serum', the slogan of Kelloggs—'the food that fights ageing', and *Marie Claire* magazine (no. 71, July 2001), which featured an 'anti-ageing special' with the title, 'The A–Z of anti-ageing', and carried the message 'how to win the war against [lines and wrinkles]'. Or consider the message contained in Erica Brealey's (2003) book, *Ten Minute Anti-Ageing*, with the accompanying statement 'want to beat the ageing process and turn back the clock? Take just ten minutes out of your day to recapture vitality and youth!' Contrast this with recent health promotion messages about promoting good health and fitness in later life which contains no 'anti-ageing' vocabulary and uses the concept of fitness as being healthy for the body, regardless of age.

Gerontological research provides ample evidence of the wide and varied levels of negative attitudes and treatment showed by young people, and older people themselves, towards ageing. Studies related to ageism have generally examined how the attitudes and beliefs of younger people contribute to denying older people opportunities and equitable treatment. For example, Giles et al (1992) demonstrate how young people process and respond to the speech of older people in stereotypical ways. In another study, Ryan et al (1995) show how younger people at an interactional level use patronising verbal and nonverbal communication towards older carers. Sawchuk (1995), who undertook an extensive analysis of advertisement campaigns and other marketing strategies, concludes that at a public level many marketing discourses perpetuate and reinforce negative stereotypes of old age. Studies that have focused on older workers have consistently found that they often face ageist stereotypes that define them as increasingly marginal in the workforce (Maule et al 1996). The most significant barriers and deterrents are managerial biases that construct older workers are too costly, too inflexible and too difficult to train (Imel 1996). Such findings are emerging not only from western countries but also from former communist states. For example, Gerasimova (1996), who interviewed older women from St Petersburg, found that the major difficulties reported by her sample were age-discriminatory social policy and gerontophobic stereotypes. Reports of discrimination against older workers appear to be related to employers' interest in 'downsizing' their workforce (Encel 1995).

Health researchers have also examined how misconceptions about the ageing process can have a detrimental effect on the health of older persons (Grant 1996). Walker et al (1996) argue that ageist stereotypes underlie many of the services designed for older people with a disability, with the focus centred mostly on care and less on support of the older person to fulfil their potential. Numerous studies have also reported how therapists accept socially validated negative stereotypes of later life. For example, Woolfe and Biggs (1997) found that some counsellors were less likely to use a psychodynamic approach with older persons, and this decision could result in the underestimation of later-life potential. Social workers were reported to spend less time and had fewer contacts with older oncology patients than younger patients, with the result that social workers may not be effectively assisting older patients to cope with important health and social issues (Rohan et al 1994). Examining audiotaped interactions between physicians and young and older patients, Greene and her colleagues (1996) found that there was greater disparity between the goals of the doctor and older patients, and less joint decision making with older patients. Doctors tended to be less egalitarian, patient, respectful, engaged and optimistic with the older patients. What these studies perhaps show is how easy it is for social arrangements in society to make it possible for ageism to be so prevalent, yet for the behaviour to be seen as obscure and non-intentional (Bytheway 1995).

Language, as we will further argue later, also provides us with evidence that older people are socially constructed as 'different'. For example, the vocabulary of physicians has come under some scrutiny. It has been found that physicians use the word 'gomer' (acronym for Get Out of My Emergency Room), to describe an older patient who is an unresolvable admission to the emergency room; 'lolonad' (acronym for Little Old Lady in No Acute Distress), to describe an older woman brought to the emergency room late at night with chronic conditions made worse by a failing memory; and 'Haldol Manor' (Haldol is a sedative agent) a phrase assigned to disruptive older patients and incontinent patients living in nursing homes. Konner (1987) observed in his study that doctors see death embodied in older people, and their use of humour serves to compensate for the failure of modern medicine to save older people. Konner (1987, p. 287) made this observation:

> At the end of the discussions one senior physician shook his gray head, sighed, and smiled. 'As George Burns says,' he mused aloud, 'not many people die after ninety.' This was to become a favorite remark during morning rounds for the rest of the month, uttered ritually by the residents in chorus, whenever we left the bedside of a patient over ninety. The more hopeless the patient, the funnier the line.

To highlight the value judgment inherent in this comment, Shield and Aronson (2003, p. 89) remark: 'Of course today in the twenty-first century, more and more people die after ninety, and increasingly numbers of people live past 100. So who is the joke on now?' It should be of no surprise to us that geriatrics is a speciality with low appeal. Shield and Aronson (2002, p. 110) comment: '[Physicians] involved in the training of physicians lament how difficult it is to persuade young [medical practitioners] to enter geriatrics because it is seen as depressing and not well-paid. What a sad commentary considering the demographics.' The same is true of other health professions.

Activity 1.1

Read a local newspaper and popular magazine on women's or men's issues. What articles/stories appear about older people? What 'stereotype' messages are stated or implied about older persons?

Ageism in nursing

Nurses constitute the largest health professional group involved in the daily provision of care to older citizens. According to Stevens (2003, p. 23), the involvement of nurses in the care of the aged in Australia resulted from a 1877 inquiry into the care being received by those in asylums at the time, many of whom were there because they were aged. A decade after this inquiry, Nightingale-trained nurses were appointed to provide care in government asylums. Their appointment did not go unchallenged. There was a body of opinion opposed to the 'extravagance' of such a move 'when untrained staff would suffice' (Stevens 2003, p. 23). Well over a century later, the nursing profession, governments and providers of aged care throughout western societies are still having the same debate about the level of education and training required by nurses in order to provide quality care to older persons.

Though nursing has a long history in the provision of care to older persons, the profession is not immune to the manifestations of ageism, which is demonstrated in two main ways. In the first instance, there are the ageist attitudes demonstrated by nurses towards older clients. In the second instance, there are the ageist attitudes directed towards older practising nurses. As we will discuss below, as the nursing workforce ages, such attitudes towards older nurses have the potential to become an important issue for the profession to confront.

Ageism in nursing stems from negative stereotypical beliefs held by nurses about older persons and the ageing process, and results in negative attitudes towards aged care practice (Pearson et al 2002). Another linked factor in the ageist attitudes of nurses is the youth focus of much of western society. The nursing profession draws most of its students from high school leavers, and it is logical to assert that the majority of these students would enter the profession steeped in the culture of youth, to be confronted, very early in their student clinical practice, with the spectre of ageing and the often challenging care needs of the aged.

Yamamoto (1994), writing in the Japanese nursing context, identified the increasing numbers of people over the age of 65 who are entering acute care hospital settings, where many nursing students experience their first contact with the sick or frail aged. The attempts of schools of nursing to limit the exposure of students to older clients until they have a body of knowledge in aged care, and have achieved greater life experience and maturity, are thwarted by the increasing numbers of older people being treated in acute care hospital settings.

It could be argued that having students experience their first nursing care of older people in such a setting is advantageous to the development of more positive attitudes, an argument based upon the more pleasant practice environment more commonly to be found in acute care hospital settings. The environment in which first contact occurs can negatively impact upon student attitudes to aged care. It is for this reason that Rowland and Shoemake (1999) have urged that careful consideration be given to the selection of sites for clinical placements in aged care. Careful selection of aged care placements, and a balance between work with the well aged and the frail aged, is necessary to reduce student exposure to conditions that predispose to the development of ageist attitudes.

Aged care facilities often evoke negative feelings in students, based upon a number of factors including the presence of offensive odours, the lack of demonstrable physical recovery, the sometimes limited meaningful interpersonal communication and the challenging behaviours associated with dementia. Student nurses frequently perceive older people negatively, using terms such as 'dirty', 'silly', 'demented', 'boring', 'self-centred' and 'grouchy' (Rowland & Shoemake 1999, Davis 2002). Students are occasionally heard to refer to aged care placements in negative and at times derogatory terms.

The image of aged care amongst nursing students is too often that of a 'dead end' practice setting, the clinical setting that a nurse enters into when unable to cope in more acute clinical areas. Nurses' attitudes to aged care are negatively shaped by education that focuses on the problems associated with ageing rather than on promoting positive images of ageing (Decker & Sellers 2002). Aged care is also often poorly served in nursing curricula by being integrated into other curriculum areas (McCracken et al 1995). The result of this integration is that, rather than being seen as a unique speciality area, in the same way that other nursing areas are seen, aged care is seen as a low status area, requiring no specialised nursing education or skills. Davis (2002) argues that while pre-service education can break down ageist attitudes, interest in working with older people and reduction of ageist attitudes is not positively impacted by 'increased knowledge of gerontology alone'.

There is little appreciation amongst professional nurses and nursing students of the complexity of aged care and the specialised skills required to be an effective aged care nurse (Chenoweth 2003). Nurses tend to judge the importance of a particular area by the clinical tasks associated with that area. The high technology areas are rated as more important because they are perceived to require higher order psychomotor skills. However, while aged care usually does not involve high technology, it does involve the need for excellent assessment and communication skills and the planning, coordination and prioritising of care. These are the very skills that professional nurses need in all practice settings, but are also the skills that are often the least highly valued, especially by students of nursing. As long as this lack of appreciation persists, aged care nursing will continue to be viewed negatively within the profession.

The devaluing of aged care amongst nurses is reinforced by the lower pay rates of aged care nurses. The worth of work to society, rightly or wrongly, is largely reflected in the remuneration attached to the work. When aged care nurses are paid less than their colleagues in acute care areas the message is clear—caring for the aged requires limited training or education and limited skills and, more significantly, neither aged people, nor the nurses who care for them, are highly valued, a point illustrated by the aged care sector case study discussed below.

Jessica—an outdated way of thinking

Jessica, a 67-year-old woman, came into hospital for a mastectomy after diagnosis of a malignant lump. She was observed to be withdrawn and a little teary. The nurse who had admitted Jessica talked with her and reported at handover that Jessica was worried about the impact the imminent loss of her breast would have on her self-concept and could have on her new partner. The nurse reported that, given Jessica's concerns, she had suggested that Jessica discuss her concerns and the possibility of breast-conserving surgery with her doctor before the surgery.

The nurse was reprimanded by two of her colleagues, both of whom argued that at 67 the loss of a breast was not as traumatic as it would be in a younger woman, and 'anyway, at her age there probably isn't much there for her to lose or for her partner to look at', and 'Fancy a woman of her age having a new partner, she should be past that stuff'. As Chapter 4 argues, such comments are ageist and clinically inappropriate.

A second aspect of ageism in nursing arises from negative attitudes towards older nurses by their younger colleagues. In Australia, the average age of the nursing workforce increased from 39.5 years in 1993 to 41.6 years in 1999 (AIHW 2003) and has undoubtedly increased further in the intervening years. In the United States the same ageing of the nursing workforce is evident, the average increasing from 37.4 years in 1983 to 44.5 years in 2000 (Letvak 2002). The ageing of the nursing workforce brings out ageist behaviours in colleagues. Letvak (2002, p. 2) writes of research showing that older nurses are subject to 'bullying, undermining and persecution'. These behaviours arise out of wrongly held beliefs that older nurses are unable to carry the physical load of nursing, are rigid and dated in their practice and unable to cope with new technology. There is no evidence to support these beliefs but there are consequences of the beliefs being held, one of them being the loss of older nurses from the workforce, further compromising numbers in the workforce along with an associated loss of experience. Glass (1998) has written of the prevalence of horizontal violence ('violence' committed by nurses to nurses) in nursing, the ageist attitudes and behaviours directed towards older nurses in the workplace being but one form of this horizontal violence. It could be thought that ageist attitudes in nurses are a reflection of a culture in which advancing age is not respected, but the literature, to date, does not support this thinking. Studies have shown that in some cultures where age is traditionally respected, nurses still manifest ageist attitudes (Sharps et al 1998, Gattuso & Shadbolt 2002).

Case study: Ageism in aged care

It should be obvious that the aged care sector is both affected by, and reflects, the ageist attitudes of society in general. As we have discussed, aged care has long been considered a low status area of nursing. There is ample evidence that nurses would prefer to work in acute care settings, and often find themselves working in aged care because it suits family commitments or because they are unable to gain suitable employment elsewhere (DEST 2003).

In the discussion below, the relationship between the low status of aged care work, the lack of education and training, and the reproduction of ageist attitudes and practices in the industry is explored. It is argued that the challenge of addressing ageism in aged care organisations is one of learning. How do workers learn ageism, and how does it become a naturalised cultural practice? How can this be changed?

Learning in aged care, as in all workplaces, happens not only through formal training programs, although these play an important role, but also through experiential learning on the job. It is in this informal learning through experience that the cultural practices of workplaces are learned and reproduced. This learning usually takes place unconsciously so that by the time ageist practices are recognised in nurses' behaviour they are deeply embedded and difficult to change. It is only by understanding the processes of this informal learning that we can intervene to create better learning in aged care organisations so that ageist attitudes and practices can be changed. At the same time it is also important to facilitate a process whereby aged care workers can explore how society's ageist attitudes affect their work and how they might act politically, even in small ways, to change these attitudes. The case study from which the following examples are taken is of an umbrella organisation, 'Careco', that manages a number of not-for-profit aged care services and facilities. These include Community Aged Care Packages (low care), hostels (medium care) and nursing homes (high care). The research project, an ethnographic study of workplace learning in aged care, was undertaken over a two-year period in collaboration with aged care workers. The research methods included quantitative data collection in the form of a survey and qualitative data collection through semi-structured interviews and focus groups with care workers. The interviewees included new and one-year trainees, experienced workers without formal training, qualified supervisors and managers. They were asked about how they learned to do their work when they began working in aged care, and the continuing learning they have undertaken since. Many of the experienced workers referred to earlier work in a range of different facilities so the following quotes apply not only to Careco, but are illustrative of a range of different aged care workplaces.

Throughout the research it became apparent that the whole industry of aged care is constructed within the ageist attitudes of our society. Aged care workers are both subjected to, and participate in, the construction of ageism. This begins with the choice to work in aged care:

> I remember really clearly one lecture [with] about 230 uni students in the auditorium and they did a run of who would like to go into what fields . . . I was sort of interested in rehab . . . and a few people put up their hands—about 12—and I put up my hand [for aged care and] the whole auditorium laughed . . . I found that really interesting, that it was seen as a bit of a joke area.

This newly qualified nurse had already worked as an assistant-in-nursing (AIN) in aged care to put herself through university study. She made a positive choice to specialise in aged care despite the low status. According to Nay and Garratt (2002) it is critical that such nurses remain in aged care to provide positive role models for new staff. Many other interviewees reported that they chose to enter the field because of the personal satisfaction the work provided. Positive reasons for choosing to work in aged care including liking older people, finding the stressors in long-term environments less disturbing than in the acute sector, the specific challenges of aged care, being required to improve standards, offering professional care that has been perceived to be lacking, and enjoying the fun and history associated with nursing older people (see also Nay & Garratt 2002). The effects of ageism, however, continued once they began their employment. One of the major impacts of ageist attitudes reported by interviewees is the constant struggle for adequate resources. In for-profit organisations a user-pays economy prevails and workers feel they are required to process the residents as if they were working in a factory. There is an ever-present danger that profit rather than care is the motivating factor in such facilities. This has a direct affect on the quality of care. For example, care workers are under extreme pressure to process the largest number of residents in the shortest possible time, whether it be showering, feeding or putting to bed:

> You went on, you had X number of showers to do by morning tea, X number of toiletings, X number of repositionings. So it's very task oriented and seeing to the physical needs, not the emotional needs of the people. It's all about doing what you have to do in that minute.

When such conditions prevail, care workers learn to treat aged care residents in instrumental ways, regarding them as objects of work stress rather than as people. This dehumanising process is a fundamental characteristic of ageism.

In not-for-profit aged care facilities, resources are so squeezed that there is an intense daily concern with every level of expenditure, to the extent that care levels are severely affected. These care workers internalise discourses that there are not enough resources for proper caring and that the aged person is a burden. Their learning about care work is negative:

> So my learning was very negative in that the staff I was working with [were] probably the main people I was learning [from] and the messages that were being reinforced were . . . 'we don't have the money to provide any care, they don't care about the older person', 'we've just got to make do with what we've got'. And it was very substandard [care] . . . poor linen, poor conditions, no manual handling equipment, and this is in 1996, this isn't twenty years ago.

When there is no time to consider the individual emotional needs of residents, the aged person becomes an object. Workers reported being unable to spend the time to talk with people, having to deny their basic needs for nurturing and regarding residents as 'attention seeking' when they legitimately require care. Some aged care workers expressed their awareness and distress about this dehumanising process:

> The way people can be treated as an object rather than as a human being; even if they're in a totally vegetative state they still have that right to be covered up and have a hug sometimes, just patting them . . . there were times where I felt that they were just not being treated with dignity and respect.

They also realise that within this dehumanising context both the aged care worker and the aged person are devalued:

> If you treat someone as a lump of meat it demeans you as well as them . . . you still have to treat them as human, as a whole human being. Otherwise you are demeaned by the whole thing and you lose your integrity and your self-respect.

Under these conditions the devaluing of the aged person becomes a naturalised part of the culture of the workplace which, for the resident in care, is their home. This correspondingly results in institutionalised and dehumanised responses from the people in care.

In the past, training in care work has been minimal, especially for entry level care workers (Somerville 2002). As a feminised occupation the high level of complex skills and knowledge required for care work have been undervalued and regarded as a natural part of the female characteristic of nurturing, Hence much of the care work in aged care has been learned on the job.

When care work is learned on the job under the conditions described above, many workers internalise the ageist attitudes and practices that have become naturalised in the aged care setting. A non-nursing professional operating from an outsider perspective expressed surprise at the naturalised acceptance of the lack of education in dementia care:

> I just made the assumption that if a nurse was working in an aged care facility they had some understanding of dementing, dementia, how to nurse an aged person, as compared to nursing somebody in a hospital who had a broken leg or cancer or something, and a lot don't. They haven't had specific training and it blows me away . . . I'll see nurses speaking with these adults in a manner that I wouldn't

speak to anybody, would never have spoken to my mother in that manner, [it's] just demeaning and as though they were children. And I really don't understand it, given that I was sure that they must have some understanding that these people really need to be spoken to as adult to adult, whether they have a dementing illness or not. So that's the first thing and I think that's cultural.

Dementia care is a highly complex and difficult skill requiring substantial underpinning theoretical knowledge. It has been shown that 'nurses who have skills and knowledge related to working with people who have dementia . . . describe their work in more positive terms than staff who feel that they do not know how to cope' (Nay & Garratt 2002). This instance highlights the ageist assumption that caring for people with a dementing illness does not need to be learned. When dementia care is not learned the resulting care practices are ageist because this becomes the easiest way for the untrained care worker to work out what to do. In this way, ageist assumptions that there is no need for education and training reproduce ageist practices. When such attitudes and practices are naturalised within an institutional setting, they become 'cultural', the 'way things are done around here'. Cultural practices are endemic and difficult to change.

In Careco, new entry level care workers are trained to value themselves and their work and they are trained in dementia care. However, when these workers begin their work in the facilities they often learn more powerfully from experienced workers who inadvertently pass on ageist attitudes and work practices because of the conditions described above:

> But the lady I spent the first three days with had a big thing about time—getting things done on time, everything's time—and that really bluffed me because I [felt] 'Okay, we have to care for these people, we're looking after these people' and what I [was seeing] was treating them like they're not humans . . . because we're in and out with them we're not talking to them . . . in one instance I got in trouble for giving a resident a drink of water. [My supervisor] said, 'Well they've just had lunch, she doesn't need a drink,' and to me that's not caring.

From these and other interviews about workplace learning more generally, it is clear that the first week, the first three months and the first twelve months are critical phases in a new worker's workplace learning. Worker subjectivities are established during this period and after this time become entrenched and thus difficult to change. In work that involves a high level of tacit, embodied learning, much of the learning needs to happen in the workplace, and is likely to be far more powerful than learning from training and from books. If new workers try to do things differently and challenge the practices of more experienced workers, peer pressure will be applied and they soon learn to conform. The question then becomes how to reinforce the positive learning of new trainees, and how to change a culture in which ageist practices are naturalised and reinforced by external societal attitudes.

Many interviewees reported making a positive choice to enter aged care and to remain there, despite the low status of the work. It is important that the positive stories these workers tell are made available to new workers in training and that the status of aged care work in general is promoted through the commitment of such workers:

> I just love being able to have relationships with people and being able to get to know them, and I always felt that I could make a difference to their lives, and the other thing that really attracted me was that nobody liked it. Nobody wanted to be an aged care nurse because it wasn't where the glamour was . . . you were only valued as a nurse if you were in the high tech areas and doing the whizzbang stuff, and I just rejected that whole concept completely because I got so much reward out of my relationships with the residents and it was just so rewarding personally to be able to go there, do a good day's work and know that, even as an RN [registered nurse], let alone a manager . . . you could make such a difference to people's lives.

It is clear from the interviews that one of the main ways that new workers learn positive non-ageist practices is by working beside experienced workers who have deep and positive experiential knowledge about how to do their work well. Many of the workers interviewed reported highly positive experiences of learning from one or two key role models. They remembered them many years later:

> There were a couple of really good RNs that I remember working with as an AIN and I learnt a lot from them about the way they worked with residents and the way they communicated with residents. I ended up doing night duty towards the end [pretty well] permanently. I worked with an amazing AIN as well who was just phenomenal. She just had the ability to make someone comfortable

and to do the right things for the right sort of people . . . [when] someone wanted something and they couldn't express it, she knew [what it was]. I learnt a lot from her.

These role models are not necessarily valued for their paper qualifications but for the life and work experiences that have made them excellent care workers. New workers learn from these role models about how to care in ways that value the aged person and combat naturalised ageist practices. It is possible to construct a work situation where all new workers are placed for a period of time with particular experienced workers who are *valued* and *rewarded* for this role.

Successful experiential learning from such key role models also tends to reproduce further positive learning in a generational process. A nurse who described learning from such role models also reported how she loved dementia care, the most complex and challenging of care work:

I love dementia care and I love the challenge, even if I'm not successful, even just that interaction, that . . . I can put all my strategies in place to see if I can assist this lady to do something that ordinarily we can't get her to do. I think that people with dementia are often cared for extremely badly.

This nurse now consciously provides a positive role model herself, specialising in dementia care, and able to model and teach new workers:

It's really important what education they get to form their attitudes early on. As an example, I've recently had some incident reports about aggression with a resident . . . from the same staff member . . . 'this resident does not like showering; this resident does not want to take her clothes off to get in the shower; this resident doesn't like dressing' . . . I can see that [this staff member] is struggling with 'How does this work?', 'Why is this person becoming aggressive?' and her answer at this stage is 'Because she doesn't like doing it'. It's almost a bit of a blame mentality and I'm working with that staff member to try and say, 'Look . . . maybe try it this way or maybe think about it differently' . . . the support that [new staff get at this] facility is very lucky in that to care for residents with dementia you've got to be really flexible. So if they don't want their shower that morning then okay, they mightn't have it that morning.

This nurse works with care and compassion with the staff and the residents in her facility and teaches them by example to value both themselves and others. She focuses on the need for formal education and for supportive workplace learning. Her approach, however, includes even more than this. It is not enough to provide an education and be a patient and supportive role model—it is also important to change the system. She has radically changed the practices of aged care in her facility. New flexible practices have been introduced in place of a dehumanising system that caused many residents, especially those with dementia, to become distressed. This is a practice of critical advocacy.

A small part of the solution to ageism in aged care is to rotate new care workers in an organisation through the facility to learn from the experience of working beside those workers who model non-ageist practices. It is important that this happens early in a trainee's working life because the tacitly embodied practices associated with ageism are so difficult to change once they are learned. New trainees need support to continue with non-ageist practices when they move to a different facility. They need to be encouraged to develop a practice of critical advocacy, to be able to identify the presence of ageism and to act to challenge it. This applies first to the practices within their own workplace, and then to understanding the way aged care workplaces themselves are constructed within the ageist practices of our society. Naming is a process of radical change.

Activity 1.2

What are the challenges facing the health professions with regards to ageism? What education/learning strategies changes would you suggest that could overcome some of these challenges?

Discourses on older people and ageing: Some theoretical considerations

One of the strategies for eliminating ageism and promoting positive ageing is to consider the ways in which we talk about ageing, both in our everyday lives and within the professions of aged care and gerontology. The French philosopher, Michel Foucault (1975), argued that there is a very strong correlation between three key features of our working lives: the ways we talk in our workplaces; the organisational structures in which we work; and the hierarchies of power and authority within organisations. The same holds true on a broader scale in society in general. That is, there is a strong relationship between the popular discourses of the day, the ways our social institutions are structured and the social relations of power. For example, strong anti-refugee sentiment in the popular press impacts upon politicians who make refugee policy, and this in turn impacts upon the everyday experiences of refugees in their new society. Further, the relationships between these factors are not linear but cyclical, with each factor acting upon the other. Put in another way in relation to gerontological issues, if older people are disadvantaged and disempowered in our society then we can look, as we discussed earlier, to the ways in which people talk about older people and the institutions that service them in order to understand the means by which they are disempowered. Thus the search for discourses on ageing is a key strategy for understanding how it is that older people may be disadvantaged and discriminated against in our society. Importantly, understanding how discourses work provides a key to changing them. Thus we are able to effect social change by changing the ways we talk.

Discourses can be thought of as story-lines or narratives on a particular subject. They attain authority in various ways. One way that a particular discourse can attain influence is by riding on the back of other influential discourses. So, for example, if we argue that positive ageing is fair and just, then our analysis would be that the discourse of positive ageing attains authority or legitimacy on the basis of its links to discourses of equity and social justice. If we agree that fairness is important we will be interested in, or open to being convinced by, the discourse of positive ageing. In a society where there is widespread support for the liberal policies of multiculturalism and tolerance of difference, we are more likely to be open to arguments about the specific needs of various ethnic groups of older people. If we live in a racist, sexist and homophobic society in which it is possible to discriminate on the basis of race, gender or sexuality, it is likely that we will be unmoved by the plight of black, lesbian, older women, for example. Fortunately there are legislative protections for minorities in most western societies; unfortunately there are still numerous infringements of these legislative rights, and challenges to the values of inclusion and social justice that underpin them. Thus, despite legislative protections, the struggle for age-integrated social institutions and practices and for the inclusion of all remains a challenge.

This raises another important quality of discourses: they are contested and changing. Indeed, it is interesting to consider the historical changes in discourses on older people and ageing, and what these changes reflect of the changes in social values and contexts. For example, the term 'older citizen' is what may be termed a discursive shift from the term 'old citizen'. This shift can be argued as signalling that ageing is now considered a relative rather than absolute term, that is, one is not old, but merely older than others. This seemingly small discursive shift signals a number of significant changes, including a recognition that we are all ageing; that age, like beauty, is in the eye of the beholder; support for the notion that 'you're only as old as you feel' and so on. Indeed, the argument about the relativity of the term is supported by an analysis of changes in government policy. What was officially considered a chronological old age a century ago is now significantly higher due to better health and longer life spans. In Australia, for example, although the 'old age' pension is available now to men at age 65 and women at age 61, research on workplace age discrimination identifies 45 years as the common age when one becomes 'old' in the workplace (Encel 1998, p. 48). Thus the notion of 'old age' is a social construct and one that is rapidly changing (Worthington 1998). At times such discursive shifts reflect social changes, at other times they can lead to changes. That is, sometimes changes in the way we talk follow social change (for example, changes in the law), and at other times lead to social change. Hence, when we suggest that gerontology professionals 'watch their language' we are suggesting not only that various vilification laws need to be adhered to, but that careful use of particular discourses will lead to important shifts in workplace practices, as we will discuss later.

Current discourses on ageing

What then are the major discourses on ageing used by health professionals, policy makers and governments today? The search for discourses on ageing and an analysis of the ways in which they are changing requires attention to a number of factors, including identifying the assumptions underpinning what we say and the effects of what we say. Our words reflect our basic ideas, feelings and beliefs in addition to reflecting our own social positioning in the world. In turn, our words shape beliefs, feelings, social positioning and the material realities of the world. Another important feature of discourse analysis is that it needs to be done constantly. That is, we need to pay constant and frequent attention to both *what* we say and the *effects* of what we say: we need to keep vigilance over our utterances. Just to complicate the situation further, discourse analysis needs to pay attention not only to what we *say*, but also to what we *don't say*. Sometimes what we don't say conveys more meaning than what we do say. If we don't speak up against something, then by our silence we can be seen to affirm it. If we allow the continued use of terms such as 'old', it could be argued that we are perpetuating a form of disrespect. Think about some of the everyday discourses on ageing in your society. What is said and what is not said?

When we argue for more positive attitudes to ageing in this book what is implied is that currently there are some influential negative attitudes towards ageing that need to be addressed. When we say one thing we are often, by implication, also saying something about the opposite. Thus when we talk about 'older citizens' we are at the same time implying something about 'younger citizens'. Indeed, addressing the thing and its opposite is a basic framework of western thinking and speaking. We call this type of thinking a binary logic. When we describe an injustice we are also implying something about what justice looks like. When we argue for ethical care of the frail we are implying something about unethical care.

What are some of the key binaries in use in gerontology and what debates are associated with them? A binary that has remained unchallenged until relatively recently, particularly within contexts of institutional care, is that of elderly/sexually inactive and young/sexually active. As Chapter 4 argues, such a binary has failed to recognise the sexual life and desires of older people. Similarly, the binary of institutional versus home care has in recent years been broken down through innovative community care programs. In addition, the binary of retiree versus worker is being challenged by the notion of 'active retirement' in which older people undertake various types of productive labour and retain active lifestyles.

What then are the more influential discourses on ageing in our societies, what assumptions underpin them and what social impacts do they have? First amongst the more influential discourses on ageing in contemporary times are the discourses that underpin this book, specifically those relating to positive ageing. In the United Kingdom a national policy called 'Our Healthy Nation' (United Kingdom 2001) seeks, amongst other strategies, to promote age diversity in communities and workplaces and the formation of healthy neigh- bourhoods where 'everyone is valued equally, regardless of race, age and gender' and 'where people are responsible citizens and support each other'. The policy recognises the links between worklessness, poverty, poor mobility, poor mental health and social exclusion for various sectors of the community, including older citizens, and seeks to redress their marginalisation within a broad-based approach to social inequality in the nation's health and well-being. Within the policy, the 'Age Positive' strategy emphasises the value of older citi- zens to the community through a focus on potential, skills and ability rather than age. Positive ageing in general terms is a discourse that links to a number of influential discourses to do with healthy lifestyles, anti-discrimination and inclusion, productive and active lifelong citizenship, ethical work practices, fairness and social justice, and the need to disrupt some of the ideas that have constructed the ageing in negative or abject terms.

The discourse of positive ageing is attaining widespread influence in official, professional and popular discourses. Official discourses, for our purposes, include those of governments, particularly those underpinning various policies and programs. In New Zealand there is currently a national policy in support of 'positive ageing' (New Zealand Ministry of Health 2002) that seeks to work 'alongside older people as members of families, whanau and the community', and that seeks to enable older people to 'age in place' through an integrated continuum of community-based care. The policy also endorses culturally appropriate services that recognise the diversity amongst older citizens. The current government discourses on ageing in most western countries include a discourse on 'healthy agency' for older people, 'agency' here meaning the ability to act on the world, thus attempting to disrupt the discourse of the depend- ency of older people. For example, Canada's National Framework on Aging (Minister of Public Works and Government Services Canada, 1998) sets out general principles for seniors to experience longer, healthier and economically better lives than seniors of pre- vious generations. Likewise, the Public Policy and Aging Report, prepared by the National Academy on an Aging Society (1999), makes the point that policy decisions can result in 'tomorrow's elderly' population experiencing improvements in health status. Although we visualise dependency as the loss of personal freedoms, governments have a vested interest in limiting the degree of dependence of its citizens on government-funded services. To this end the Australian government has focused in its *National Strategy for an Ageing Australia* (Bishop 1999a) on cost-effective care, and on supporting and increasing the role of non-government carers of the frail and elderly. That is, there is a shift in government discourses of ageing from public to private responsibility. The official discourses of 'health care' for the frail and elderly include an emphasis on access and equity, affordability, sustainability, quality, choice and responsiveness to various equity groups. Emphasis is on health 'maintenance' rather than 'care', an important discursive shift that supports the discourse of the agency of the ageing. The 'BetterCare' program established by the Australian government to provide for the professional development of aged care workers is part of a discourse of accreditation and standards that signals a desire to further legislate against the abuses and neglect of older people and to 'professionalise' the aged care workforce. Systems of accreditation are a means of surveillance and control in contexts where deregulation has led to abuses of rights and poor standards, a context that many in Australia have described as being in a state of crisis.

The discourse of crisis is echoed by the World Health Organization (WHO 1988), although running counter to this is the discourse of opportunity. WHO argues that the rapidly ageing world offers both negative and positive possibilities for governments and societies. In support of the discourse of positive ageing WHO emphasises enjoyment rather than endurance in ageing, prevention rather than treatment, ability rather than disability, independence rather than dependence, and so on. In general there is an observable shift in official discourses on ageing away from a preoccupation with services for older persons to an emphasis on social processes.

Research discourses in recent years are also characterised by a shift in gaze away from the people who are ageing to the processes of ageing, particularly those processes that are positive on both an individual and community level. *A Review of Healthy Ageing Research in Australia* (Kendig et al 2000) identifies a number of shifts in gerontology research. Contrary to engendering sympathy for the plight of older Australians (discussed earlier as compassionate stereotyping), the review argues that the discourses of elder abuse so popular in the media could perhaps have contributed to constructions of older people as frail and lacking in agency and potency. When principally portrayed as victims of abuse, it becomes a challenge for older people to portray themselves as vital and productive members of society, reminding us of the power of discourse to construct material realities. In an analysis of the economic implications of Australia's ageing population, the discourse of 'ageing gracefully' was prominent, and linked to a fear of the economic burden of an ageing population, including costs associated with health care, personal safety, transport, housing, recreation and community support (Minichiello 1995).

Assumptions behind discourses

Having identified some of the major discourses on ageing in some western societies, it is now necessary to consider why it is they have emerged and the assumptions underpinning them. One of the major lessons that Sigmund Freud (1961) gave to the world, a lesson useful for our analysis of the discourses on older people and ageing, is that it is a feature of humanity that we both love and hate each other. Although we would like to consider ourselves as freedom loving, egalitarian and democratic, we are in fact deeply ambivalent about our fellow humans (Phillips 2002). It is a curious feature of human nature that we can both love and hate the same object. Further, as sociologists have discovered, our feelings of love and hate, affection and disaffection, arise around axes of social difference—around issues of gender, ageing, sexuality, ability and disability, ethnicity, religion, place, nationality: indeed, any marker of social difference. Thus, it is possible for us to be deeply ambivalent about our others. It is perhaps a shocking fact that we can both love and hate the very young and the very old, as the statistics on child and elder abuse attest. Our observations about these features of human emotion are, of course, not arguments that this should be so. Rather, the theory of human ambivalence gives us a way of exploring the very real problem of abuse in our society. What remains to be explained is how this ambivalence emerges, why it emerges around specific objects, and what impact it has.

If we take as a case the violence towards older people, we need to ask, Where does the hatred come from? One answer (which Freud would agree with) is that it comes from a sense of fear. Just as the very young are dependent on everything in the world, the frail elderly are a reminder of the failure of our own omnipotence, the failure of our control over our environment. Further, the elderly are a reminder of mortality, a symbol of the loss of potency, libido, passion and desire, for each of these losses is also within our-selves. We struggle with these qualities in ourselves and don't wish to be reminded of them. Frail elderly people, it could be argued, are frequently constructed as 'abject' peoples. The notion of abjectivity is a key concept explored by Kristeva (1982) as a way of explaining the social effects of Freud's argument about our deep ambivalence. The abject, she explains, is 'that part of ourselves that the self seeks to expunge in order to make the self more sociably accept-able'. That is, the abject is an aspect of ourselves that we don't want to accept or recognise: in this instance, our potential to be frail and elderly. Thus, if we fear loss of control over our environ-ment, we will expunge from our lives all reminders of this. If we fear death, we will be uncomfortable around reminders of death.

Who are society's abject peoples—those who are expunged from our lives and our social consciousness? In eighteenth-century England the very poor were considered abject peoples and were banished to the far colonies on convict ships. In colonial Australia, the United States and Canada, the Indigenous and First Nations peoples were considered abject peoples to be herded into reserves far from cities or on the margins of white towns. It has been argued that today's 'old age homes' are a reminder of the ways in which we banish abject peoples. Such an argument against the institution-alisation of the elderly, while compelling when we remember the history of the institutionalisation of marginal peoples, tends to ignore the very real needs of frail and elderly people for daily social support. Thus today's debates around institutionalisation tend to be complex and contradictory, the contradictions reflecting our deeply held fears and ambivalences around difference, and in this instance, reminders of our own mortality. What are the key debates within aged care and gerontology today, and in what ways do they reflect historical ten-dencies and deep ambivalences? What are the contradictions in what we say as health professionals and what factors help explain these contradictions?

What are the traces of ambivalence in discourses on ageing? There are three common clues to be found within language that indicate ambivalence towards the ageing; the first is called 'essen-tialising'; the second is 'othering'; the third is 'superannuating'. Essentialising about particular groups means to over-generalise about them and to focus on the group commonalities rather than the differences within the group. Thus when we characterise older people as frail or in need of care we forget that many are strong, some are at times both frail and strong, and many are neither. We tend to over-generalise about older people, to forget their many differences, the diversity of interests, passions and life experiences amongst them. Thus in gerontology research a reliance on averages denies variation. The OECD (1996) advocates a re-examination of assumptions that ill-health is a defining feature of older age. Defining features are examples of over-generalisations or essentialisms. They ignore diversity. There are, of course, many subgroups within older citizens in our societies, all of whom have different histories, desires, social situations and needs.

The second clue to ambivalence is the process of othering, in which older people are always portrayed as other to ourselves. We think in terms of self and other as very different, perhaps as opposites. What we are, they are not, and vice versa. If I am young and vibrant and active, my older others are the opposite of this. If I perceive myself as central to the social world, I will consider older people as marginal to it. Othering has the effect of distancing. Social distance is one of the major problems facing older people. In many societies the term 'seniors' is used to describe older people. Indeed, in Australia 'seniors cards' are available for everyday discounts and special considerations. In Canada there is a Federal Department of Aging and Seniors. In what ways is the term 'seniors' a form of othering of some sections of our societies? Does the term 'seniors' work in both positive and negative ways for certain groups? The danger of talking about (rather than with) older people, representing their interests, saying what it is they want or need, categorising them, although necessary in some contexts, is that it tends to perpetuate the process of othering by denying older people their own voice and choice. The age integration of social institutions, such as in the UK policy of age integration in neighbourhoods and workplaces, is one means by which the young–old, self–other binary can be dissolved.

The third strategy through which ambivalence becomes institutionalised is superannuating, which means that we assume older people belong in another time. If we belong in the contemporary world, they belong in the past. The term 'old-timers' exemplifies the superannuating of older people, the denial of their vital place in the contemporary world.

All these discursive strategies, essentialising, othering and superannuating, have the effect of dehumanising older people. When we dehumanise certain groups it makes it easier for us to deny them basic human rights, to treat them with disrespect and to devalue their experiences and desires. Each of these strategies perpetuates a form of violence towards the ageing, perhaps not in the overt form of violence which marks the body, but in a disavowal of their humanness which arguably is just as damaging. It is important therefore to identify each of these strategies in our language and to begin to develop alternatives.

Often our language lags behind what we know to be a problem. It is not inconceivable that in time we will realise that there is a violence in the terms 'older' and 'ageing' and we will invent new language to deal with this. The work of discourse analysis for gerontology professionals thus involves both critique and invention. It involves frequent self-reflection and collective review of two key questions: What is the effect of what we say? and, How can we say things differently and in ways that lead to better outcomes?

Activity 1.3

Find a recently released government policy document on any aspect relating to older people. Analyse the language used to describe older people and/or ageing. What are the positive or negative implications behind these discourses?

Conclusion

It seems rather obvious to say that the history of getting old is the history of all living things. From the moment the spark of life quickens, the organism moves inexorably towards death. When we use the clock to measure this we call it 'ageing'. However, identifying living things by the clock is not really very helpful. We may be able to say that a person has lived for 50, 60 or 70 years but it tells us little else about them. It says nothing about their skills, their health, their interests, their wealth. Butler (1975) makes the point that chronological age is a way of marking the passing of time but is not an indicator of a person's physical, emotional or psychological abilities. He goes on to note that psychological indicators show that older people exhibit greater variations from the mean than any other age group. In fact, he suggests, the older people become, the more unlike each other they become. Unlike 'typical' 2-year-old behaviour or physical development, there is really no 'typical' 72-year-old behaviour or physical condition. Despite this, many groups in society use the measure of 'time' as a marker of 'type', as if it were the only way to identify people. Thus time has become a stereotype for identifying people at whatever age, and decisions are made on the basis of it. Changing this way of thinking will be a challenge. Who will bring about this change and how will it unfold and be negotiated are key questions.

At this point in western societies, few older people have themselves developed an anti-ageist consciousness (Walker & Minichiello 1996). That is, many members of this marginalised group have not yet become conscious of the effects of stereotyping and discrimination and their inferior ascribed spoiled identity; they have accepted the negative characteristics associated with later life because they see it as a normal part of 'being old'—as Biggs (1993) argues, to the detriment of their potential selves. In an Australian study, Minichiello and his colleagues (2000) found that older people come to accept living with ageism by adopting a philosophy of 'not making waves', trying to 'get on with life' and ignoring unpleasant interactions. Here are some examples of how the older person adjusts her life to deal with the discrimination and hardship of 'being old' in society:

> . . . to accommodate for inadequate pensions older people move into shared accommodation, struggle to manage, or 'scrape and save' to get things they need. Informants who said they were pushed or bumped in the street adopt the strategies of not going out so much, taking a walking stick for defence whenever they go out, not saying anything to the person and ignoring the aggressor. Those who are treated rudely or impatiently in shops simply disregard this behaviour. Informants describe instances in which they have simply stopped participating in certain activities because access is poor. They withdraw from situations in which they are treated as old or unwanted, or in which they would have to assert themselves and ask for special treatment in order to enable them to continue with an activity (Minichiello et al 2000, p. 272).

Walker and Maltby (1997) make an important observation worth discussing here. They note that in the 20th century many older people have been political leaders (for example, Ronald Reagan and the Soviet leaders of the 1970s and 1980s), but senior citizens as a group have been far less active in politics than their counterparts. One study in Europe reported by Walker and Maltby (1997) asked whether 'older people should stand up more actively for their rights' and found that over 80 per cent agreed with this statement. There is a view amongst the public that older people have not been politically active to date.

However, there are signs that older people are on the political move and developing an awareness of being discriminated against because they are 'old'. Political parties and new age-based groupings are being formed and the politicisation of ageing issues is squarely on the public agenda. Charters of rights are being passed in the European parliament and in the United Nations, expressing the individual and social rights and aspirations of older citizens (see, for example, the Declaration of the Rights of Older Persons (Butler 2002)). In the field of education we are seeing the rapid spread of Universities of the Third Age, designed to reintegrate older people into the world of higher education. As noted by Walker and Maltby (1997, p. 115), this development is of the greatest importance because 'it is aimed at overcoming the education deficit experienced by many older people, especially older women'.

Demographers and political scientists are predicting that the unprecedented numbers of the baby-boomer generation will be exerting powerful social and political influences in the decades to come. Ken Dychtwald (1999) in *Age Power: How the 21st Century Will Be Ruled by the New Old*, predicts that as a result of the demands of the baby boomers, markets will change—clothing designs, travel accommodations, automobile design and investment planning, to name a few. The ageing baby boomers will be computer literate (see Chapter 11), well educated, and have economic resources that were not available to previous cohorts of older persons. As Chapter 2 shows, they will be living longer and healthier lives. They will be much more informed consumers who will exhibit different communication interactions with service providers, including health professionals, and insist on choice, on being informed and being provided with quality service. Consider the following statistics provided by Dychtwald (1999), in his argument that the 50 and over population represents a new age-power.

For example, in the United States this group:

- controls more than $7 trillion in wealth or 70 per cent of the total wealth;
- has a high level of home ownership (more than 79 per cent own their homes);
- represents 40 million credit-card holders;
- purchases 40 per cent of all new cars;
- has the greatest net worth assets of any age group.

These powerful statistics, with their impact on the economy and market forces, along with the growing determination of older people themselves to address the consequences of ageism on their lives, will result in a revolution of change in the decades to come. With this change will come opposition, liberation, opportunities and new ways of thinking about later life in society.

2

The role of health promotion in healthy ageing

Rafat Hussain, Rodrigo Mariño, Irene Coulson

This chapter provides an overview of the definition and measurement approaches for some of the key terms such as 'quality of life' and 'active ageing', followed by a discussion of the link between ageing and health promotion using a variety of examples from past research into these issues. The principles and issues in provision of health promotion for older adults are discussed to assist readers to develop skills in developing health promotion programs for older population subgroups.

Why are ageing, quality of life and health important to us all? Throughout the world the ageing process unifies us as a human race and defines us all. The fact that the world's population is ageing is a triumph for the human race. We all age, and collectively we yearn for quality of life and good health in later life. Because human beings must grow older, the ageing process and health is an issue that concerns us all. Health is largely determined by cultural factors, economic status, gender, personal values, race, age and geography (WHO 2002). The traditional definition of health, the absence of disease or disability, is inappropriate for older persons. While older persons can experience disability, they can still achieve improved quality of life and good health. Definitions of health for older people must include 'health and well-being as inseparable from identities and experiences accumulated throughout the life' (Kendig 1996b, p. 369b). Kendig goes on to say that health for older people should be viewed from the perspective of their friends, adult children and health professionals, and provides a holistic understanding of older people's health actions. Health defined in this manner may provide clues as to how older people are actively ageing, and are organised and motivated to align themselves with healthy ways of life (Kendig 1996b).

The term 'active ageing' was adopted in the late 1990s by the World Health Organization (WHO 2002) in exchange for 'healthy ageing' because it was more inclusive and recognised factors in addition to health care that affect individuals and how populations age. Active ageing is defined as 'the process of optimizing opportunities for health, participation and security in order to enhance quality of life as people age' (WHO 2002, p. 12). The active ageing approach shifts strategic planning from a needs-based approach to a rights-based approach by recognising the rights of older people for opportunity and treatment in all aspects of life, thus promoting healthy lifestyle behaviours. WHO states that the determinants of active ageing include economic, social, personal and behavioural determinants, physical environment and access to health and social services. There is evidence to show that these predictors can determine how older people and populations age. Moreover, as people age their quality of life is largely determined by their ability to maintain autonomy and independence (WHO 2002).

Quality of life is often measured as an individual's behaviour and/or level of functioning; it can also be defined and measured as how individuals perceive their health status or well-being (Muldoon et al 1998). Together, the objective and the subjective dimension provide a broad-ranging context, incorporating in a complex way a person's physical health, psychological state, independence, social relationships, personal beliefs and relationships to salient features in the environment (WHO 1998a). How quality of life is perceived by individuals and addressed by health policy and services will be one of the greatest challenges this century will need to address.

Approaches for measuring successful ageing

There are two different approaches for measuring successful ageing, the biomedical model and functional status. The biomedical model tends to largely measure health as absence of ill health. Among the indices to measure health include the concept of healthy life expectancy, including disability-free life expectancy (DFLE) and disability-adjusted life expectancy (DALE) (Murray & Lopez 1997; Robine et al 1999; Mathers et al 2001). DALE provides an estimate of expected number of years to be lived in an equivalent state of full health. There are now over 199 countries for which DALE data is available (Mathers et al 2001). One of the consistent trends seen across most developed and developing countries is gender differentials: women not only have a higher life expectancy than men but also have a higher prevalence of chronic conditions and disabilities, particularly in old age (Henrard 1996; Robine et al 1999).

From the individual's perspective, to age successfully requires not only a low risk of disease and disease-related disability but also high mental and physical functioning and active engagement with life (Rowe & Kahn 1997). To maintain physical and mental functioning requires a focus on the concept of functional capacity. It can be argued that old age cannot be totally free of disease and disability—hence functional status allows us to measure the ability of older persons to perform activities that are essential to their sense of well-being and quality of life (WHO 1998b).

A recent study that used both quantitative and qualitative measures found that when successful ageing was defined as an optimal state of overall functioning and well-being, few people met the criteria (von Faber et al 2001). However, older people themselves view successful ageing as a process of adaptation. Using this perspective, many more people could be considered to have aged successfully (von Faber et al 2001). The concept of self-rated health has been shown to have validity. A large cohort-based study of older people in Manitoba found that self-rated health was both an important predictor of mortality over a twelve-year period and was also a useful predictor of successful ageing (Roos & Haven 1991).

Health promotion and ageing

Increasingly WHO is recommending a life course perspective for achieving successful and healthy ageing. For health systems to adopt this perspective as a means for achieving active ageing requires policies and strategies that lend themselves to integration for health promotion, disease prevention and provision of affordable and accessible curative health care services, especially at the primary care level. We use the concept of health promotion both as a philosophy that empowers people to take control of their health and as an over-arching strategy that brings together preventative and curative health care services to enable people to have healthier lives. Epidemiological evidence indicates that old age should not necessarily be equated with poor health, provided serious efforts are made to modify the role and impact of extrinsic risk factors (Reed et al 1998). To lower the risk of disease, the emphasis must be on early and lifelong prevention addressing the main risk factors that play a key role in accelerating the process of chronic disease morbidity and mortality (Kilander et al 2001). Preventive health strategies need to be enacted at all three levels—primary, secondary and tertiary.

Primary prevention strategies promoting healthy lifestyles will be most effective when initiated at the earliest opportunity. Whereas the benefits of primary prevention would be greatest when initiated amongst younger age groups, there is considerable benefit to be obtained by enacting preventive strategies across all age groups. For example, falls are a major cause of morbidity and mortality amongst older persons (Rivara et al 1997). Certain types of physical activity have been shown to be beneficial for reducing the incidence of falls in old age (Campbell et al 1997; Wolf et al 2001). In this instance, primary prevention needs to extend beyond the promotion of physical activity to identifying other medical risk factors that increase the risk of a fall, and to changes in environmental conditions that exacerbate the risk of falls (Haber 1999; see also Chapter 11). Simple preventive measures such as reorganising of furniture, provision of handrails and appropriate night lighting can also lead to a marked reduction in the incidence of falls among the elderly (Carter et al 1997; Turkoski et al 1997).

Another example is primary prevention in oral health. Today, more than ever before, older adults are keeping their natural teeth, and improvements in oral health status will continue into the future. This will bring about important changes and challenges to health promotion initiatives. Much of the work of current oral health promotion is aimed at altering or maintaining the individual's oral hygiene practices. However, traditional oral health education might be ineffective amongst people with diminished cognitive status, decreased visual acuity, or loss of strength or function of hands, each of which may alter an individual's ability to maintain their oral hygiene successfully (Erickson 1997). Thus, maintaining a good oral health status will mean different approaches, from new requirements for oral hygiene aids (for example, toothbrushes designed for a better grip) and development of new therapeutic agents (such as fluorides), to different societal attitudes towards oral health (losing teeth is not a part of the normal ageing process). All these elements should be considered as part of oral health promotion.

Secondary prevention provides opportunities for early diagnosis and early treatment of disease and conditions, as well as for health promotion (ACGP 2002). Secondary prevention includes screening programs to prevent the progression of treatable diseases, such as diabetes, hypertension, osteoporosis and various forms of cancers (ACGP 2002). Secondary prevention for cardiovascular disorders assumes a significant importance for elderly populations (Campbell et al 1998; Holt et al 2000). Screening programs for cancer have been shown to be effective in limiting disease progression for conditions such as breast cancer, the leading cause of mortality amongst women (Blanks et al 2000; US Preventive Service Task Force 2002), and cervical cancer (Anttila et al 1999; Taylor et al 2001). Although lung cancer remains one of the leading causes of death in the developed world, preventive measures are aimed at the primary level (smoking cessation) rather than screening.

Health promotion through tertiary preventive strategies is also needed to prevent the progression of disabilities in older people. Disabilities not only reduce the quality of life; severe disabilities are also a major risk factor for institutional care (Guralink et al 1995; Gill et al 1996). Physical activity can reduce disability in older persons through reduction in the functional impact of the disease (Leveille et al 1999). Resistance or aerobic exercise can reduce pain and disability from conditions such as arthritis, a major cause of disability (Ettinger et al 1997). Progressive hearing loss is a common disability in old age that has not only a physical dimension but also a social one. Older people with hearing loss are likely to limit social contact and community participation (Kempen et al 1998). Similarly, poor oral health in old age is not simply a risk factor for malnutrition; oral health is critical to appropriate physical, emotional and social functions (Fiske et al 1998). Clinical data also demonstrates that oral health problems are related to local and systemic morbidity (Chauncey et al 1985). For example, aspiration of oral secretions and their bacteria is increasingly being recognised as an important factor for pneumonia (Gift 1988), and periodontal disease is now considered to be an important risk factor for cardiovascular disease (Katz et al 2001). Provision of appropriate assistance in the form of hearing aids, vision correction and management of oral health problems can all be viewed as examples of tertiary prevention aimed at limiting disability and improving well-being and the quality of remaining life.

A related aspect of preventive strategies for health promotion is focusing on mental health issues that promote active engagement with life. While there has been considerable focus and attention on determinants and management of dementia in older people (Cooper & Holmes 1998; Kales et al 1999; Lyketsos et al 2000), other aspects of promoting mental health have not received adequate attention. Many older people face considerable emotional stress and psychological distress in the form of inadequate social support networks due to loss of family members and friends, and reduced contact with society due to retirement (Kaplan 1997). Older people are also more vulnerable to violence and abuse (Lachs et al 1997; Comijs et al 1998). Elder abuse encompasses not only physical violence but also psychological, financial and sexual abuse, as well as neglect, which may take the form of intentional or unintentional failure to fulfil a caregiver role (WHO/ International Network for the Prevention of Elder Abuse [INPEA] 2002). While there are no precise estimates of the prevalence of depression amongst older persons, it is considered to be an underlying cause for triggering or accentuating functional limitations in later life (Robinson 1998). There is increasing evidence of the negative impact of depression on mortality and morbidity in old age (Bruce et al 1994; Kaplan et al 1994; Carrington Reid 2003). While women tend to have higher rates of depression than men in general, in the older age groups it has been found that men have higher suicide rates than women (Pearson & Conwell 1995). A longitudinal study aimed at assessing predictors of successful ageing found that good mental health, increased physical activity and higher community involvement were together more significant predictors of successful ageing than when studied separately (Strawbridge et al 1996).

Health promotion strategies that focus only on promoting physical health as part of active ageing but fail to be cognisant of the need to enable older people to be sexually (see Chapter 4), emotionally and psychologically active and healthy are likely to achieve a minimal return in the form of improved health status of older persons.

Activity 2.1

List at least four health conditions that are amenable to primary, secondary or tertiary prevention. Against each condition list one or two appropriate health promotion strategies.

Principles of health education and health promotion in older adults

This section provides an overview of the factors that impact on the learning abilities of older adults in relation to health education and health promotion. It includes a review of the literature, with suggestions that might optimise learning performance in older populations. Contrary to the myth that it is too late for older adults to benefit from changing lifelong habits (Jarvis 2001), studies show that lifestyle modifications have been successfully implemented even amongst the very old, provided the effect of co-morbidities is not overwhelming (Kicklighter 1991; Young 1996; Burbank et al 2000; Chernoff 2001). Furthermore, the most commonly reported reason for not undertaking health promoting and disease prevention measures by older adults (diet, exercise, stress management, tobacco avoidance, etc.) was 'not being told to' by the primary health care provider (Resnick 2000). With the growing number of older adults worldwide, it is especially important to educate both the health providers and the general public, particularly older adults themselves, that older adults are unique individuals with exceptional needs, who are capable of change and are able to learn new, or to maintain acquired, healthier lifestyles. Failure to change or poor performance might be related to a range of non-cognitive factors (Taub, quoted in Kicklighter 1991) such as:

- health status
- poor learning conditions
- lack of confidence
- poor motivation
- task relevance

- age-related physiological changes:
  (a) visual changes
  (b) hearing changes
- fatigue, [and]
- distrust of research or health services.

Kicklighter (1991) suggests that programs aimed at older adults may need some modifications to compensate for non-cognitive factors and to enhance their learning capacity—for example, visual acuity, peripheral vision, tolerance to glare and ability to adapt to dark and light might diminish with age. Suggested changes include avoiding dark rooms and preferring rooms with good light, but without glare. Printed materials should use large fonts (36-point), be well spaced and printed in primary colours. In particular, the author indicates that blues, greens and violets should be avoided, preferring red, orange, brown and black. Hearing impairments are the most common chronic condition in populations over 65 years (National Center for Health Statistics 1999). They are reported by 23 per cent of persons aged 65–74, 33 per cent of persons aged 75–84, and 48 per cent of persons aged 85 and older in the United States (Daly & Katzel 1997). These conditions range from tinnitus to complete deafness (Chávez & Ship 2000). Because of these conditions, older participants in health education sessions might misinterpret words and sentences during conversation, which may lead to anxiety, hostility or withdrawal. Table 2.1 includes some suggestions that may compensate for hearing and visual impairments.

Retrieval of information may also become slower with age, and older people may experience an age-related memory loss called benign senescent forgetfulness (Gift 1988; Beers & Berkow 2000). This may require special attention to methods of communication, for example, allowing extra time to respond so participants do not feel rushed (Kicklighter 1991).

The importance of lifelong learning is well established in the literature and in recent decades has received increasing attention (Kicklighter 1991; Young 1996; Chernoff 2001; Jarvis 2001). However, despite the experiences in health promotion and the amount of health promotion material available, several authors have concluded that there is little literature providing sufficient details to guide practice (Rogers et al 1992; Kreidler et al 1994; Brice et al 1996; Haber 1996; Kay & Locker 1998). They conclude that few studies provide strong evidence on how best to provide

Table 2.1: Suggestions for improving communication with participants who have hearing and visual impairments

Suggestion for improving communication	Hearing	Visual
Make certain hearing aids are in place and working properly	x	
Know how to assist participants with hearing aids if necessary	x	
Speak slowly	x	
Use short simple sentences	x	
Ask questions slowly with adequate response time	x	
Avoid asking more than one question at a time	x	
Avoid sudden change of topics	x	
Speak clearly and loudly, but do not shout or over-exaggerate the words	x	
Minimise outside noise	x	
Reduce glare		x
Make certain that participants wear glasses when necessary		x
Printed material should be well spaced, and in large, bold or contrasting letters		x
Avoid dark rooms	x	x
Use gestures and non-verbal cues when appropriate	x	x
Face the participants and make eye contact	x	x

Sources: Kicklighter 1991; Chávez & Ship 2000

health promotion and disease prevention services to older adult populations. However, to ignore opportunities for health promotion and disease prevention in these groups is unfair, as such neglect is likely to increase inequalities in health standards, and may lead to even greater demands for curative and oral rehabilitative services by older adults.

Health promotion, health education, health maintenance and healthier lifestyles all depend on individuals completing certain behaviours (Burbank et al 2000). Because traditional education might be ineffective in changing an individual's lifestyle, what follows are some elements to take into consideration when planning and developing health promotion programs.

Key elements for adult learning

Relevance

Programs with the greatest chance of success are those programs that are relevant to individuals (Kay & Locker 1998; Chernoff 2001). A good first step towards assuring relevance is to understand the issues surrounding the social meaning of health experiences. Participants should be encouraged to articulate their own health-related perceptions, concerns, needs and conceptualisations about health and health promotion activities (Stead et al 1997).

Taking into account the individual's experience

Adult learning does not occur in a vacuum. Older learners bring experience to the leaning process, which is a resource to be used (Erickson 1997). Thus, new information has to be related to what is already known. Older learners have to be given the opportunity to challenge material, discuss contents, discard known information and request additional information. In examining health care information through the lens of personal experience, some may reject any evidence that contradicts long-held beliefs and values, or is foreign to their cultural framework (Rubenstein & Nahas 1998). It would be more worthwhile for health educators to work towards modifying these beliefs than to challenge them (Haber 1996).

Realistic and measurable goals

Health promotion activities should include active participation by recipients in program planning, implementation and evaluation (Young 1996; Dahlin-Ivanoff et al 1998; Rubenstein & Nahas 1998; Chernoff 2001; Koelen et al 2001). This will also ensure that health promotion activities will be based on the target group's own goals and needs (Young 1996; Koelen et al 2001), and is likely to increase the participants' sense of program ownership, which is one of the key goals of health promotion. Motivation to learn is enhanced when learners feel they are progressing, thus it is important that they have a clear understanding of the desired goal and the means to achieve it. Older adults are able to evaluate their own progress against predefined criteria, therefore ongoing feedback about their progress towards set goals is likely to yield positive results.

Group-based interaction

Interactive educational efforts, like group health education sessions, have been regarded as an effective approach for older adult learning (Drossaert et al 1996; Little et al 1997). There is empirical evidence of the effectiveness of this approach in achieving health promotion goals in the areas of physical activity (Stead et al 1997), macular degeneration (Dahlin-Ivanoff et al 1998), breast cancer (Solomon et al 1998), diabetes and nutritional information (Kicklighter 1991) and oral health knowledge, attitudes and behaviours (Mariño et al 2002). However, it must be kept in mind that there may be topics, such as safe sex, body image, bad breath and obesity, that participants feel embarrassed or hesitant about discussing in peer groups (Little et al 1997).

Furthermore, older adults make up a highly heterogeneous group. When culturally and linguistically diverse older adults are considered, materials and discussions have to be in the person's own language. As already noted, traditional cultural/ethnic beliefs should not be challenged, but incorporated and reinforced or modified as needed (Haber 1996). While communicating with people who have dementia or are confused can be difficult and frustrating, Jarvis (2001) indicates that those with dementia can still keep learning while their condition progresses, provided their personhood is valued.

Key recommendations for group discussions in health education include:

- Health education should be conducted using a combination of group discussions and printed material. All verbal or printed information provided should be easily accessible, non-intrusive and relevant to the older adult participants.
- Ideally, these sessions could take place at a venue where the older adults usually go (civic clubs or clubs for the elderly, churches, etc.).
- The size of the group has to be one that allows interaction between the participants (5 to 10 participants per group).
- Language level should be:
  - appropriate for the target group
  - non-technical
  - concise
  - factual and specific.
- The group facilitator must be able to establish direct visual contact with participants.
- Each session should be brief (20–30 minutes) with one main topic and two or three major points. During the session, major points should be reviewed and repeated and questions clarified.

- Any printed material should:
  - be used to reinforce the session's main topic and major points, so that the participants can refer to them at home when less stressed
  - be written in large fonts
  - printed on matt, non-glare paper
  - use appropriate ink colour
  - use diagrams and other visual images that include familiar people, settings and symbols.

Sustainability

Sustainability is another important outcome for health promotion programs. This is significant because positive changes in knowledge, attitudes and behaviours, can only be achieved in the long term through sustained efforts (Koelen et al 2001). O'Loughlin et al (1998) conducted a thorough review of health promotion interventions and proposed additional key elements to ensure sustainability of interventions amongst older adults. These included volunteerism (programs run by non-paid staff were more likely to remain viable), support by a peer 'program champion', alignment with the organisation's goals and mission, and modifications during implementation.

Case study: Oral health promotion program for older migrant adults

The following case study describes the framework, process and results of a community-based oral health promotion program designed to address the needs and barriers to oral health care of Italian and Greek adults living in the community (Mariño et al 2002). It involved active, independent-living adults, 55 years and older, who participated in clubs for older persons.

The study included both qualitative and quantitative research components. The qualitative component comprised a series of focus group discussions conducted by bilingual researchers in the participants' native language at social clubs frequented by the group. A total of 172 older adults participated in the focus group discussions. The purpose of the group discussions was to obtain a better understanding of issues surrounding the social meaning of the oral health experiences of this group; to identify the participants' views, perceptions and concerns about oral health; and to inform the development of the instruments for data collection for the quantitative stages of the project.

For the quantitative phase a standard oral health examination and a structured interview were conducted. The interview included items concerned with socio-demographics, self-reported oral health status, utilisation of oral health services, oral hygiene practices, and oral health attitudes and knowledge. In addition, a number of previously validated scales were used to collect information including quality of life (Ware et al 1995, 1996; Slade 1997), and nutritional status (Lipski 1996). The oral examination consisted of an assessment of mouth soft tissue conditions, dental status, periodontal status and an assessment of oral hygiene. The total number of older adults who participated in the project was 734, which included 374 Greeks and 360 Italians. Participants were enrolled in the study over a period of approximately eighteen months. At the end of this stage, clubs were assigned to control and test clubs.

The oral health intervention, known as ORHIS (for Oral Health Information Seminars/Sheets), had two components: oral health seminars and oral health information sheets. The seminars consisted of a series of oral health sessions offered at fortnightly intervals. The session included groups of 8–10 older adults, who during 20–25 minutes at their social club worked through the oral health issues within the group, facilitated by a bilingual research assistant.

This format was developed following suggestions emerging from a thorough evidence-based literature review on health promotions in older adults (described earlier in the chapter), and suggestions on the format made by the participants themselves during the focus group discussions. Topics selected were those that the participants identified during the group discussions as relevant to their needs and for which they wanted information and new skills, as well as those identified by the findings from the oral clinical examination and oral health interview. The topics covered the nine areas that often comprise oral health promotion programs: expected oral changes in old age, dental caries and periodontal disease, what to do with remaining teeth, oral cancer, denture care, dry mouth, importance of receiving oral health care, oral health and diet, and how other diseases may affect oral health. The final content of each ORHIS was derived using an iterative process as delineated in Figure 2.1.

A script for the session and a first version of the ORHIS for each selected topic was prepared prior to the first discussion cycle. The first

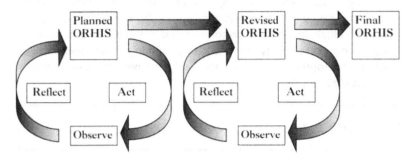

- Focus groups
- Clinical information
- Questionnaires

Figure 2.1: The ORHIS development process

session introduced the participants to the topic. Participants had the opportunity to challenge material and discuss contents. At the end of this cycle the research team met, and a second script and version of the ORHIS was prepared. The second cycle addressed deficiencies identified in the first round and noted any outstanding issues on the topic. The second version of the ORHIS was distributed and discussed among groups participants. The outcome of the second cycle was used to develop the final ORHIS for that topic. All the final versions were written in the native language of the participants and formed part of a set that was given to all participants, in an appropriately designed folder.

The evaluation was conducted into two parallel phases, one quantitative, the other qualitative. Together these two sources of data provided a more comprehensive view of the success of the health promotion intervention. The qualitative evaluation of the study involved fourteen group discussions with 150 older adults across the two ethnic groups. Participants showed strong support of the project and valued its approach, the methodology (education seminars), the preparation of simple printed material, and the distribution of dental materials relevant to each individual seminar. The quantitative evaluation involved a post-intervention measurement of change in oral health status/knowledge and behaviour. Five hundred and forty-two older adults participated in the quantitative evaluation. Analysis of the data (pre- and post-intervention results) indicated a strong effect of the intervention in terms of improved oral health knowledge, and attitude towards oral health care. There was also a significant increase in the proportion of participants in the experimental program who undertook a dental visit or treatment as a result of the intervention, compared to the control club group.

The approach used by this project (Mariño et al 2002) indicates that oral health related improvements can be achieved which can enable older individuals to increase control over oral health which in turn can assist in enhancing quality of life. Such a community-based approach might be appropriate for a wide range of health promotion programs amongst older adults.

Activity 2.2

What are the key elements of health education and promotion that can be used for older people?

Activity 2.3

In a health promotion program for older adults, what type of strategies would be appropriate to improve communications with participants with age-related visual and hearing changes?

Case study: Preventing vascular dementia in older persons through promoting healthy lifestyle behaviours

International research shows that vascular dementia (VaD) is the second most common dementia after Alzheimer's disease (Hamdy et al 1998; see also Chapter 5). While VaD is often associated with high blood pressure and cerebrovascular disease (Lis & Gaviria 1997), it is largely preventable. The major preventative VaD health promotion strategy is to target the risk factors predisposing to this condition in those who are cognitively and physically intact, as it offers the best alternative to costly aggressive treatment of the condition itself. The strategy includes taking responsibility for health through early screening and management of hypertension, cardiac arrhythmias and diabetes, while reducing cholesterol in itself can lower the incidence of VaD (Dartigues et al 1997).

In this section we describe a study conducted by Coulson, Mariño and Minichiello (2001) and Coulson et al (2002) that examined the relationship between knowledge and practice of healthy lifestyle behaviours in the prevention of VaD in Australia and Canada. The study was derived from 296 participants in Australia and 281 participants in Canada, recruited from senior citizen agencies. A survey consisting of 35 lifestyle knowledge items was utilised to reflect the six conceptual dimensions (Table 2.2) of the Health-Promoting Lifestyle Profile (Walker 1997). The second part of the survey included 52 items developed from the Health-Promoting Lifestyle Profile, a validated measurement tool that asked about lifestyle behaviours within the six conceptual dimensions.

The study found that increasing knowledge of VaD by itself may not ensure healthy lifestyle practice because the correlations between lifestyle knowledge and lifestyle behaviours were generally low. This was particularly the case with lifestyle behavior and healthy nutrition. The main finding, consistently found for Canada and Australia, was a higher healthy lifestyle score for those who expressed greater self-assessment of health status, higher knowledge of interpersonal relationships and medical knowledge and lower stress levels. The disparity between knowledge and practice should not be surprising and confirms that health education, while not sufficient to modify health behavior, is necessary to behavioural change (Steptoe et al 1997).

Participants in the study indicated that the Australian and Canadian Food Guides were difficult to follow because the number of food servings were too large to consume, and found that the guides were not user friendly for older people. For example, the print was small and difficult to read. In addition, anecdotal notes revealed that participants found it difficult to read labels on food or understand the meaning of the information related to nutritional value. Moreover, affordable programs are urgently needed that encourage exercise to improve appetite and maintain body weight and provide assistance to those who do not have the resources to purchase nutritional foods.

The study revealed a large proportion of the participants knew about the importance of contacting a health professional for health problems or obtaining a second opinion, but many did not practise this behaviour. 'Poor communication with health professionals may be related to poor access to health services, inability to pay, and negative attitudes about

Table 2.2: Health-promoting lifestyle profile: Six healthy lifestyle dimensions

Health self-responsibility	Observing one's own body and attending to its messages, seeks advice from appropriate persons when indicated.	*Sample question: Question health professionals in order to understand their instructions.*
Nutrition	Awareness and benefits of a nutritious diet, consumes a nutritious diet, aware of medications and side-effects.	*Sample question: Eats 2–3 serves of fruit each day.*
Physical activity	Maintenance of a regular physical exercise program and consults with health practitioner to advise on appropriate exercise program.	*Sample question: Follows a planned exercise program.*
Stress management	Ability to achieve peace of mind when chronic, major life events or acute daily hassles occur, utilises effective stress management and coping mechanisms.	*Sample question: Takes time for relaxation everyday.*
Interpersonal relationships	Seeks support and intimacy from friends and family, attends and participates in support agency activities, participates as a volunteer, participates in education programs, seeks professional counseling when needed.	*Sample question: Spends time with close friends.*
Spiritual growth	Ability to identify a sense of purpose in life, satisfied with self and others, has established goals for the next six months, shares wisdom and knowledge with others and is content with life.	*Sample question: Believes that my life has purpose.*

Source: Walker 1997

health professionals by older persons' (Coulson et al 2001, p. 282). Health promotion strategies should consider how senior citizens could take a more active role in promoting active ageing programs. For example, senior citizens should act as role models in leading exercise programs, instead of young people. In addition, participants knew the importance of physical exercise and leisure activities, but did not practise this behaviour. The results showed that higher knowledge of physical activities was a strong indicator of a higher healthy lifestyle score (Coulson et al 2001). The results concluded that well-being later in life involves more than good physical health—it involves people being content, and experiencing meaning and purpose in their lives.

The results confirmed that while many older adults knew that relaxation and stress management were important for the maintenance of health, many did not practise or know how to practise stress management techniques. Research needs to be undertaken to explore how older adults can learn relaxation and stress management techniques. Policies and programs can then be developed that promote these techniques, thus contributing to wellness in the lives of older adults. In addition, results for both countries revealed that a large proportion of participants did not recognise the importance of maintaining fulfilled relationships, nor did they have a network of caring people. The literature supports that the absence of satisfying relationships can result in loneliness and depression (Walker 1997).

The case study confirms that health promotion education by itself does not ensure healthy lifestyle practice for older adults, as correlations between lifestyle knowledge and lifestyle behaviours in all cases are generally low. The goal of committing to healthy lifestyle behaviours must be maintained throughout the life span if we are to reduce disability and VaD in the population. Regardless of age, older people must be taught that it is never too late to improve lifestyle practice and add quality years to one's life.

Conclusion

Healthy ageing requires proactive health promotion strategies that are enacted at primary, secondary and tertiary level, and also include accessible and affordable curative care services. It is important that the philosophy and principles of health promotion are used to guide policies and programs that are not limited in their scope to maintaining or improving physical health and/or provision of reha- bilitative services, but more importantly, are used to enhance the overall quality of life of the ageing population. The multi-dimensional nature of a healthy ageing approach requires an emphasis on improv- ing the psychological and emotional well-being of the ageing population, in addition to improving their physical health. Moreover, good health promotion programs require both awareness of, and commitment to, meeting the needs of all older adults including sexu- ally and culturally diverse population sub-groups.

Few studies provide adequate guidelines on how best to provide promotive and preventive information and services to the ageing population. However, examples of innovative approaches focusing on effective health promotion can be found in literature. Some of the experiences in health promotion with older adult groups highlighted in this chapter would indicate that the provision of an environment that facilitates group learning, followed by printed material, appears to best meet the social and learning needs of older adults. Also, the use of community resources would improve the cost-effectiveness of the interventions. Nonetheless, further research is required in order to improve health promotion practice. This would provide the 'know how' necessary to re-orient health services (Koelen et al 2001). Without this knowledge and understanding, designing health promotion interventions, which are responsive to the specific concerns of the older adults, will continue to remain a challenge.

3

The experience of ageing: Influences on mental health and well-being

Colette Browning, Yvonne Wells,
Andrew Joyce

The experience of ageing in our society is influenced by many factors—including biological, behavioural, psychosocial and economic—as well as the physical environment and access to health and community services (see Chapters 1, 2 and 11). These determinants impact on the physical and mental well-being of older people and underpin the concept of active or healthy ageing as outlined by the World Health Organization (WHO 2002). The relationships between these factors are multidirectional. Psychosocial factors such as adjustment to late-life transitions (for example, widowhood) or the availability of social support can influence physical and mental health. In turn, physical ill health impacts on mental ill health (for example, depression and anxiety) and social connectedness.

The focus of this chapter is to examine what influences mental health and well-being in later life. Promoting mental health and well-being is central to achieving positive ageing. We focus in particular on the influences of social factors and life transitions. For the purposes of the current discussion, indicators of mental health include depression and anxiety and indicators of well-being include positive and negative mood or affect (happiness/unhappiness). Social influences on mental health and well-being highlighted in this chapter are social support, social activities and social networks. The life transitions examined include retirement, widowhood and caregiving. Before we examine specifically the influences of social factors and life transitions on well-being, we will consider the evidence for the impact of ageing per se on mental health and well-being. The two case studies later in the chapter highlight variability in well-being in old age and the different influences on well-being. You should consider these case studies as you read this chapter.

Does growing old affect mental health and well-being?

As in most western countries, the main disabling conditions for older people are physical conditions, such as arthritis and circulatory problems (see Chapter 2; ABS 1999a). About three-quarters of people aged 65 and over have a physical condition as their main disabling condition, while mental health problems in the oldest-old (those aged 80 years and older) are significant. Mental health problems are the main cause of disability for about 15 per cent of people aged 80 years and over (ABS 1999a). For women aged 65 and over, anxiety disorders are the most prevalent mental disorders, followed by affective disorders and substance use disorders. For older men, anxiety disorders are the most prevalent followed by substance use disorders and affective disorders (ABS 1998).

Age-specific suicide rates tend to decrease across adulthood for both men and women (AIHW 2000). For women the rates are below 10 per 100 000 of population. For men, rates decrease from around 40 per 100 000 of population in the 20–29 age group to around 20 per 100 000 of population in the 70–79 age group. A group of particular concern, however, are men aged 80 and over, where age-specific suicide rates are in the order of 30 per 100 000 of population.

The aforementioned figures give us a picture of the clinical end of well-being in older people in many western countries. Much research, however, has been directed at the effect of ageing on mood or happiness. It has been well documented that socio-demographic influences such as age, marital status and income account for only a small amount of the variability in happiness between individuals (see Ryff 1989 for a review of the literature). Early theorists assumed that the weight of negative life events in old age, such as declining physical health and the loss of social networks through death of friends and spouses, would lead to a greater prevalence of unhappiness (Mroczek & Kolarz 1998), but studies of age effects on wellbeing have not consistently supported this contention. Carstensen (1992) has argued that well-being may improve in old age due to better regulation of emotions as we grow older. Her socio-emotional selectivity theory argues that because older people see their future options as less open than do young people, they construct their social lives to maximise positive mood or happiness. Other theorists have argued that personality is the key determinant of happiness at all stages of the life span and that this construct, shown to be relatively stable across the life span, may be more salient in determining well-being in old age than ageing per se (Costa et al 1987). More recently Ryff and Keyes (1995) have argued that the determinants of well-being are multifactorial and include situational factors (such as health status), personality factors and socio-demographic factors.

Mroczek and Kolarz (1998) posed the question: 'Does age affect well-being over and above the other factors shown to influence wellbeing?' Many of the studies investigating happiness measure positive and negative affects using a set of 10 or 12 questions. For example, participants are asked: 'During the last month how often have you felt sad?' (negative affect) or 'During the last month how often have you felt cheerful?' (positive affect). Mroczek and Kolarz (1998) reported two studies of people aged 65 and over that found differences in the age–affect relationship depending on the age group examined; for example, Ryff (1989) found that affect balance increased across young, middle-aged and old cohorts. Costa et al (1987) reported the results of a follow-up study, conducted in 1981 to 1984, that retested well-being in a sample who were aged 25 to 75 years in 1971–75 and found stability in positive and negative affect for all age groups over that period. At retest, older age was associated with lower negative and positive affect.

In order to clarify the complexity of the relationship between age and affect, Mroczek and Kolarz (1998) examined the interaction between age, personality, socio-demographic factors, contextual factors (stress and health), and positive and negative affect. The participants were aged 25 to 74 years and were surveyed using the Midlife Development Inventory. This inventory includes measures of affect; socio-demographic measures including age, gender, education and marital status; extraversion and neuroticism; measures of work and relationship stress; and self-reported health. They found a negative relationship between age and negative affect in men but not in women. Negative affect was lowest amongst older men; for women there was no relationship between age and negative affect. Being single was associated with high negative affect regardless of age, while older married men showed less negative affect than young married men. Thus only married men showed a negative relationship between age and negative affect. Mroczek and Kolarz (1998) postulated that marriage may provide men with the social context where they learn to reduce negative affect. The relationship between age and positive affect in men was linear. However, although personality moderated the relationship, older introverted men were more likely to show higher levels of positive affect than young introverted men. In women the relationship between age and positive affect was characterised by an accelerating curve.

How do social networks and social support affect mental health and well-being?

Social well-being or social health has been loosely defined and conceptualised at an individual level, incorporating interpersonal interaction and participation in social organisations (Bowling 1997). Social support, social activity, social networks and loneliness are components of social well-being that have been linked to mental and physical health outcomes. For older people, low levels of social activity, poor social support, poor social networks and loneliness have been linked to increased risk of mortality (Berkman & Syme 1979; House et al 1982; Kaplan et al 1988; Glass et al 1999); to increased levels of depression (Hraba et al 1997); to a greater likelihood of entering a nursing home (Russell et al 1997), and to lower feelings of self-esteem and life satisfaction (Ishii-Kuntz 1990; Felton & Berry 1992). Thus improving the social lives of older people has the potential to increase positive mental and physical health.

As previously noted, Carstensen et al suggest that older people pro-actively manage their social relationships to maximise emotional gains from a more limited social network (Lang & Carstensen 1994). Lang and Carstensen analysed data of a sub-sample of 156 community-dwelling and institutionalised people from the Berlin

Ageing Study (BASE). The age range was 70–104 years. Participants were asked to free recall social partners and to rate the emotional closeness of these relationships using three concentric circles, the inner circle representing 'very close', and succeeding larger circles representing less emotional attachment. Lang and Carstensen (1994) found that there was a reduction in the size of social networks across the age span. However, the reduction was greatest for the outer circles and there was very little reduction in the number of people mentioned as very close. Family was heavily represented in the inner circle and friends in the outer circle. Those people with nuclear family were more socially embedded than those without nuclear family and they had a higher average of close emotional relationships. For people without a nuclear family, those who had three close emotional relationships felt equally as socially embedded as those with a living nuclear family.

According to Lang and Carstensen (1994), the data suggests that older people were actively managing their social situation. If mortality and morbidity were determining their social network then there should have been equal reductions across the four levels of emotional closeness. As the percentage of social partners above the age of 75 was equivalent in each circle it was not the case that the outer circle represented age-matched friends and the inner circle was composed entirely of younger family members. People without a nuclear family were able to include friends and other relatives as close emotional partners. The outstanding problem from this study is making developmental conclusions from cross-sectional data; Lang and Carstensen acknowledged that longitudinal findings would strengthen their claims.

Lang et al (1998) followed up the Lang and Carstensen (1994) study using a larger sample size, although again the study was not longitudinal. Their analysis was based on the full sample of the BASE study, 516 older people, 156 of whom were used in the 1994 study. Lang et al (1998) used all 516 participants to investigate the contribution of personality versus social context in shaping the size of participants' social networks and their average level of emotional closeness to people within their network. Personality was measured with items assessing extraversion, neuroticism and openness to experience. Social context referred to whether the person had nuclear family members or no nuclear family available. The personality measures were related to network size with extraversion and openness to experience positively related to network

size and neuroticism negatively related to network size. Only neuroticism was related to average emotional closeness to network
members. However, social context was a more powerful predictor
of emotional closeness than neuroticism. Those with a nuclear
family had larger networks and higher averages of emotional closeness. The complement of 360 participants used in the 1998 but not
the 1994 study was analysed to cross-validate the 1994 study and
the same pattern of results was found. The inner sanctum of emotional closeness did not decrease over the age span, unlike the
outer circles.

General measures of social support have also been related to
mental health. Larson (1978) reviewed 30 years of literature on predictors of well-being for older Americans and concluded that social
activity, along with health and socio-economic status, have shown
the strongest relationships with well-being. Henderson et al (1998)
found that social isolation, as measured by a scale representing
social support, and amount of contact with family and friends, was
related to incidence of psychotic symptoms. Hraba et al (1997)
concluded that social isolation, operationalised as a lack of social
support, was a mediating factor between age and depression.

Hays et al (1998) studied different elements of social support as
predictors of different components of depression. They found that
receiving instrumental help was related to an increase in depressed
affect; this is consistent with other studies that have found a positive relationship between support received and depressed affect
(Leathers et al 1997). Those not receiving help were in better psychological health. The increased levels of help being received by
people with depression might represent other people responding to
signs of depression (Leathers et al 1997; Hays et al 1998). When
only people requiring assistance were studied, it was found that
bereaved older adults with high levels of information, and tangible
emotional support had less psychological distress than people
scoring low on those support indices (Krause & Markides 1990).

Hays et al (1998) also found that satisfaction with social interaction was related to lower scores for somatic complaints and
depressed affect. Availability of a confidant was one of the
strongest and most consistent protective predictors of depression.
Negative life events were the strongest predictors of depressed
affect but were not a consistent predictor of the other components
of depression. Size of the social network was a protective factor
from depressed affect and interpersonal problems. Giving instru-

mental support was related to an increase in interpersonal problems, although it protected against lowered positive affect. These research findings were consistent with previous findings that depression is characterised by a number of events and experiences that each have a modest effect.

Other studies have examined the relative contribution of frequency and quality of social contact with self-esteem and other indices of emotional well-being. Lee and Ishii-Kuntz (1988) found that frequency of contact with friends had an effect on emotional well-being through the creation of feelings of social integration. Feelings of loneliness impacted most strongly on emotional well-being. Another study by Ishii-Kuntz (1990) compared satisfaction and frequency of contact with psychological well-being. Perceptions of frequency and quality of social interaction were compared with affective and cognitive measures of well-being. The perceived quality of interaction, such as how satisfied people were with the time they spent with family and friends and how satisfied they were with activities with friends and family, was significantly related to well-being and controlled for any relationship between well-being and frequency of contact.

Ranzijn and Luszcz (1994) found both frequency of contact with adult children, and satisfaction with that contact, to be related to well-being in older people. The analyses were conducted separately for people living alone and those living with others (Ranzijn & Luszcz 1994). For people living alone, both frequency and satisfaction with contact predicted morale and depression. When the entire sample was included, both frequency and satisfaction predicted morale but only satisfaction was an independent predictor of depression. There are many factors important in well-being, of which parent–child interactions are just one contributor. This concurs with the conclusions of Hays et al (1998) that there are many different factors contributing to depression. Ranzijn & Luszcz (1994) argued that the high levels of social contact evident in their study limited the predictive validity of parent–child interactions and that a sudden decline in contact would reduce well-being.

Lawton et al (1999) investigated the relationship between objective and subjective indicators of family contact, friends contact and activity participation with positive affect and depression. They hypothesised that each subjective indicator would be related to positive affect but not depression. This view stemmed from the dual-channel theory that the sources of psychological well-being differ for positive and negative affect. External stimuli, such as time spent with friends and time spent on activities, would enhance positive affect but not influence negative affect, whereas intrapersonal factors, self-esteem and personality factors would influence negative but not positive affect. They also hypothesised that friends contact and activities participation would influence positive affect directly and indirectly, through their effects on friends quality and time quality respectively. Family contact would have no such relationship. The subjective measures of friends quality and time quality were related to positive affect but only the one objective measure of activity participation was related to positive affect and not friends contact. Family contact and quality did not show independent relationships with positive affect in the structural model. It was reasoned that the obligatory nature of familial relationships and their mixture of both conflict and support could have contributed to the findings of no relationship between family contact and affect. The authors suggested that perhaps a minimum level of family contact is required for positive affect and a relationship with positive affect can only be detected when the sample consists of participants below such a threshold. The lack of a relationship does not equate with the positive value of family mentioned by the participants. It would seem that families have the potential to offer strong benefits for emotional health.

Joyce (2002) analysed data from the Health, Behaviours and Outcomes of Older Adults Study, a longitudinal study of older people living in the community. This study tracked changes in people's health status, social and psychological well-being, health behaviours and service use from 1994 to 2000 (see Kendig 1996b for a description of the outcomes of the study at baseline). Joyce (2002) tested which components of social well-being were important for emotional health, tracked changes in social well-being indicators over time, and examined whether changes in social well-being predicted changes in emotional health as measured by positive and negative affect. A number of measures of social well-being were included in the analyses. The amount of contact with family and friends was measured, as well as the types of social activities engaged in, perceived social support and perceived adequacy of social activity.

Joyce (2002) found that social activity, social support and

social contact were all significant predictors of positive affect, and that none of the social well-being variables predicted negative affect, after controlling for physical health and demographic variables. Social activity and social support independently predicted self-perceived social activity adequacy. Consistent with the findings of Lawton et al (1999), social activity made an important contribution to emotional health. Social activity levels were related to positive affect and participants lower in social activity were more dissatisfied with their usual social activity. An implication of the research linking social activity with quality of life (Larson 1978; Lawton et al 1999) and quantity of life (Berkman & Syme 1979; House et al 1982; Kaplan et al 1988; Glass et al 1999), is that older people low in social activity participation would benefit from increased socialisation. Kendig (1996a) found that there was a group of older people who were low in social activity participation and who were motivated to increase their social activity levels. Close to a fifth of the sample wanted to be more socially active.

Joyce (2002) also tracked changes in social well-being indicators over six years and examined whether changes in social well-being predicted changes in emotional health. Only a small percentage of the sample showed shifts in emotional health, functional status, or self-reported adequacy of social activity participation over the study period. There was some indication that changes in perception of social activity levels was a predictor of change in emotional health. There was no detectable relationship between change in levels of social contact and change in emotional health. This was consistent with research showing that satisfaction with social contact is a better predictor of well-being than amount of social contact (Ishii-Kuntz 1990). Changes in functional status did not impact on positive or negative affect and the majority of those that did become more dependent did not change their social activity perceptions. Both negative and positive affect remained stable over six years, which is consistent with a study of positive and negative affect among 203 older participants over a four-year time gap (Kunzmann et al 2000). The baseline data for this study provided a picture of a healthy and content older population (Kendig 1996b) that was similar to the profile captured by a similar study of older people in Adelaide, Australia (Ranzijn & Luszcz 1994). The longitudinal analyses conducted by Joyce (2002) in Melbourne, Australia, revealed that these high levels of emotional well-being were maintained across the survey period.

How do life transitions affect mental health and well-being?

Transitions are significant events in people's lives. Although occurring over a short period of time, they may have lasting effects on health and well-being (Parkes 1971; McCallum 1986). Transitions can occur at any point in the life span. The transitions of mid-life and later life include retirement, widowhood, becoming a grandparent or a caregiver, acquiring disabilities and moving to a residential facility. Individuals vary in their capacity to adapt, but for many, transitions provide an opportunity for a new beginning. McCallum (1986) presents a general transition model describing how transitions impact on well-being. He postulates that transitions can lead to adjustment difficulties that in turn impact on well-being. The type of resources (for example, psychosocial and instrumental) needed to meet changed environmental demands, and perceptions about the transition (for example, desirability and adequacy of resources), both influence adjustment and well-being independently.

Some writers have specifically included personal characteristics as moderators of adjustment in their models of transitions (Schlossberg 1984). Examining intrinsic personality characteristics, such as self-efficacy and hardiness, is warranted because such traits are believed to enhance one's adaptation to life transitions and one's ability to persist in challenging roles such as being a caregiver.

Hardiness is one of the best-studied personality characteristics in older people facing transitions. People who perceive themselves as being in control of their lives, and to a large extent having control over the events in their lives, are amongst what Kobassa (1979) calls 'hardy copers'. A transition is perceived by hardy copers as just another hurdle to jump along life's raceway. They are willing to take responsibility for their actions and do not blame others for the transitions that inevitably come into their lives. Other personality characteristics featured in the literature on transitions and older people include dispositional optimism, self-efficacy or self-esteem, and—on the negative side—neuroticism, which has been defined as an underlying tendency to experience emotional distress.

In this section we look at three life transitions: retirement, care-giving and widowhood. The roles of personality, social support and social networks in adjustment to these transitions are highlighted.

Retirement

Retirement is a life transition that has become an increasingly complex process and more difficult to define over the last generation. People may not move directly from full-time work to full retirement—they may move to part-time work or become unemployed or a discouraged job seeker (Bishop 1999a). For many people, however, rather than signalling the end of a productive life retirement now presents new opportunities for a more active and satisfying life.

Retirement can be viewed as a process rather than a discrete event (Shaw et al 1998). Atchley (1974) proposed several phases of retirement, beginning with a pre-retirement phase in which the person forms attitudes towards their anticipated retirement. The retirement event itself may be marked by celebrations. Immediately following the retirement is the honeymoon phase, which is characterised by vacations and new interests. There may be a rest and relaxation phase, perceived as a period of brief respite from the obligations of work, or individuals may institute a retirement routine to maintain activity levels. The honeymoon phase may be followed by a period of disenchantment—they may feel 'let down' or experience undesirable circumstances such as poor health or restricted finances. Finally, there may be a period of reorientation, in which people adjust their expectations to accommodate realistic lifestyle goals and establish a stable, satisfying retirement routine.

In their cross-sectional Australian study, Sharpley et al (1996) found evidence amongst male retirees of a honeymoon effect during the period seven to twelve months after retirement and of a period of disenchantment thirteen to eighteen months after retirement. The adjustment of the women in their study was more even, characterised by a decrease in depression during the first two years of retirement.

Although retirement in most western countries has traditionally been viewed as complete withdrawal from the labour force at the age of 65, the age at which people have been retiring has been going down over the past 25 years. In Australia, for example, between the ages of 60 and 64 only 47 per cent of men remain in the workforce, down from almost 80 per cent 25 years ago (Rosen-man & Le Broque 1996). While women tend to retire earlier than men, the trend for women appears to be for increasing workforce participation in their fifties and sixties (see Chapter 6).

The Australian Bureau of Statistics (ABS 1997) study of retirement and retirement intentions found that the most common reasons for women ceasing their last full-time job were: to get married (19 per cent); pregnancy/to have children (18 per cent); to look after family, house or someone else (12 per cent); and their own ill health or injury (12 per cent). In contrast, the most common reasons amongst men were: ill health or injury (33 per cent); reaching compulsory retirement age (20 per cent); they were too old or had reached an appropriate age to retire (17 per cent); or retrenchment (12 per cent).

Early retirement appears to be less under individual control than retirement at later ages. Cornish (1997) found that 81 per cent of Australian men and 64 per cent of women who retired early over the period 1992–96 did so for 'induced' reasons such as employment problems, health problems (of both self and others) and compulsory retirement policies.

Wells and Kendig (1999) found that recent retirement was not detrimental to health or well-being, although activity levels were lower amongst the recently retired. However, retirement may be associated with reduced mental health or well-being in a minority of people. One study found that slightly over 10 per cent of retired people do not enjoy retirement or are undecided (Rosenkoetter & Garris 1998).

The experience of retirement depends on myriad factors, including both the individual's experience of work and the way in which they left work. For people in extremely stressful or dissatisfying work environments, retirement may represent an escape from the burden of work and an opportunity to engage in valued leisure pursuits (Shaw et al 1998). Not surprisingly, people whose retirement is involuntary, or who relinquish work sooner than expected, are more likely to experience a poor adjustment to retirement (Braithwaite & Gibson 1987; Hardy & Quadagno 1995; Rosenkoetter & Garris 1998). On the other hand, people who retire because they want to, because they wish to do other things, or in response to financial incentives, are more likely to be highly satisfied in retirement (Quick & Moen 1998).

High levels of personal resources can ease the transition to retirement. For example, people with better health and those with higher incomes are most likely to be satisfied with retirement (Seccombe & Lee 1986; Ford et al 1992; Calasanti 1996). People who have been retired for less than three years are especially likely to benefit from their retirement if they meet life challenges flexibly and with tenacity (Trepanier et al 2001). In addition, it is not surprising to find that retirees with high self-efficacy—a confident attitude about their ability or competence to survive life's challenges—also report better psychological well-being (Sharpley & Yardley 1999; Wells & Kendig 1999). Compared with mature-age workers with high self-esteem, those with low self-esteem are more likely to have a negative attitude towards their retirement and are less likely to plan for it (Mutran et al 1997).

Developing a satisfying lifestyle in retirement is also important. Satisfied retirees remained active, have plenty to do with their time, and continue to have friends with whom they associate on a regular basis (Rosenkoetter & Garris 1998). Social attachments outside work should preferably be formed in advance of retirement to avoid poor health consequences (Solem 1987). Joyce (2002), in a study of older people's social lives, quotes a 60-year-old male informant illustrating the importance of social attachments in the adjustment to retirement:

> I can still remember a number of senior people who suddenly found it very difficult because there wasn't anything else in their lives . . . Well actually it was a strong enough impression on me that it scared me off early retirement. And I guess what I've done now is . . . doing some part time work which I've done for five years . . . I've got hobbies and friends and things I want to do . . . I find being involved with people and [the] discipline and the mental challenge [is] a very important part of my life (2002, p. 75).

Married people express higher levels of retirement satisfaction than do unmarried people (Seccombe & Lee 1986). But marriage may be a mixed blessing. Shaw et al (1998) suggest that after retirement a new balance in the relationship must be established, based on a new set of routines and patterns of communication. A recent analysis of the Cornell Retirement and Well-Being Study (Jungmeen & Moen 1999) found that being recently retired was positively associated with increased morale for men, especially when their wives remained employed. In contrast, becoming retired was linked to increased depressive symptoms for women, especially when their husbands remained employed.

Lorraine—a loss of direction

Lorraine is aged 62 years and retired from a part-time job as a legal secretary two years ago. She has been divorced for five years and has not re-married. Until a year ago she was enjoying her retirement and had completed many projects around the house and garden. In the last year, however, she has been feeling bored and misses the regularity and stimulation of her job. She cares for her grandchildren occasionally and has regular contact with her adult children, which she enjoys. She has one close friend who she sees occasionally for lunch. 'I feel as fit as I ever have but am now wondering what I will do for the next 20 years or so. I am going to die of boredom if I do not find something to occupy my time.'

She has had an armchair interest in environmental issues since the local community successfully blocked the building of a waste dump in the local quarry, which has now been turned into a lake and parklands. Her son has suggested she join the local Landcare organisation but she is reluctant to do so as she does not know anyone involved in the organisation and does not believe she has the skills to contribute. She has always considered herself introverted and has difficulty in new social situations.

Activity 3.1

When reading this chapter consider the example above in terms of the impact of retirement on well-being and the influence of individual predispositions on social engagement. How might you encourage Lorraine to link with a community group? Would this be desirable?

Caregiving

Caregiving is another important life transition that affects well-being. Governmental policies encouraging community care and reducing institutionalisation have shifted the responsibility for caring for frail and disabled older people from formal services back to family caregivers. However, family care is not always the best option. Caregiving can sometimes exhaust the caregiver's resources. The relationship may not always be loving or responsible, and in extreme cases may entail elder abuse or neglect.

The view that older people are a burden on younger generations, and the fear that the weight of this burden will increase as the population ages, are largely unjustified. While older people are the most likely to require care as a result of illness or disability, they are also the group most likely to be providing care to one another, and may also continue to be caregivers as parents or grandparents. There is often interdependence between older persons with varying levels of disability or chronic illness. The greatest source of help for a majority of older adults with a disability is their spouse (Wells 1996). In 1998, around one in six Australian caregivers (401 000 people) were aged 65 and over; the majority of these (69 per cent) were caring for their partner (ABS 1999b). Similar caregiving patterns emerge in other western countries (see Chapter 8).

Little is known about the process of becoming a caregiver. For adult children of older people, often middle-aged themselves, the transition to caregiver is an extension of filial responsibility and is strongly gendered: adult daughters are three times as likely to become caregivers as adult sons and only half as likely to relinquish care (Dwyer et al 1992). In contrast, the gender imbalance in spousal caregiving is minor (Wells & Kendig 1997), with slightly more men than women likely to be the principal resident carer after age 60 (McCallum & Geiselhart 1996). While the transition to caregiving within a marriage usually arises from feelings of mutual affection and obligation, mutuality and balance in the relationship may be disturbed in the process.

A great deal of literature on caregiving is focused on the undesirable aspects of care provision rather than the positive or rewarding outcomes. Since most studies have employed non-representative samples of caregivers recruited through services or support groups, the literature probably depicts an unnecessarily pessimistic view of caregiving in later life (Wells & Kendig 1997). The well-being of caregivers is important: caregivers who perceive their role as unrewarding are more likely both to experience depression and to engage in behaviours that are potentially harmful to their spouses (Williamson et al 2001).

Becoming a caregiver for a spouse or parent is often associated with an increase in symptoms of depression (Marks et al 2002). Undesirable impacts of caregiving may include feelings of burden and restrictions on a caregiver's employment, family life and social participation. Long-term consequences may include poorer health and increased rates of depression, anxiety, guilt and distress (Biegel et al 1991). There is little doubt that providing extensive care for a disabled spouse is associated with elevated symptoms of depression and anxiety (Cannuscio et al 2002). High stress and depression are reflected in physiological markers as well as in self-report (Gallagher-Thompson et al 2001).

Nonetheless, the majority of caregivers carry out their caregiving tasks without experiencing detrimental outcomes (Schofield et al 1998). One recent study (Cohen et al 2002) reported that 73 per cent of caregivers whose mean age was 64 could identify at least one positive aspect of caregiving. Positive feelings about providing care were associated with lower depression scores, lower burden scores and better self-rated health. Positive consequences may include feeling closer to the person who requires care, and increased self-efficacy and feelings of satisfaction in fulfilling a valued role (O'Bryant et al 1990; Wright 1991; Hinrichsen et al 1992).

Caregivers who bear a high caregiving workload and those who are caring for a spouse with dementia (rather than a physical condition) are likely to experience high levels of stress (Stull et al 1994). Other risk factors for high burden and depression in caring for a frail or elderly spouse include female gender, poor health, and dissatisfaction in the pre-existing or current relationship with the care-recipient (Brodaty et al 1990; Miller & Cafasso 1992; Miller et al 2001; Rankin et al 2001). The longer the caregiving lasts the more likely caregivers are to experience stress or depression, or to feel burdened (Proctor et al 2002).

Access to coping strategies and satisfactory social support may ameliorate the effects of stressors, or act as a buffer between stressors and outcomes (Biegel et al 1991). For example, caregiving stress is less likely to translate into depression for caregivers who perceive that they have social support (Majerovitz 2001), and having satisfactory opportunities for leisure is important for the health of caregiving husbands (Shanks-McElroy & Strobino 2001). Having alternative roles (such as employment or family roles) may act as a resource or as a source of extra stress, depending on the degree of conflict between the roles (Edwards et al 2002).

There is growing evidence that personality traits are an important contextual factor in the development of caregiver stress. Not all of the research is specific to older people as caregivers but includes samples of adult children as caregivers. It has been shown that women who are caring for parents while simultaneously occupying the roles of mother, wife and employee cope better if they are more optimistic: dispositional optimism moderates or buffers the effects of stress on depression (Atienza et al 2002). Caregivers of disabled older adults who are hardy copers report less dissatisfaction, depression and fatigue (Clark & Hartman 1996; Clark 2002). In contrast, caregivers with high levels of expressed anger report a high level of burden (Vitaliano et al 1991).

Adult child caregivers who are more extroverted are more likely to place the care recipient in institutional care (Pot et al 2001). However, this traditional measure of personality does not appear to influence caregiver distress or sense of burden (Reis et al 1994; Renzetti et al 2001). On the other hand, caregivers who have high scores on a measure of neuroticism see themselves as more burdened than those with low scores, are more likely to have health complaints, are less likely to be able to garner social support to help them face the demands of their situation, and report more symptoms of depression (Hooker et al 1992; Reis et al 1994; Markiewicz et al 1997). Caregivers with more neurotic traits are more likely to appraise caregiving demands as stressful, and these appraisals in turn impact on mental health outcomes (Hooker et al 1998).

Some types of caregiving are more likely to be associated with beneficial impacts than others. For example, women who provide non-residential care (that is, to someone in another household) to a biological parent or someone who is not related to them report more purpose in life than non-caregiving women and are likely to acknowledge beneficial impacts of caregiving on their well-being (Marks et al 2002).

Caregivers may also experience transitions out of caregiving through widowhood or institutionalisation of the care-recipient. Caregivers who report high levels of burden are more likely than those with low burden to institutionalise the care-recipient within five years (Hebert et al 2001). The impacts of widowhood and care-recipient institutionalisation on former caregivers vary (Canadian Study of Health and Aging Working Group 2002). While caregivers who experience high levels of caregiving strain are more likely to report high bereavement strain (Bass & Bowman 1990), they are both less at risk for increased depression on bereavement and more likely to report that they have reduced their health risk behaviours, than spouse caregivers who were not particularly strained in providing care (Schulz et al 2001).

George—positive and negative impacts of social contact

George is aged 82 years and lost his wife six months ago after her long battle with dementia. He had cared for her at home for ten years, but in her last year she was admitted to a high-care residential facility. George cooks for himself and receives home help for cleaning and general house maintenance. Despite his caregiving role, George has maintained contact with his two closest male friends. Through respite care he was able to play golf with them once a week. This provided him with a necessary buffer against the stress of caregiving. Lately he has been socialising with them at the local club. George still grieves for his wife but has decided to live his life productively. 'I have always taken a positive view about life's challenges and will do so until they wheel me out in a coffin.'

He still drives but limits this to going to the local shops and golf club. Since his wife died, his daughter has been calling and visiting regularly and is anxious about his well-being. However, George is unhappy with his daughter's 'meddling'. She is particularly worried about his driving although George has not had an accident in 20 years. He is happy with his social contacts with his friends, which he can control, but feels his daughter is treating him like a dependent child.

> **Activity 3.2**
>
> Consider the example of George in terms of the potential positive role of social activity in his well-being and, conversely, the potential negative impacts of unwanted social contact. How might you improve the communication between George and his daughter?

Widowhood

By the age of 65 it is likely that an individual has experienced a number of significant losses of persons close to them. These are most commonly the loss of their parents, but may also include the loss of a spouse, siblings and friends, or less commonly the loss of a child. Widowhood is experienced by both men and women and is a transition that is often both abrupt and severe, and causes a great deal of personal distress. In Australia, 14.7 per cent of men aged 65 and over and 45.6 per cent of women aged 65 and over are widowed (ABS 1999a), figures that reflect the situation in other western countries.

Grief reactions to widowhood are healthy. Characteristic feelings associated with healthy grief include shock, sadness, numbness, sorrow, yearning, fear, anger, anxiety, helplessness and abandonment. The widow or widower may experience intrusive memories of the deceased, and have difficulty making sense of what is happening. A recent qualitative study differentiates four major phases: numb shock, emotional turmoil, disorganisation and despair, and acceptance (Hegge & Fischer 2000). Physical symptoms may include tightness in the chest, palpitations, oversensitivity to noise, poor sleep, lack of energy and poor appetite. Widowhood is associated with increased use of alcohol, but only within two years following bereavement (Perreira & Sloan 2001).

Earlier studies found that people whose spouse died had an increased risk of mortality in the following years (Parkes 1987). This result has not been replicated in more recent studies. However, a recent analysis of suicide rates in the United States by race and marital status found that widowed men and women were more likely than married men or women to commit suicide. This association was much stronger in younger than in older age groups. Amongst older people, having been widowed increased the risk of suicide by a relatively small margin (Luoma & Pearson 2002).

The most common negative outcome following widowhood is loneliness (Lund et al 1986). Other consequences can include lower social participation, lower life satisfaction and higher consumption of psychotropic medication, including anti-depressants and sedatives (Wells & Kendig 1997).

Grief associated with bereavement is not given a psychiatric diagnosis unless it remains persistent or chronic for twelve months or more. Research with recently widowed older Australian men found that only 8.8 per cent exhibited bereavement phenomena at thirteen months post-bereavement (Byrne & Raphael 1994). Rather, most widows and widowers eventually make a satisfactory adjustment (McCallum 1986). While some theoretical viewpoints have insisted on the importance of 'grief work', recent research indicates that intense preoccupation with the death in the first few months predicts a less satisfactory adjustment two to three years later (Wortman & Silver 1990).

Becoming a widow or widower may also entail some positive consequences. For some, widowhood provides an opportunity to begin a new life, and feelings of self-efficacy may increase (Arbuckle & de Vries 1995). Some widows enjoy a new-found freedom in not having to look after someone else (Davidson 2001). One recent study found that widowed persons experienced a sustained increased in informal social participation following the loss of their spouse, and their level of social participation was comparable with those who were continuously married (Utz et al 2002). These older people used social activity as a coping strategy to deal with negative impacts of widowhood. Joyce (2002) provides an illustration of how an older widow 'got on with her life' following the death of her husband:

> Partly I think it is because my husband would have expected it of me. He thought I could do anything, and he was quite positive. He took care that I should know exactly how to . . . well of course I had to do all the financial things when he was at sea and have the car serviced and all those things, so I think the fact that I was alone like that conditioned me. Well then of course we had the last years together but early in the piece I used to think well, he would

have expected me to get off my bum ... because he always thought of me as being very capable.

The personal consequences of widowhood depend on a range of factors at different levels: macrosocial conditions (such as gender-based allocation of social roles); dyadic characteristics, including marital quality; and individual-level attributes, such as gender and coping skills (Carr & Utz 2001–02).

Adjustment following widowhood is affected by factors such as the suddenness of the bereavement (especially if by accident or suicide); financial pressures; low support from family members immediately afterwards and low support from friends further down the track; high commitment to the role of spouse; long-lasting pre-bereavement caregiving strain; the presence of unresolved issues from a previous bereavement; and a history of past psychiatric problems (Kavanagh 1990; Martin-Matthews 1996). Another informant quote from Joyce (2002) illustrates the negative consequences of loneliness associated with widowhood.

> Oh it's terrible, it's terrible, I am just learning. I was a hopeless cook, I was spoilt, really, she did everything. But you've got to survive, it is not the best, you're not very happy at all, you're not very happy at all ... getting worse [loneliness] ... yeah getting worse ... oh yes it is very lonely, lonely and unhappy but I'm getting used to that. I have two daughters, they both have good jobs, no grandchildren ... oh it has gotten worse, see you've got to have some reason to get up of a morning ... If I had grandchildren it might be different I could live for them, look after them ... Oh it just seems to be getting worse that's all, hasn't been any reason ... motivation, yeah lack of motivation.

A few studies have found higher levels of distress amongst widowed women than widowed men. The usual explanation for this is that widowhood causes more financial difficulties for women than it does for men (Umberson et al 1992). In contrast, several studies have shown that bereavement is generally a more severe transition for older men than for women (Fry 2001; Lee et al 2001). Reasons for the increased difficulty experienced by men may include their lower frequency of church attendance, a stronger dislike of domestic labour and lower ability to assist their children (Lee et al 2001). It has been speculated that sudden spousal deaths are more likely to be anticipated by older women than by older men because of men's mortality disadvantage. Older women may go through a rehearsal for widowhood as they observe their peers experiencing the loss of a spouse.

However, a recent study showed that forewarning of widowhood did not affect depression, anger, shock, or overall grief six and eighteen months after being widowed. Rather, prolonged forewarning was associated with high anxiety in the surviving spouse (Carr et al 2001). Whether or not forewarning exacerbates or mitigates the impacts of widowhood appears to depend on whether the surviving spouse felt strain in caring for the ill spouse—noncaregivers and non-strained caregivers may both experience an increase in depression following the death of their spouse, while strained caregivers do not (Schulz et al 2001).

The relationship quality before bereavement may affect the course of adjustment. Widowed individuals with harmonious marriages experience the lowest health after widowhood (Prigerson et al 2000). Surviving spouses who were highly dependent on the partner who died are likely to experience higher levels of yearning for their spouse, whereas those whose relationships are conflicted experience low levels of yearning (Carr et al 2000).

While factors such as health, income, education and social resources are important resources in coping with the loss of a spouse, the widowed person's existential beliefs about the meaning of life, optimism for the future, and aspects of religiosity and spirituality have been shown to be even more helpful (Fry 2001). An Australian study of the impacts of widowhood on women found that the use of humour was an important coping mechanism (Feldman et al 2000). Few studies on the impacts of personality characteristics on the capacity to deal with widowhood have been published. However, optimism is known to be an important resource for psychological well-being within the first two years of the death of a spouse (Fry 2001).

Implications for services and programs for older people

There is strong evidence that satisfying social lives are important in the mental health and well-being of older people. Recent policy initiatives by some governments have recognised this relationship

(Andrews 2002) and some programs and services have been established to address social isolation. We have also seen that life transitions such as retirement, caregiving and widowhood can influence the social lives and well-being of older people both positively and negatively. Can we prepare for these events?

Retirement planning programs are becoming increasingly common. Sharpley and Layton (1998) found that having prepared for retirement, emotionally and socially, predicts successful adjustment. However, in Australia only 37 per cent of retired men and 22 per cent of retired women say that they actively prepared for retirement (Wolcott 1998). This is a common pattern among many OECD countries (see Chapter 6). Higher proportions of working men (70 per cent) and women (63 per cent) between the ages of 50 and 70 years say that they are actively preparing for retirement. However, this preparation is largely financial (Wolcott 1998).

There has been an increasing awareness of the importance of supporting family caregivers through community services. However, few caregivers use any services or formal supports (Schofield et al 1998). Recent meta-analyses of the literature have indicated that interventions to support caregivers of people with dementia are effective. Caregivers rated interventions as beneficial, and clinically significant outcomes in reducing symptoms of depression and, to a lesser degree, anxiety, anger and hostility, have been demonstrated (Schulz et al 2002, Sorensen et al 2002). Psycho-educational and psychotherapeutic interventions show the most consistent short-term effects on all outcome measures (Sorensen et al 2002).

Community service provision may actually increase the likelihood of institutionalisation for a care-recipient (Cohen et al 1993). It is unclear whether this indicates a benefit of closer monitoring of persons in need of higher levels of support, or an enforced reduction in such persons' levels of independence. In any event, many caregivers see their responsibilities as continuing when their relative is placed in residential care.

Comparatively few interventions are available to assist widows and widowers. There are no country-wide voluntary associations of widowed people, as there are of caregivers, and fewer organisations devoted to providing services to widowed people than there are to people planning their retirement. Studies of bereavement counselling and bereavement support group meetings have demonstrated that these interventions can assist widows and widowers (Caserta &

Lund 1993; Potocky 1993). Men and women who have elevated symptoms of distress a year after the death of their spouse can be helped by being directed towards more unfamiliar coping strategies—men towards emotion-focused coping and women towards problem-focused strategies (Schut et al 1997).

Influences on social activity and well-being that are often neglected are those related to access to services and programs. For example, accessible and affordable transport is a key concern for older people in terms of their ability to engage with their communities, not only to access services but also to support greater social interaction. Joyce (2002) found that the activities and interests of older people provided the context for socialising and many of these interests were dependent on mobility. One participant in this study said that having access to transport was her most important social need. Others stated:

> I just like to be with people . . . even here, if I work in the morning, I get sick of it and I'd just hop in the car and go down . . . Just have a coffee or go to the beach . . .

> . . . transport is a big problem . . . I still drive, so I can go anywhere, I don't have to stay home Friday, Saturday, and Sunday. I could go somewhere but not everyone can; [of] the people . . . in our day care I doubt if there is one that drives . . . they have got to depend on somebody taking them somewhere so mobility is a big problem.

Conclusion

Well-being is an important part of the goal of 'healthy' or 'successful' ageing, concepts that are now being promoted strongly by governments and researchers (Browning & Kendig 2003; Rowe & Kahn 1997). In order to address the needs of older people and promote positive mental health we must recognise the multiple determinants of well-being in old age including; personality, health status, gender, marital status, satisfaction with social contacts and adjustment to life transitions such as retirement, caregiving and widowhood. In addition, maximising well-being in old age requires attention to the importance of mid-life experiences and attitudes as precursors to the experience of ageing.

But is healthy ageing achievable for all? With increases in

longevity worldwide we now have a large cohort of people who will survive into their eighties and beyond (the old-old or the fourth age) and it is this group who, according to Baltes and Smith (2003), are most vulnerable to the impacts on well-being of declining health and functioning. We need to know more about the values and motivations of people who have reached the fourth age and what matters to them in late life in terms of dignity, respect and life satisfaction. An ageing society tests our individual and collective responsibilities in creating environments that maximise well-being for all ages.

4

Sexuality, sexual intimacy and sexual health in later life

Victor Minichiello, Samantha Ackling, Chris Bourne, David Plummer

The long-held assumption that older people are asexual is no longer tenable (Minichiello et al 1996a). To perpetuate such misconceptions can only be considered ageist, particularly when current political discourses acknowledge older people as citizens with equal rights, needs and privileges. Yet it is not easy to correct the myth of the asexual older person, given the cultural predisposition to favour youthfulness and to associate sexual attraction with being young (see Chapter 1). Another indication of the tendency to understate the sexual interest of older people is the limited space given to this topic in popular and scientific culture. Until recently, few studies treated sexuality in later life as a legitimate subject for investigation, despite longstanding scientific, religious and medical preoccupations with sexuality. For example, in a study labelled the 'definitive study of sex' in the United States (Michael et al 1994), not one of the 3432 respondents was over the age of 60! Moreover, the waves of studies on sexuality in the era of HIV/AIDS by and large ignored older people (Donovan et al 1998). Even a recent study of health relationships in Australia, which surveyed a representative sample of 10 173 men and 9134 women, claiming to study 'the sexual practices of the Australian population' and for the first time provide 'an extensive and reliable portrait of the sexual health of the Australian population', it did not include anyone over the age of 60! (Smith et al 2003). That older people are outraged by their exclusion from such studies can be best described by the following letter to the editor:

The support of mythology about older people becomes increasingly annoying. Many policy makers and researchers make decisions about older people based on fanciful ideas rather than facts. The latest group to assume that older people do not exist are researchers from La Trobe University. They were given a great deal of government money for 'a study to examine the sexual practices of the Australian population' but excluded people over 60. Since publishing their results and receiving criticism for ignoring people over 60, they have announced that this will all be remedied by their new study, which will actually include people up to the age of 65.

As a person who has lived longer than either of these studies will allow, I find it offensive that these researchers make the presumption that people who have retired are sexless and presumably no longer citizens. Experience of life brings scepticism. Is it any wonder that older people find it difficult to believe those who have little idea about Australian society, let alone what the activities of a major component in its population might be, sexual or otherwise?

There is a well-known poem that sums up how older people are treated:

As I was going up the stair
I met a man who wasn't there.
He wasn't there again today.
I wish to God he'd go away.

Older people are not going away. Very soon, there will be more people over 50 than under. What will the researchers, policy makers and governments do then?

An older person
(*The Daily Examiner*, Letter to the Editor, 13 March 2004, p. 6)

Should we be surprised by such omissions? Gerontologists have over the past century documented many negative beliefs that prevail in western societies about older people. One of these is the myth of the 'asexual older person'. Cultural stereotypes about the sexuality of older people are grounded in general negative attitudes towards older people, prevailing views being that older people are offended by sex, that sexual interest and activity is inappropriate in older people, that older people are unable to engage in sex, that sex is a health risk, and that older people are physically unattractive and therefore sexually undesirable (Schaivi 1999). It is not difficult to find media stories that reflect and reinforce these views. Robinson (1983), for example, found that reporters writing about the sexual interest of older men and women portray the topic as humorous, ridiculous, repugnant or an appropriate subject for patronising comments. A major newspaper reported on the front page the results of a survey that found that older people are sexually active with the following headline: 'Sex and the aged: Survey surprise!' (*The Australian*, 26 October 1995).

There can be little doubt that the sexual activity of older people is shaped by the extent to which our culture defines their sexual needs and attitudes, attitudes which they then internalise. Some sociologists argue that the sexual behaviour and attitudes of individuals are fundamental areas of social control, and where older people are concerned are shaped by the fact that sexual behaviour is no longer linked to reproduction (Minichiello et al 1996a). We cannot ignore that the attitudes of many older people in western societies have been influenced by the Victorian sexual standards that prevailed earlier in the 20th century, attitudes that differ from the social and sexual culture of present middle-aged individuals. For example, masturbation was described in a medical advice book for home treatment written in 1912 as a 'secret vice', with identifiable illness features. The authors used the sub-headings 'causes of', 'effects of', 'prevention of', 'signs of' and 'treatment of' to describe this 'condition' (Richards & Richards 1912). Few people today would use such language to describe masturbation! Some researchers have speculated that older people's lack of knowledge about sexuality may be due to their limited access to education about sexuality in their youth (White & Catania 1982), a topic we will return to shortly.

It is also useful to understand the historical framework that has perpetuated the myth that older people are asexual and that sexual expression is linked specifically to reproduction. This belief evolved primarily from religious rhetoric and formed the basis of social control regarding 'appropriate gender roles' (Covey 1989). Some argue that a framework that is formed on the basis of reproductive sex is exclusionary and caters only to heterosexual, pre-menopausal relationships (Minichiello et al 1996a), a narrow view that is dismissive and serves only to disempower older people's sexual expression. It also does not allow for the diverse forms of sexual behaviour occurring in this age group to be acknowledged and described.

Just what do the terms 'sexuality' and 'sexual intimacy' mean, and how do they correspond to older people's sexual lives? Hillman (2000) provides broad definitions: sexuality is defined by a combination of emotional intimacy, sexual behaviour, sensual activity and sexual identity; sexual intimacy refers to the interpersonal relationship between people who may or may not engage in sexual activity, with an emphasis on the emotional experience and subjective feelings of closeness, both definitions being useful in understanding the trajectory of sexual experiences across the life span.

Much of the current literature reflects the generally conservative attitudes of individuals born either before or during the 1930s. This research has been essential in providing evidence that people are, and continue to be, sexually active in later life. This cohort may not be representative of the next generation of 'older people', however. Ageing populations in western countries are made up of the baby boomers who experienced the sexual revolution of the 1960s and 1970s. Anecdotal evidence suggests that this next generation will be less inhibited, more likely to experience multiple partners during their adult lives, and perhaps be more open about exploring different types of relationships and ways of gaining sexual satisfaction and intimacy.

In quoting Shere Hite (1976), author of the *Hite Report: A Nationwide Study of Female Sexuality*, Gross (2000) supports the notion that we should call sex 'something else', and that it should include 'everything from kissing to sitting close together'. One of the obstacles to accepting such a broad definition of sex is the male myths surrounding sex, particularly amongst the older generation. As Gross (2004, p. 1) notes, 'Sex, with or without Viagra, is to be initiated and managed by the male, and his definition of sex is focused intensely on conventional intercourse, meaning penetration by an erect penis'. Yet as Gross and others have argued, should older males look at sex in new ways they may lessen their anxieties about erections and ejaculation. Dr Richard Cross, a medical educator from the Robert Wood Johnson Medical School in New Jersey, makes an equally important comment:

Why do older men need an erection? This is a holdover from the era when sex was seen as dirty unless for making babies. Do older men and women really want pretend procreation? No, of course not. What they want is closeness, exciting touch, recognition that sexual interest, desire and activity last throughout life and need to be adapted in new ways as biology slows them down in later years (Gross 2004, p. 5).

Recent research conducted by the American Association of Retired Persons is suggesting that attitudes are changing and that older men do not necessarily equate youth with sex. In fact, older men and women find people of their age physically attractive (Gross 2000). Olivia Goldsmith's novel-movie, First Wives Club, makes the point that the so-called 'candy store' phase of the attraction of an older man to a younger woman is not as ideal as it is meant to be. As Gross (2004, p. 7) so nicely explains:

What begins to happen is that the experiential and cultural gap between the generations starts to shadow the 'hot sex' era the older man thinks he is in. Since even the aerobics instructor who replaces the first wife in the movie has to get out of bed some time, the need for conversation develops. Then, both in the movie and in real life, the older man realises she doesn't get his jokes (she's never even heard of Milton Berle), and she thinks the Great Depression is back there with the Crusades in medieval history along with the great experience of his life, World War II. In my research, if she's as young as male fantasies often suggest, she can't even remember the Vietnam War, he discovers.

Recent studies of older people and sexuality reveal some interesting findings. First, attitudes are changing. For example, Arluke et al (1984) conducted a content analysis of romantic and sexual advice in books for older people published before and after the 1970s, covering a 30-year period. They found a less negative attitude towards reporting sexual activity in later life, but still a reluctance to promote dating and sexual relationships. Another more recent study found that the attitudes of health care educators towards sexuality in later life was positive, although there were deficiencies in their knowledge (Glass & Webb 1995).

Second, older people hold a mix of attitudes about sexual issues. It is true that the current generation of older people generally hold more conservative views than younger people (Hillman & Stricker 1994). For example, a study that examined the beliefs of three age groups towards sexuality found that the older group (65–79) evaluated themselves, and were judged by the other age groups (18–25 years and 40–55 years), to be less knowledgeable about sex, less desirous and less capable of having sex (Cameron 1970). Generally speaking, the literature reports that the attitudes of older people towards sex and their sexual experience have been found to vary by gender, marital status and religion (Hillman & Stricker 1994; Schiavi 1999). For example, in comparing the sexual attitudes of two age groups over and under the age of 65, Snyder and Spreitzer (1976) found that religiosity, gender and marital status were significant predictors of sexual attitudes in both groups. Another study reported that prior sexual history was a strong predictor of sexual attitudes (White 1982). A more recent study developed a predictor model that, in 86 per cent of cases studied, was able to successfully determine whether the older respondent would be in a sexual relationship (Minichiello et al 2004). The factors significantly related to sexual relationship status were: age; living with a partner or spouse; satisfaction with their own health; knowledge of sexual issues; perceptions of the importance of sexual expression to well-being; and number of sexual partners. Studies have also reported a positive correlation between greater sexual knowledge and more permissive sexual attitudes, and that religion emerges as a salient factor in influencing sexual attitudes (Steinke 1994). There are also gender and age differences. Older men have been reported to value sex more than older women, and those aged 80 and over to perceive sex as less important (Minichiello et al 1996b).

Research to date

Empirical research into the sexual lives of older people began in the 1950s, with findings that men and women over the age of 60 were still sexually active and physically capable of engaging in sexual intercourse (Kinsey et al 1948, 1953; Masters & Johnson 1966; Pfeiffer et al 1968, 1969; Pfeiffer & Davis 1972; George & Weiler 1981). While it seems beyond dispute that sexual activity can change with age, and that the importance attached to sex by older people, or at least to penetrative sex, generally recedes (for an excellent summary of the relationship between ageing and sexuality see Rossi, 1994;

Schiavi & Rehman 1995; Schiavi, 1999), this is quite a different matter from equating ageing with being asexual. As early as the 1950s Kinsey and his colleagues (1948, 1953) and later, Masters and Johnson (1970), documented the importance of sexuality throughout life with their large-scale population-based studies. These studies were able to document both that sexual activity declines gradually over time for both women and men, and that sexual interest declines more slowly than sexual activity. Further research continues to validate the sexual lives of older people. For example, Diokno et al (1990) found in their study of 1956 older community-dwelling residents aged over 60 that 73.8 per cent of married men and 55.8 per cent of married women continued to be sexually active. Janus and Janus (1993) found of 441 participants aged 65 and older, 69 per cent of men and 74 per cent of women continued to have sex at least weekly. Mulligan and Moss (1991), in their survey of 1249 randomly selected male veterans, found that sexual intercourse for men with partners decreased from a mean of once a week for men aged 30 to 39 years to once per year for men aged 90 to 99 years. They also found that erectile capacity decreases significantly with age. A more recent large study found that, although age correlated consistently with both reduced sexual activity and erectile difficulties, a substantial number of older men continued to be sexually active when supported by positive attitudes towards sexuality (Bortz et al 1999). Interestingly, but perhaps not surprisingly, Martin (1981) found that recalled frequency of sexual behaviour in earlier years emerged as a significant predictor of current sexual frequency.

However, it is important to note that no consensus exists as to what is considered a normal or ideal frequency level of sexual activity or interest in adults over the age of 65 (Matthius et al 1997; Schiavi 1999). Reasons for this lack of consensus include whether or not individuals have partners or are married, their gender (women tend to outlive men, which may cause a shortage of available opposite-sex partners) and, most importantly, the restrictive descriptor of sexual activity as intercourse. While some studies have attempted to broaden descriptors of sexual behaviour to include masturbation, oral sex, fantasy and the use of vibrators (Bresher et al 1984; Janus & Janus 1993; Johnson 1996; Bortz et al 1999), an inclusive definition of sexuality and sexual intimacy is still difficult to find.

Ageist attitudes towards older people, particularly in reference to sexuality, are abundant and enduring. Specific examples of such

---

Older persons' views about intimacy

Lorna Beal, 73, threw herself into grandmothering when her first husband died of cancer after 30 years together. She became content on her own. Then she met Arthur, 82, through mutual friends and 'we just gelled'. A year later they were married. No one gave Lorna away. She met Arthur halfway down the aisle, and he accompanied her to the altar. For an awful moment guests thought the bride had got cold feet, but twelve years on they couldn't be cosier.

Gwen Scott and her partner, Alan Noble, are doing their own thing. 'Someone asked me recently, "Are you and Alan an item?" I suppose we are. We're an item,' she winks. She is 70; he is 76. Pictures of his first wife, Glenice, who died from breast cancer six years ago, hang on the wall beside more recent snaps of Gwen.

'People asked me, "Why don't you move in with Alan?" I told them I didn't want to. I want my own space. I like to have my time to myself,' Scott says, echoing feminist rhetoric that was out of her reach as a wife and mother of two children in a conservative provincial community. When her husband of 35 years died from leukaemia in 1986, Scott spent twelve years on her own and came to relish her independence. 'I was showing him how to bowl and I never thought he'd end up as a companion, but it blossomed straightaway.'

Source: *The Weekend Australian Magazine*, 31 August–1 September 2003.

---

attitudes can be found in jokes that perpetuate these ideas. For example, 'old is . . . when you can't remember the last time you had sex with your husband and your husband can't remember either' (Bytheway 1997, p. 63). Often humour used in this way focuses on decreases in sexual attractiveness and drive as well as mental and physical losses (Grant 1996). Unfortunately, such humour only perpetuates the myth that sexuality is intrinsically linked to youthfulness, with the underlying ideology that youthfulness represents excitement, independence, physical prowess and attractiveness (Hillman 2000). Ironically, there is evidence to suggest that the onset of menopause allows some women to feel more sexually liberated as they no longer have to worry about the risk of pregnancy (Riportella-Muller 1989). Nevertheless, a subtle shift is beginning to occur with prominent newspapers articles that are positive and empowering, portraying older people's sexuality as affirming and normal (Legge 2002). The case study above describes the experiences of some older people, and such positive expressions of intimacy in later life are increasingly being reported in popular culture.

Biomedical issues

In both men and women, physiological changes that can impact on sexual activity may occur. For example, as men age a decrease in testosterone levels generally occurs, and while this does not directly affect sexual functioning it has been attributed to a decline in libido (Meston 1997). To experience an erection more direct stimulation for longer periods is often required. The ability to achieve orgasm remains, although contractions may be fewer with less intensity and ejaculation may also have less volume (Zeiss & Kasel-Godley 2001). For women, changes predominantly occur due to the loss of estrogen after menopause. Changes may include thinning of the vaginal lining and a reduction in vaginal lubric-ation that may lead to pain during intercourse. Orgasmic response remains, however, as with men, intensity of contractions may be reduced. There is some suggestion that maintaining sexual activity reduces the chances of these physiological changes in both men and women (Meston 1997; Zeiss & Kasel-Godley 2001).

Coping with physiological changes can be distressing, but medical technology can assist. The use of lubricants and hormone replacement therapy can reduce vaginal dryness. A range of inter-ventions for altered erectile function is also available and includes hormone treatment, vacuum devices, implants and surgery (Schiavi 1999). One of the drug treatments for impotence is widely known as Viagra. Launched onto the global market in 1998, it became the biggest selling drug in the world within two weeks (Tucak 2002). Treatment is in the form of a tablet, which works by dilating blood vessels in the penis, thus increasing blood supply and facilitating erection. The tablet must be taken at least

30 minutes prior to sexual activity and the effects can last up to four hours (Pfizer 2002). Perhaps one of the reasons men have embraced the use of Viagra with such enthusiasm is its ease of administration. Other drugs available on the market such as Caverject require a direct injection into the penis that can be difficult and painful to administer. A tablet is simple to take and no one need know, thus maintaining privacy and self-esteem.

Practitioners also need to be aware how a patient's state of health may affect sexual activity. The recent medical literature shows that illnesses and surgery can have a measurable impact on sexual function of older persons, and can lead in some cases in sexual dysfunction. Schiavi (1999) provides evidence to, show that:

- the onset of Parkinson's disease can result in low sexual desire in as much as 44 per cent of patients;
- sexual dysfunction is a well-known complication of prostate surgery and that transurethral prostatectomy, a common procedure for patients with benign prostatic hyperplasia, can result in rates of erection impotence of 5–40 per cent and retrograde ejaculation can occur in up to 80 per cent of patients;
- after a myocardial infarction 10–70 per cent of patients report a diminished frequency and quality of sexual activity and loss of sexual drive.

Some medications can also adversely affect sexual performance. Crenshaw and Goldberg (1996) note that most of the top-rated drug categories administered to patients over 65 years of age are commonly associated with sexual dysfunction. For example, bendrofluazide is associated with a frequent rate of erection complaints; in most cases, sexual problems are resolved after discontinuation of the medication (Schiavi 1999).

In treating sexual dysfunction in older patients, practitioners need to be careful that their assessments incorporate a psychosocial approach, for example, evaluating relationships and personal self-worth. This is essential to avoid overly medicalising sexual problems, which shifts the focus from the individual and the context of their life purely to genital function. A medical assessment should also look beyond the requirements of penetrative sex and include other non-penetrative activities, for example, masturbation, oral sex, kissing, touch, romance and companionship.

Psychological issues

Healthy sexual expression generally requires a good relationship, irrespective of age. A recent study of women conducted by the Kinsey Institute found that the best predictors of a woman's sexual satisfaction were based on her overall emotional well-being, and the emotional relationship with her partner (Hillman 2000). This is supported further by Kingsberg (2002, p. 431), who states 'regardless of the length or nature of the relationship, its quality is enhanced by emotional intimacy, autonomy without too much distance, an ability to manage stress, and to maintain a positive perception of self and the relationship'. These are important factors particularly when positioning sexual problems within a psychosocial schema. In a study of 23 older women aged 61–90, Jones (2002) quotes one of her lesbian participants discussing her partner's problem with vaginal dryness. Initially the participant implies that this is a response to ageing; she then changes her mind and says instead that vaginal dryness is about being with the right sexual partner.

There is a need to establish differences between physiological and psychological factors that impact on sexuality for men. In the past, the focus of men's sexuality has concentrated primarily on the capacity of the penis to perform. This view has been exploited with the introduction of Viagra as the 'sexual salvation' of ageing men (Kingsberg 2002). Psychological changes in men are frequently attributed to natural physiological changes brought on by the ageing process. Often these changes are perceived as negative and are associated with depression and a loss of well-being. Metz and Miner (1998) suggest a more positive definition, proposing a mellowing of attitudes, expansion of the meaning of intimacy, increased reflectivness, spiritual growth and integration.

Studies to date on male sexuality have focused predominantly on sexual performance, ignoring satisfaction as an independent measure. The way in which men respond to sexual change depends on how they integrate these changes into their overall life. Some may experience little or no effect on their well-being, others will react with distress and impaired self-esteem and doubt (Schiavi 1999). Precisely how individual men react to these changes will be determined by their beliefs, knowledge and the attitudes that have shaped them as individuals. For example, Minichiello and his colleagues (1996a) found that many older people hold the view that 'it is difficult for older people to express themselves sexually' and 'older people are more likely to be disapproved of for showing sexual interest', a context which may put older people 'in the closet', so to speak. By this we mean that societal attitudes may make older people feel uncomfortable, guilty, ashamed or deviant for being sexual, with the consequence that this may silence them.

The sociological context

Society's impression of older people as sexually unattractive is reinforced in a culture dominated by youthfulness. Youth is symbolised by vigour, beauty and procreative power; the stereotypes of ageing include impotence, ugliness and sterility. These attitudes maintain the myth of the asexual ageing adult. Indoctrination of these ideas has been systematically shaped by our social institutions, religion advocating sex is for procreation, and the media perpetuating the association between youth and attractiveness. These tenets form the basis of our beliefs and knowledge, which shape the way in which older people perceive themselves. They also perpetuate and reinforce expectations which may be maintained by the next generation.

Sexual attractiveness in women is often judged by their physical attributes (Hillman 2000). Women's magazines place an emphasis on preserving youth by advocating the use of skin care and hair dye designed to disguise the effects of ageing (Kellett 2000). The simple act of shopping, often seen as a domain of enjoyment and an opportunity to reaffirm femininity, can become an unpleasant chore, as it reinforces undesirable changes in appearance and function. Clothing manufacturers do not allow for arthritic hands by providing clothes with Velcro patches or larger fasteners. Imagine trying to shop for a dress when you have a dowager's hump, and every dress you put on is either to short in the rear, or too tight across the back for comfort, neither of which allows you to feel feminine or attractive (Hillman 2000).

Men also experience insecurities about their masculinity as they age. Often the penis and its ability to function is central to what the literature refers to as masculinity. As Hillman (2000, p. 139) states, 'in nearly all cultures, the functioning of the male phallus is tied intimately to a man's sense of self, body image and implied social worth'. This phallocentric model begins at a young age and continues throughout the life span. The notion of developing and sustaining a masculine identity through one's sexual conquests is longstanding, and while this can be affirming and empowering for men who do not experience sexual dysfunction, for those who do it can be debilitating (Marsiglio & Greer 1994). Culturally, as we become more accepting and knowledgeable of older men's sexuality, the challenge will be to reconstruct men's sexuality to include broader definitions of sexual intimacy and to make a shift away from phallocentric models.

Often people fail to appreciate how the social context can influence behaviour. Older men and women may have different experiences, opportunities and expectations with regard to sex. Is it because they are biologically different, or because social factors are at play here? Let us consider how gender differences in life expectancy may affect the sexual experiences of a population.

Demographic data indicate that there are many more women over the age of 65 than men (Minichiello et al 1992). If marital status or living with a partner is a measure of 'increased opportunity structures' for sex (Turner & Adams 1988), then heterosexual older women have more limited opportunity for sexual expression. Facing an increasingly disproportionate sex ratio as they age, heterosexual women are more likely to experience widowhood and fewer possibilities for remarriage (Robinson 1983) and, as evidence suggests, celibacy due to the loss or illness of a partner (Kellett 1991). Older women may also find alternative expressions of sexuality, such as masturbation, sex outside marriage or polygamy, difficult to reconcile with historically and culturally influenced life-long beliefs and values.

Gender differences with respect to both sexual behaviour and attitudes of older people were identified in the sexual health survey conducted by Minichiello and his colleagues (1996b). The results revealed that of the six independent variables, which included gender, age, marital status, ethnicity, self-reported health and spiritual belief, gender was the only independent variable associated with all five dependent variables—reported number of sexual partners, currently involved in a sexual relationship, perceived importance of sex, changes in sexual interest and changes in sexual activity. Minichiello and his colleagues found that older men were five times more likely than women to report having many sexual partners in their lives, and older women were twice as likely as men to report having never had any sexual partners. Older men were twice as likely to be presently in a sexual relationship, and older women more likely to report that sex is not important at all in later life. The study also found a significant association between gender and changes in sexual interest. Over two-thirds of the older women reported a decrease in sexual interest and one-third indicated that their sexual interest had remained the same since 40 years of age. In contrast, less than half of the older men reported that sexual interest had declined and half of them reported that their level of sexual interest had been maintained. The results show no main effect for age or marital status, indicating that women regardless of their age or marital status were more likely than men to report a decrease in sexual interest.

Gender differences were not restricted to sexual behaviour. Significant differences in knowledge and attitudes between older men and women were found. For example, partly because sex has been constructed by popular culture to be 'men's business', women held less knowledge about sexual issues. Older women were less likely to be aware of sexuality as a lifelong need, that prescription drugs and depression had an effect on their sexual interest or that sexual relationships offered psychological and physical benefits. Yet women held slightly less conservative attitudes toward sexuality issues. For example, older men were significantly more likely to agree with the statement 'Homosexuality is wrong'; older women were more often neutral in their responses to this item.

Another social context to consider is the investment made by society to improve the knowledge level of older people with regards to sexuality and sexual health, a point touched on earlier in this chapter. With the discovery of HIV/AIDS and the realisation that prevention is the most effective way to contain the virus, a host of education campaigns was developed to improve people's knowledge of sexual safety—but implicit in these education programs is an ageist tone, as older people are not seen as an appropriate target population. We should not be surprised to learn that when researchers study the knowledge level of older people about sexual matters, they have found it to be low. Using a Sexual Health Knowledge and Beliefs Index (SHKB), which included statements about the relationship between sexual activity, depression and medication; the physical and psychological benefits of sexuality in later life; and, the influence of past sexual activity on a person's sexual activity in later life, Minichiello et al (2000) found that from a possible score of six their sample had a mean score of 2.45. Only

3.9 per cent of respondents answered all six items in the affirmative, while 17.4 per cent of the sample answered none in the affirmative. Between 41–50 per cent of the respondents answered five items in the affirmative. As expected, the older the person the less positively they scored on the SHKB index. The lack of attention to providing older persons with lifelong education about sexuality is concerning because studies have consistently found older people to have insufficient knowledge about sexuality (Minichiello et al 1996).

Research reveals a positive relationship between greater sexual knowledge and positive attitudes towards sexuality (Luketich 1991). This raises an interesting question: if studies show that older people retain interest and physical ability for sexual expression, and particularly if we accept that sexuality is an important component of human existence, then why are older people so seldom the target of supportive services and education on sexuality? Some gerontologists have argued that this contradiction can be explained partly by our youth-oriented culture, which fails to recognise or accept that older people are sexual (Minichiello et al 1996a).

Activity 4.1

Interview an older person about their views on sexual intimacy. What have you learnt? Were any of your assumptions challenged?

Women and sexuality in later life

Hillman (2000) correctly comments that there has been far less research on women's sexuality, and in particular, older women's subjective experiences of their sexuality. This gap in the current literature needs attention. However, we do know that studies consistently report that older women are two times less likely than older men to engage in sexual activity such as sexual intercourse (Minichiello et al 1996b). We also know that it is the lack of the availability of a partner for older women, and persisting gender differences in patterns of socialisation, sexual behaviour and attitudes that appear in adolescence which partly explain gender differences in later life (Minichiello et al 2004). More recent studies and the popular press document that older women engage in a variety of sexual activity, including using devices for self-masturbation, hiring escorts, using the Internet for locating pornographic sites and for finding partners (Hillman 2000; Strombeck 2003).

As noted earlier, there are some physiological changes related to sexual function and ageing in women worth further discussion. For example, as the result of changes in hormone production the size of the uterus, cervix and ovaries is reduced by up to 50 per cent. As Hillman (2000) notes, decreases in estrogen can result in a thinning of the vaginal lining, a loss of vaginal elasticity and a decrease in vaginal lubrication, making intercourse a painful and unpleasant experience without the use of appropriate intervention. Not surprisingly, studies show that up to 30 per cent of middle-aged and older women experience pain during intercourse. Older women have an overall lower usage of condoms and recent concerns have been expressed about this practice and the potential HIV risk due to vaginal trauma because of reduced elasticity (Bourne et al 2002).

Hillman (2000) also notes that as women age their risk for both breast cancer and cervical cancer increases. Yet older women, up until recently, were less likely to have mammograms compared to their younger counterparts. Practitioners need to be more vigilant in asking older women if they are sexually active, as the virus responsible for many cases of cervical cancer may be transmitted through sexual contact. Practitioners also need to be aware that there are some simple methods that can assist older women to be sexually active and remain healthy. For example, masturbation on a daily basis can increase blood flow to the vaginal area, which promotes increased lubrication.

Other studies reveal that hormone replacement therapy assists in dealing with the physiological changes induced by a lack of estrogens and is effective in combating vaginal atrophy and dryness (Belchete 1994), and that topical lubricants can make intercourse less painful and more enjoyable.

Sexual diversity

There is now greater recognition of the variability in the sexual practices of men and women. Like the rest of society, health professionals are interacting with a more openly self-identifying population of older gay and lesbian people. Consider the following statistics. Woolf (2003, p. 1) reports that there are between 1.75 and 3.5 million older gay men and women in the United States and that 'this is approximately equal to or two times greater than the number of older adults living in nursing homes'. Twenty-seven per cent of the population of San Francisco is gay or lesbian. There are some 9301 same-sex couples living in New York City. The Australian Bureau of Statistics reports similar figures in census data on same-sex couples living in Australia because for the first time the government office collects information on this issue (ABS 2001).

Despite this context, the issue of homosexuality has been, until recently, ignored in gerontological publications; for example, a major British text (Pifer & Bonte 1990) included only one reference on the topic, and a major American gerontology text devoted only one paragraph to gay and lesbian ageing in a book of over 450 pages (Binstock & George 1990). This is somewhat surprising because homosexuality as a topic has been extensively researched in both the social and medical literature. A number of studies have investigated the relationship between adjustment and levels of acceptance of gay identity (Bell & Weinberg 1978), but few studies have attempted to examine how gay older men cope with later life (Lee 1987).

A number of researchers have suggested that later life adjustment is not affected by sexual orientation per se, but is made problematic by society's negative attitude towards homosexuality (Lee 1987; Minnigerode & Adelman 1987). These studies report that gay men must deal with problems related to stigma which continue to affect adjustment in later life. For example, an American study found that adjustment to ageing was significantly related to satisfaction with being gay and the sequence of early gay developmental events (Aldelman 1991). High life satisfaction, low self-criticism and few psychosomatic problems were significantly related to both high satisfaction with being gay, and to gay experimentation prior to self-definition as homosexual or lesbian. The data also showed that high life satisfaction appeared strongly related to five factors. These were high self-acceptance of homosexuality; concealing sexual preference in the workplace; low involvement with older gay people; early age of awareness; and decrease in the importance of homosexuality in later years.

Three landmark studies specifically examined the relationship between adjustment to later life and being gay (Berger 1982; Vacha

1985; Lee 1987). Berger's (1982) study refutes some of the stereotypes about older gay men, showing that they are not lonely, unwanted or isolated. However, Lee (1987) reported a correlation between self-concealment and greater life satisfaction and more negative attitudes towards growing old and being gay. Likewise, Vacha (1985) illustrates that the discrimination that comes with ageing is compounded by the discrimination of being gay. Although a few of Vacha's informants expressed gerontophobia, the majority interviewed accepted their sexual identity and old age. He found the following recurring themes in the lives of these gay older men: the importance given to sex at all stages of a gay man's life; non-acceptance and harassment by families, police and doctors; the need to deny their homosexuality in their early lives and the influence this had on establishing and maintaining a long-term partnership; and the frequent use of drugs and alcohol. The majority of the informants had lived through the danger of being fired from jobs, receiving dishonourable discharges from the military, being rejected by families and assaults by other men. On the positive side, Vacha observed that because these men had survived difficult times in their lives they seemed unusually buoyant and sure of themselves in their old age.

As Tirrito (2003) points out, it is important for health professionals to accept the position that sexual orientation should not influence the ability of a client to receive services or be eligible for assistance. In fact in some countries it is illegal and discriminatory to do so. Like women, who face the double jeopardy of gender and age in later life, gay older people face the same problems as all older persons as well as the prejudices of homophobia. As Tirrito notes, the problems of isolation, loneliness and lack of access to help during illness or a crisis, especially, may be made worse due to the fact that few people working in aged care have training in 'gerohomosexuality'.

Woolf (2003, p. 2) identifies some issues of particular concern to the older gay man or lesbian:

> First, the health care system has been traditionally unresponsive to recognizing the existence of homosexuality as an alternative lifestyle. Thus, services are aimed at a heterosexual population. Quam presents the example of a woman who is diagnosed with breast cancer and afraid to tell her physician that she is a lesbian. This inability to communicate honestly with a health care

professional can only negatively impact treatment. Second, homosexual partnerships are often not recognized to exist even though the individuals may be been involved in life-partner situations for many years. Often, partners are not allowed to visit their loved ones in the hospital, not allowed to participate in health care decisions of their life-partner, are not allowed to live together in retirement facilities, or are even barred or excluded from funeral arrangements. This discounting of primary relationships can have a tremendous, painful effect on the gay men or lesbians involved . . . [L]astly, the individual who 'comes out' or explores the same-sex orientation for the first time as an older adult has few resources to meet people or adjust to their reorientation.

Consider the results obtained from a study that provided older gay men with the opportunity to discuss issues with regards to accessing health services: Hays et al (1997, p. 119) found that most reported difficulty talking to doctors about their sexuality and 'went along' with doctors assuming that they were heterosexual widowers. They noted that few general practitioners (described as 'straight') initiated any discussion concerning sexual health matters even when they knew their patients were gay. When the informants took the initiative in discussing sexual issues, most received what they considered to be ageist reactions to their concerns, particularly those issues relating to sexual performance:

The doctor says, 'Well you know you're in your late sixties and you're on you own now, so does it really matter?'

He said to me, 'Oh you don't want to worry about that, why would you want to worry about that now?'

It is therefore not surprising that older gay and lesbian people rarely reveal their sexuality to their doctors. Changes to the sexual health discourse as a result of HIV/AIDS may now make it easier for practitioners to raise sexuality matters. However, there are issues worth noting here: many older people have internalised some of the prejudicial attitudes towards homosexuality and may require assistance with more positive views about themselves and their homosexuality before they are comfortable discussing their sexual difficulties.

Older people and HIV

HIV (Human Immunodeficiency Virus) causes a lifelong infection that can weaken the body's immune system. The most advanced stage of HIV infection, called AIDS (Acquired Immune Deficiency Syndrome), occurs when the immune system is severely compromised, allowing the development of life-threatening diseases, infections and cancers. AIDS can occur about ten years (with a range of one to 20 years) after initial infection with HIV. Antiretroviral treatments now extend the period during which people with HIV remain without symptoms of immune suppression or AIDS. These treatments suppress the activity of the virus and delay immune suppression or, if treatment is started later, allow immunity to be restored. Anti-HIV treatments have allowed people with HIV to continue working and live active social lives.

The impact of HIV/AIDS on the lives of older people has been less well studied than for younger people, although important differences are emerging. The number of older people with HIV/AIDS is increasing because of the delayed recognition of older people with HIV and people receiving treatment for HIV are living longer (Manfredi 2002; National Institute of Health 2003). Twelve per cent of people diagnosed with AIDS in the United States are aged over 50, while the number of people over 50 with HIV (without AIDS) is significantly higher, and includes many people who have never been tested (Centers for Disease Control 2002a). An Australian study that examined the profile of 2621 people over 50 years of age who attended a public sexual health clinic revealed that over half had a past sexually transmitted infection (STI) and did not know their HIV status at registration, even though they were sexually active (Bourne et al 2002). Even more concerning, 45 per cent of the women and 37 per cent of the men never used condoms when having sex.

The lack of awareness of personal HIV status in older people is perhaps not surprising because they know less about the disease than younger people (Garvey 1993) and have not been specifically targeted with HIV education (Donovan et al 1998). Also, many doctors are less likely to discuss sex and drug taking with their older patients because they assume patients will be too embarrassed to discuss these sensitive topics, or are not having sex or using drugs. Other studies, however, clearly indicate that older people are willing to discuss sexual activity and receive more sexual health information (Minichiello et al 2000; Gott 2001). Doctors, like some older people, can also be uncomfortable with sex and drug taking. Targeted training of doctors in sexual and drug history taking may be required to ensure adequate exploration of this important aspect of all people's health.

Patients and their health care providers may mistake HIV/AIDS symptoms for other conditions more commonly associated with older people. Typical examples include fatigue and poor memory being mistaken for 'age-related dementia' rather than advanced HIV disease or AIDS dementia; assuming a pneumonia is community-acquired rather than caused by *Pneumocystis pneumonia*; and gingivitis ascribed to poor oral health rather than HIV-related immune suppression.

Like younger people, older people may be reluctant to be tested because of fear of the stigma associated with HIV. The standards of care for HIV testing which were developed to overcome concerns about stigma and privacy should be equally available to older people but have not been developed because of ageist assumptions about sexuality and older persons. These standards include labelling of pathology tests with codes to mask the person's identity, opportunities for private consultations and strict confidentiality of information. Families, including same-sex partners, intimately involved in the care of older people will need to understand that this approach facilitates (rather than undermines) quality care of their dependents. The importance of early HIV testing to provide access to care, treatment and prevention services cannot be underestimated.

Older people diagnosed with HIV/AIDS have been shown to have poorer outcomes than younger people—an effect produced by differences in access to care, provider relationships, co-morbid conditions, health habits and age-related changes (Smola et al 2001). The limited data available on the use of combination anti-HIV therapy in older people suggests a similar success at virological suppression but a slower and blunted immune recovery compared to younger patients (Manfredi 2002). Whether this difference is related to age-related immune dysfunction that contributes to an increased susceptibility to infection ('immunosenescence') is unclear (Castle 2000).

The emerging knowledge about metabolic complications of anti-HIV therapy (Carr et al 1998; Dube & Sattler 1998; SoRelle 1998; Mina et al 2001) will be particularly relevant to older people even though they are not included in most treatment studies. The observed complications include increased rates of elevated serum lipids, body fat changes, impaired glucose tolerance, myocardial infarction and cerebrovascular disease. The common risk factors for cardiovascular disease, like hypertension, obesity, elevated lipids and reduced physical activity, peak in older people and active management of these problems is indicated in people with HIV. HIV disease alone may also contribute to blood vessel changes like atherosclerosis. Osteoporosis, common in older people, is also associated with long-term HIV disease, and may increase the risk of complications such as spontaneous fractures and fall injuries. More information is needed about HIV and non-HIV drug interactions and toxicities that may interfere with drug effectiveness and treatment adherence (Levy et al 2003).

As noted earlier, health care workers often neglect the sexuality of older people. Acknowledging their sexuality will ensure their sexual needs and safety are not forgotten. A simple way of introducing the topic of sexuality is to cover genital care when discussing skin care, and then move on to inquire about sexual activity and condom use. The use of water-based lubricants during sexual intercourse will reduce the risk of trauma of genital skin, which is commonly fragile in older people. The use of impotence treatments has enabled many older men to recommence sexual relationships at a time when the prevalence of sexually transmitted infection including HIV is on the rise. These men and their new partners grew up when the rules of dating, communication and sexual safety were different, so they will need information and education to help them adapt to the new environment. Older women frequently out-number older men, thus heterosexual women may feel pressured to engage in unprotected sex or otherwise subjugate their needs in order to secure a male partner. An honest discussion about sexuality and behaviour will be the only way to tackle such issues.

Despite the many challenges to health care of older people with HIV, models of successful ageing amongst people with HIV/AIDS have been developed (Kahana & Kahana 2001), and have been introduced for use in populations with disabilities and chronic illness. For example, the Preventive and Corrective Proactivity Model of Successful Aging (PCO) is anchored in confronting 'life stressors' like illnesses, social loss and lack of person–environment fit. While most models of successful ageing focus on sustaining physical health and functional abilities, this model emphasises social and psychological states as 'quality of life indicators', including affective states, meaning of life, maintenance of valued activities and relationships. The model involves the activation of social and personal resources to buffer the effects of the life stressors through preventive adaptations. An older person with HIV may actively promote their health by ceasing smoking or participating in physical activity. Helping friends and other people while in good health can ensure older people build social supports and receive more assistance when or if their health fails.

HIV/AIDS can affect older people in another way. Many younger people with HIV/AIDS turn to their parents and grandparents for financial support and nursing care. Similarly, they may care for the orphaned and sometimes HIV-infected grandchildren. The mental, physical, and financial drain of caring for others may be very difficult for older caregivers, especially if they have a poor understanding of the illness. Special programs have been funded by international donor agencies for developing countries where large numbers of young and middle-aged people have HIV/AIDS and are being cared for by older people. Large numbers of deaths from AIDS have caused significant changes in family structures in some of these countries.

In summary, HIV/AIDS provides a considerable challenge to the health of older people. Yet preliminary information indicates older people are resourceful and adaptable and that their responses to other chronic health problems are providing valuable solutions to the difficulties posed by HIV/AIDS.

Activity 4.2

What would you include as part of a public health education campaign designed to reduce older people's risk to STI or HIV? Would you assume that older people are a homogeneous group as part of your campaign? Or would you develop different strategies for different groups of older persons?

Diversity of issues and experiences

Life after prostate

John was 75 and enjoyed a loving relationship and a good sex life, but recently had a prostate operation. Before the operation, John's doctor had devoted a good amount of time to talking about life after 'the op'. He had warned that there might be some problems with John's sex life. Not only was the surgery known to sometimes interfere with erection, but John was also having his testicles removed to stop his sex hormones from causing the cancer to grow more quickly. John decided that the operation could be lifesaving and must go ahead . . . he could live with sexual issues if he had to. Sure enough, after he returned home, John experienced problems. But he didn't hesitate to go back to the doctor because he already felt so comfortable discussing these issues with him. Were there any medications that could bring his erections back? John's doctor asked whether John noticed any erections when he woke in the morning. John said he did, not as strong, but they were there. This answer told the doctor that there was still some function left and that time, simple treatments and a little counselling were likely to help.

Life-saving medication

Peter and Sally had a wonderful relationship and a good sex life. That was until Peter started those dreaded blood pressure tablets, and he began having problems keeping his erections. Peter immediately suspected the medication and started taking them irregularly. To make matters worse, the problems with his sex life made him even more anxious. Neither of these factors helped his blood pressure! Peter went back to his doctor, who increased the dosage of the blood pressure medication and gave him new tablets for depression. Now he lost his erections entirely! Peter changed doctors. The new doctor did things differently—inviting Sally to come to the consultation too, asking about their sex life, and prescribing new medications which wouldn't have the same impact. They all decided the depression tablets were no longer necessary.

Life after menopause? Loss, liberation, release?
Jenny, Florence and Doris met at the local seniors' club.
They had become club regulars partly because it gave them
interests but above all, because they were able to form
friendships and 'debrief' with each other. One day they
found themselves swapping stories about 'the change', as
they called it. They were surprised at how different their
experiences were. For Jenny, menopause was a crisis.
Jenny liked being young and valued the idea that she could
be a mother. She saw menopause as a loss of her
womanhood and took a long time to adjust to her 'new'
self. Florence had a completely different experience; for her
there was no longer the risk of getting pregnant and her
troublesome periods had gone too. In many ways she
found menopause liberating and with the aid of some
lubricant, her sex life actually improved! For Doris,
menopause was also liberating, but in quite a different way.
In recent years sex had become a chore, and Doris decided
to use menopause as an excuse to stop having sex
altogether. That suited her perfectly!

Sex and the unexpected
Cathy was 78. Amazingly for her, she met a new partner!
Rod was 80 and such a lovely man. Because things were
getting serious, they thought they should do the right thing
and get some tests done. They went to a clinic where the
doctor saw them together briefly and advised that tests
were not necessary at their age. They disagreed, and the
doctor reluctantly took blood samples. A couple of weeks
later they went for their results. Oddly, this time the doctor
saw them separately. Cathy was a little worried. Maybe Rod
had hidden something? What if he had HIV? As it turned
out, Rod was okay, and Cathy's HIV test was negative too.
But Cathy was surprised to find that her Hepatitis C test
was positive. Suddenly from the mists of time a few things
fell in place: her late husband died of liver cancer; she had
injected drugs at a party during the 1960s. Cathy was
totally unprepared for this outcome, and she panicked.
What would happen to her and Rod now?

A change of life
Andrew and James had been together for 36 years and had lived in the same house for 20 years. They shared everything. Then suddenly James wasn't there. He went down the street, had a heart attack and that was that! Andrew was heartbroken, but that was only the beginning. Even though James had left a will, the tax department didn't recognise their relationship and tax was imposed on the inheritance. Andrew was left with no alternative but to sell their precious house. Where would he live now? He finally decided that the only alternative was to go to a retirement village. After all, he was 75 and no longer had any other real supports. He wanted to live nearby as he couldn't face too much more upheaval in his life. Andrew picked up the phone and called the nearby retirement village. The moment someone answered, it flashed across his mind that the village was run by a church group. Butterflies filled his stomach—he couldn't cope with things getting much more difficult. How were they going to treat him?

Activity 4.3

How do the examples above challenge some of your own views about sexuality in later life?

Conclusion

This chapter has challenged some of the ageist assumptions under-pinning how society views the sexuality of older people. Below we describe a range of situations that health professionals, older persons and the community at large will increasingly encounter as sexuality in later life is more widely accepted and connected to quality of life and relationship issues. Our aim here is to provide a better understanding of the motives and diversity behind the emotional and physical contexts surrounding love and sex in later life. Sexual expression, or the lack thereof, in older people should be an informed choice, not the result of external pressures embedded in ageist assumptions applied by health professionals and older people themselves or the larger society in which they live. It is not enough, as Chapter 1 argued, for education simply to expose the myth of the asexual older person. Our re-education and policy strategies here must allow for recognition of the fact that many of the problems and barriers older people face in regard to expressing their sexual selves are created and sustained by institutional arrangements (the health care system, media, current policies, sexual health services, etc.). Sex, romance and older people are easy targets for comedy, for example. Kate Legge (2002) wrote in the *Weekend Australian Magazine*:

> The web site satirewire.com hams up the image of two old sticks with crepey skin getting tangled in colostomy bags and heart monitors. 'Being old does not extinguish the passion for having sex,' reports the web site, but 'thinking about old people having sex does.' These stereotypes reek of mothballs. Hetzel, who is an artist in her spare time, imagines a more fitting image for the future. She conjures up a red chilli to convey old age: shrivelled on the outside but peppery hot all the same.

It is clear from the evidence in this chapter that older people are not asexual. Therefore, it is important for practitioners to discuss sexual health needs with their older clients, rather than ignore them or accept stereotypes that suggest that those needs are either not important or do not exist. Comments such as 'but you are 72', 'you should not worry about such things', 'condoms or an HIV test are not required for you', 'are you married?' are not helpful to older patients as they demonstrate presumptions, if not ageist and homophobic attitudes. We strongly recommend that basic competency in talking about sexuality in later life and in documentating the sexual history of older people should be an essential skill for today's clinicians. Their competency should include a better and wider understanding of 'sexualities' as put forward by the rich sociological literature on this topic and the diverse personal and sexual needs and experiences of a range of groups, including older people who are gay and lesbian.

5

Considerations and challenges in the prevention of dementia

Irene Coulson, Rodrigo Mariño,
Vicki Strang

In most developed countries the average life expectancy is now close to 80 years, with the most rapidly increasing segment comprising those who are more than 80 (Henderson & Jorm 2000). In these countries, a 65-year-old person is expected to live eighteen more years; an 85-year-old person is expected to live five more years (WHO 2001). With these increases, and the strong association between advancing age and the prevalence of dementia, the absolute and relative number of people living with dementia will increase significantly.

The prevalence and incidence of dementia increase exponentially with age. The prevalence of dementia doubles every five years, up to 85 years of age (Henderson & Jorm 2000), affecting 1 per cent of those aged 60–64, increasing to 3 per cent at age 70 and to 20–30 per cent at 85 years of age (Prince 1997; Henderson & Jorm 2000). The prevalence amongst older nursing home residents, as a group, is estimated to be 60–80 per cent (Marcantonio 2002). Dementia is the leading cause of institutionalisation amongst the elderly in western countries and accounts for more than half of nursing home admissions (Marcantonio 2002).

In the United States, somewhere between 4 and 5 million people are affected by dementia; this number is expected to quadruple by 2040 (Binstock et al 1992; Prince 1997). In Australia, predictions indicate that from 1987 to 2031 there will be an 233–245 per cent increase in dementia cases diagnosed (Commonwealth Department of Community Services & Health 1990). Other developed countries, such as Japan, are also facing an epidemic of dementia cases as the baby boomers reach retirement age (Mayeux 1993).

Senior citizens are rightfully concerned about succumbing to the disease and are asking why there is such emphasis on prolonging life when dementia will be the final reward. This, as well as the fatalistic view that 'nothing can be done' once a dementia diagnosis has been established, causes great concern to health care professionals and governments about the ability of current systems to adequately address the care needs of people who acquire the disease.

This chapter provides an introduction into the epidemiology, the social meaning and impact of dementia on society. A discussion on the prevention of dementia follows. The chapter also highlights challenging areas for the future and areas of health services and ethical consideration. Because a great deal of information is available about dementia care, but little about the prevention of dementia, a special focus is given to preventable forms of dementia, namely vascular dementia.

The growing problem of dementia

Ageing is a privilege and a societal achievement. Thus facilitating the continuous good health of older adult populations is a major challenge to public health in developed and developing countries that will have a continuing impact on all aspects of society. The growing number of older adults places increasing demands on the public health system and on the medical and social service system. In the United States, about one-third of the total health care expenditure is directed to the care of older adults (Centers for Disease Control 2002). Dementia is one of the most serious disorders affecting older persons because of the prolonged years of suffering and the burden of costs experienced by those diagnosed, their families, and the health care system (Marcantonio 2002). With the rising incidence of dementia amongst those 65 years and older, the cost of treatment will have a major impact on the country's health care expenditure (Jarvik 2000).

Chiu et al (1992) have defined dementia as a deterioration from a known or estimated prior level of intellectual function sufficient to interfere broadly with the conduct of the patient's customary affairs of life, which is not isolated to a single narrow category of intellectual performance and which is independent of level of consciousness. In addition, dementia is manifested by some or all of the following features: memory impairment, aphasia, apraxia, agnosia, disturbances in executive functioning, and impairment of social and/or occupational functioning. The natural history of the disease varies according to the cause of the dementia; however, victims typically experience a steady, inexorable decline in intellectual function over two to ten years, culminating in total dependence; death is often due to infection (Marcantonio 2002).

Dementia is a clinical syndrome, not a specific condition, which always involves decline in the mental function in multiple domains resulting in confusion, loss of intellectual ability, cognitive and memory impairment (Nay & Garratt 1999). Several types of dementia have been identified, the most common form being Alzheimer's disease (AD), followed by vascular dementia (VaD) (Hamdy et al 1998). AD is almost twice as common as VaD in most western countries, with AD alone accounting for about 50 per cent of all dementia cases (Hamdy et al 1998). In Japan, however, VaD accounts for 50 per cent of all dementia cases occurring in individuals 65 years of age and older (Chiu 2000; Henderson & Jorm 2000; Alagiakrishnan & Masaki 2001). Additionally, VaD may coexist with AD, accounting for up to another 20 per cent of cases (Loeb & Stirling 2000). Together these two types of dementia can thus account for up to 90 per cent of cases (Marcantonio 2000).

Vascular dementia occurs when cells in the brain are deprived of oxygen by a blockage in the blood supply—the cells die, leading to symptoms of dementia. People with VaD can experience symptoms such as memory loss, difficulties with communication and reasoning, and eventually a loss of physical abilities. In VaD, the symptoms may occur in 'steps', remaining the same for long periods of time, whereas persons with AD experience a slow, steady decline. Factors associated with increased risk of VaD include: age, history of stroke, low education, hypertension, white matter lesions, history of myocardial infarction, diabetes, cerebral atrophy, cortical infarcts, left hemispheric stroke, early urinary incontinence (Hamdy et al 1998).

Studies of mortality in developed countries have shown that survival after diagnosis of VaD is less than in AD, about five years. There are some suggestions that mortality in less developed countries might be higher (Prince 1997). VaD progresses over a period of many years and is generally not diagnosed until it reaches a relatively late stage of development, presenting with an abrupt start and progressing stepwise with stabilising stages until another episode occurs.

Alzheimer's disease is difficult to diagnose and can only be positively concluded on post-mortem examination (Loeb & Stirling 2000). Brain imaging techniques make it easier to diagnose VaD, where areas of the brain are seen to be damaged due to mini-strokes (Hamdy et al 1998). The well-known Hachinski Ischemic Scale (Hachinski 1992) is a three-staged approach containing a set of criteria sometimes used to provide supportive clinical evidence of VaD. See Table 5.1.

An elevated Hachinski score of seven or higher provides support of a diagnosis of VaD (Lis & Gaviria 1997). Hachinski (1992) and Kuller (1999) argue that further studies for the prevention of VaD should be aimed at those in the brain-at-risk stage, and the most promising line of research is the prevention of risk factors.

Other assessment tools that can facilitate a diagnosis include the *Diagnostic and Statistical Manual of Mental Disorders*, the *International Classification of Diseases*, the National Institute of Neurological Disorders and Stroke-Association International pour la Recherché at L'Enseignement en Neurosciences (NINDS-AIREN) criteria and the protocols of the Alzheimer's Disease Diagnostic and Treatment Center (ADDTC) (Marcantonio 2000).

Lewy body dementia is a new addition to the types of dementia, possibly accounting for 10–15 per cent of all dementias (Henderson & Jorm 2000). Other less common forms of dementia are dementia related to anoxia of the brain (cardiac arrest); physical or chemical

Table 5.1: Hachinski Ischemic Scale (1992)

Stage 1	Brain-at-risk stage: Includes the elderly, hypertensive, smokers, diabetics, and patients with atrial fibrillation, cardiac patients and those with asymptomatic extracranial arterial disease and no cognitive impairment.
Stage 2	Pre-dementia stage: In this stage patients may have subtle cognitive impairment and includes those persons with a history of transient ischaemic attacks, silent cerebral infarctions and systemic lupus erythematosus.
Stage 3	Dementia stage: Includes those persons with VaD, atherosclerosis of extracranial arteries, cardiac embolism, intracranial small vessel disease, or other causes of stroke.

trauma (boxing or alcohol abuse); genetically linked dementias such as Huntington's disease; dementias resulting from illness such as HIV/AIDS or Creutzfeldt-Jakob disease; and dementias related to Parkinson's disease and Pick's disease (Henderson & Jorm 2000; Marcantonio 2000; Alagiakrishnan & Masaki 2001).

The social meaning of dementia

Few problems associated with advanced age produce more fear in older people than dementia. This fear is justified, according to Kitwood (1997), who is amazed at how the unique characteristics and the very essence of persons with dementia have been expunged from our health care systems, even where rigorous methods of record keeping, assessment and care planning have been in place. They gradually become non-persons in the system because little effort is made to preserve their distinctiveness. Persons with dementia, therefore, soon feel a lack of personal identity as outsiders to the illness interpret meaning for them (Kitwood 1997). They are often ignored and misunderstood, leaving them socially marginalised and experiencing a reduced quality to their lives (Kitwood 1997).

It is well known that the construction of social meaning in human beings is influenced by culture, personal values, gender, race, class, age, geography, sexual orientation and ability to make decisions for oneself. In this process, we rely heavily on language and on the social environment in which we live (see Chapter 1). In other words, we know who we are through our associations with other people and we learn how to identify ourselves by our environment and culture. When the ability of people to use language and to interpret the environment around them becomes impaired, as it does in dementia, their social context becomes understandably distorted. When people lose their ability to organise their lives and to articulate their insights and beliefs to the people around them, the societal tendency is to regard them as 'obliterated'. As an example, Kaufman (1999) shows how the narratives of older people who are dying describe how their families' wishes coincide with the biomedical wish to prolong their lives through intubation, even though they had requested a natural death.

Regardless of the form of dementia, it is imperative that the person's attributes, personality, culture, environment and the ways in which the person can be normalised and brought back into ordinary ways of relating to society, are taken into consideration (Kitwood 1997). The articulation of identity and personhood requires constant negotiation between the individual and the culture, in relation to understanding the views and needs of the sufferer. The social meaning and prevention of dementia deserves the highest priority because of the unique capacity of dementia to rob old age of dignity and quality, often bringing down at the same time spouses and other family members (Callahan 1992).

Studies are urgently needed to understand how dementia and death are understood by persons with dementia, families and health professionals, and how dignity and personhood can be preserved in dementia. Other studies should focus cross-culturally on the social and family roles of those with dementia. Careful attention also needs to be paid to the researchers' own discourse of the meaning of cognitive decline, in order to understand the social context of the dementia experience. Research must be socially situated and attuned to the power that discourse has in shaping and interpreting the social context and meaning of the dementia experience.

Preventable dementias

The question of whether dementia can be prevented continues to be debated in (Sachdev et al 1999; Coulson et al 2001). There is urgency to this debate given the escalating prevalence of dementia in the 85-plus age group, the most rapidly increasing age group of seniors <www.alzheimer.ca/english/disease/stats-people.html 2002>. Because of the traditionally fatalist view of dementia, its prevention has not been explored to a great extent in the past. Dementia care was the major focus in the 20th century, yet understanding dementia requires an appreciation of the importance of preventative care.

Vascular dementia presents the greatest scope for prevention. This is because 'unlike AD, whose risk factors are less solidly established, the risk factors of VaD are known, because they are largely the same as those identified for stroke' (Henderson & Jorm 2000, p. 26). Before addressing the prevention of AD and VaD in particular, let us briefly discuss prevention as it relates to the other less prevalent dementias.

Prevention of less prevalent dementias

If precursors to these types of dementia include factors such as brain injury from trauma, alcohol abuse or infection, the possibility of preventing the subsequent dementias exists simply by engaging in less risky lifestyle activities (Hamdy et al 1998). Preventing head trauma by wearing protective headgear when engaged in such high-risk activities as boxing and cycling, and the regular use of seat belts, could prevent dementia later in life. Minimal alcohol intake throughout the life span and the use of condoms in high-risk sexual encounters are other examples.

The prevention of dementia related to diseases such as Parkinson's disease, Pick's disease, Huntington's disease and Lewy body dementia remains more elusive. Although symptomatic treatments are available, preventing the dementias associated with these diseases is not yet understood, and no specific preventive strategies are yet available. Genetic counselling is available for persons known to be carriers of a disease such as Huntington's disease, whereby they may be advised of their risks of passing on the defective gene to the next generation (Hamdy et al 1998).

Prevention of vascular dementia

Ways of avoiding vascular dementia (VaD) are similar to avoiding cerebral vascular accidents (CVA) or strokes because the predisposing factors to both conditions are similar. VaD and CVA are both associated with high bloodpressure and both are largely preventable through lifestyle choices (Whitlock 1997). Lifestyle practices for the prevention of stroke are well known. One need only consult a local Heart and Stroke Association to receive a wealth of reading materials and access points to numerous websites about the practices most effective in preventing CVAs. Stroke has a number of modifiable risk factors. These include smoking, alcohol consumption, hypertension, obesity, diabetes mellitus and hyperglycemia, hypercholestoreleaemia and cardiac diseases, and lack of exercise (Henderson & Jorm 2000; Sacco 2001). Lifestyle behaviours related to the broader social context can also influence the onset of VaD significantly. For example, remaining actively engaged with living one's life is vital. It is well recognised that strong social networks and support are essential in maintaining and enhancing health at all ages (Clark et al 2000; Coulson et al 2001).

Positive lifestyle choices include taking responsibility for one's health, ensuring regular exercise, good nutrition, a satisfaction with self and life, interpersonal relationship support from friends and family and the ability to achieve peace of mind when chronic or major life events or daily hassles occur (Walker 1997). Tobacco and excess alcohol intake should be eliminated, although there is some evidence to suggest that the moderate consumption of red wine, with its anti-oxidant properties, enhances cerebral perfusion. Targeting and promoting healthy lifestyle behaviours is the best alternative to costly effective treatment, leading to improved quality of life for older people.

Additionally, underlying medical conditions need to be monitored. Hypertension should be controlled through the maintenance of an appropriate physician-directed medication regime. Obesity, with its strong predisposing linkages to type 2 diabetes and hypertension, should be avoided. The physician might also suggest medications with low-level anti-coagulant properties (for example, aspirin), and anti-inflammatory agents. (Hachinski 1992; Sachdev et al 1999).

Klinge (2000) believes that health care practice should no longer focus on 'complaints related medicine' but rather on 'risk orientated medicine'. Walker (1997, p. 466) suggests that 'of all the dimensions of a health-promoting lifestyle, self-actualization or spiritual growth may be most central to wellness. It involves having a sense of purpose in life, experiencing awareness of and satisfaction with self, and continuing to grow and develop as a person'.

Valuing the spiritual aspects of life and having a sense of purpose are important elements in maintaining quality of life and remaining actively involved in life. And, most importantly, the brain needs to be stimulated frequently and regularly. Research has indicated that achieving higher educational levels and/or working in stimulating occupations can act as a buffer to the onset of dementia later in life (Ott et al 1995; Plassman et al 1995). Remaining curious and continuing with intellectually challenging activities are the most desirable approaches in keeping the brain stimulated. The notion of lifelong learning takes on great significance in the context of dementia prevention.

Prevention of Alzheimer's disease

Despite the large volume of current knowledge regarding dementia, the causes of AD are still unknown. Several theories have been postulated: age, family history (or genetics), head trauma, metal toxicity (aluminium and other metals), but important risk factors for dementia may still be missing (Price 1997). There is still more to learn about causes and risk factors for AD, about the contribution that common chronic illnesses such as hypertension play in its development, and how to prevent or delay its onset. By identifying those persons at risk, interventions can be better targeted (Marcantonio 2000).

Snowdon's (2001) study found that those with brain infarcts had poorer cognitive function and a higher prevalence of dementia than those without infarcts. This study involved 678 members of the Sisters of Notre Dame religious congregation in seven convents across the United States, ranging in age from 75 to 106. Researchers were allowed unprecedented access to the sisters' personal and medical histories and undertook rigorous annual mental and physical testing. The focus of the research was to determine the relationship of brain infarction to the expression of AD.

Snowdon's findings suggested that cerebrovascular disease may play an important role in determining the presence and severity of the clinical symptoms of AD, and that AD is a consequence of a long chain of events spanning the life course. Early-life autobiographies from the convent archives were analysed to show a strong relationship between low linguistic ability in early life and a high risk of AD in later life. Other findings from the study suggest that late-life events, such as stroke, can increase the risk of AD and increase the severity of its symptoms. However, 'further research is needed before it is known whether the prevention of cerebrovascular disease can mute the clinical expression of AD' or prevent VaD (Snowdon 1997, p. 817).

Additionally, more research is needed in the next five to ten years to identify other possible risk factors and perhaps significantly alter our understanding of dementia (Sacco 2001; Alzheimer's Association NSW 2002). Recent research data, for example, has found an association between oral health, specifically periodontal health, and stroke (Sacco 2001). Better understanding of these factors could translate into new methods for prevention of diseases, as well as the prevention of dementia.

Primary prevention

Despite the evidence, health promotion strategies for older adults are not generally seen as a priority (Chernoff 2001). Furthermore, despite the known positive outcome of primary and secondary health promotion activities, only a small proportion of older adults actively engage in such activities (Resnick 2000; Coulson et al 2001). In the United States, despite the known benefits of exercise, at least two-thirds of older adults do not regularly exercise (Centers for Disease Control 2002). The establishment of intervention programs specifically designed to influence patient behaviours in these areas thus has the potential of favourable health outcomes in terms of VaD. Adherence to therapeutic regimes, however, requires substantial patient cooperation, knowledge and participation (Ventura 1984). This is even more important if we consider that the most commonly reported reason for not performing health promoting and disease prevention measures (diet, exercise, etc.) amongst older adults is 'not being told to' (Resnick 2000).

Modifying lifestyle practices throughout the life span can significantly ameliorate those factors leading to VaD. A reduction in the prevalence of both VaD and AD can become a reality if active ageing factors leading to reduced circulatory impairment and cerebral effusion later in life are incorporated into lifestyle practices in the general population. Research is now underway that is clearly directed at preventing VaD (Lis & Gavira 1997).

Evidenced-based research strategies to prevent stroke already exist and the available evidence shows that the potential impact may be substantial (Khaw 1997; Centers for Disease Control 2002). Of course, lifestyle changes are most effective when adopted early in life, but positive effects can occur at any age (Chernoff 2001). Putting preventive measures to work to ensure the continuous good health of younger and older adult populations is a major challenge to public health around the world; the prevention of VaD is the major epidemiological challenge for this century amongst public health authorities.

Secondary prevention

With dementia, as for many other chronic conditions and diseases, most current policies concentrate on secondary prevention, on strategies used to identify, treat or cure disease in the early stages or to prevent its progression (Chernoff 2001). Once diagnosed, dementia cannot be cured or reversed. Early and accurate identification of persons with very mild and mild dementia is crucial for its prognosis and to promoting quality of life for as long as possible

(Kragh-Sorensen et al 2000). Promising leads to pharmacological treatment have been developed that may slow the progression of dementia, in particular for VaD (Kragh-Sorensen et al 2000; Marcantonio 2000). Hence, 'researchers are [also] beginning to consider AD as a treatable condition' (Lovestone 2000, p. 37).

Graycar (1986, p. 8) stresses that 'in giving more time to live, science and medicine have also given more time to die'. This is particularly the case with dementia. Dementia robs the person of their individuality and autonomy, yet leaves the physical body intact, frequently condemning the person and their family to prolonged affliction. Despite this, a supportive environment has been described as a major key to the management of persons with dementia (Marcantonio 2000). This is best achieved when a person is surrounded by familiar environments, such as their home, and maintains their daily routines and regular social and physical activities (Marcantonio 2000; Alzheimer's Association NSW 2002). However, retaining a person's familiar environment has social and economic implications, for example, a caregiver requires support systems and the provision of information about how to manage different aspects of the disease process within this environment. The role of Alzheimer's societies around the world is to provide guidance and information to families about the disease and to promote quality of life for the person with dementia through research and education.

What are the future challenges?

Dementia in old age is a challenge that cannot be addressed by the public or private sectors in isolation: it requires joint approaches and strategies (WHO 2002). A worldwide movement based upon alliances between scientists, governments, caregivers and health care professionals has transformed the approach to dementia to achieve advancements in a more positive societal attitude, prevention, treatment and rehabilitation in western societies (Mayeux 1993). On the other hand, Henderson and Jorm (2000) have established that data and risk factors for dementia in less developed countries are greatly lacking. Mechanisms need to be established to ensure effective ongoing research and evaluation of proposed models of intervention for developed and developing countries. Developing methods to identify primary prevention strategies and interventions contributes to improved treatment outcomes, better health and quality of life for older adults, in addition to saving millions of dollars in medical costs.

Challenges in the prevention and treatment of dementia will continue to be demanding for researchers and society as a whole. While the prevention of dementia has now become a priority for researchers, there is still a need for society to understand its social meaning so that victims are not marginalised. Challenges in understanding the social meaning of dementia and in developing primary and secondary interventions to reduce its escalating costs to governments and families are equally important. A loved one with dementia places an emotional and economic strain on families, sometimes not taken into consideration by governments and health care agencies. The emotional cost, especially, is difficult to measure in terms of dollars, and needs urgently to be considered by health care professionals and governments.

There is a growing consensus that we can afford to grow old gracefully if governments implement policies that prevent or delay the onset of disabilities and chronic illness for as long as possible, and help older people to remain independent and economically active as they age (WHO 2002).

'Active ageing is the process of optimising opportunities for health, participation and security, in order to enhance quality of life as people age' (WHO 2002, p. 12). Active ageing allows people to realise the potential for physical, social and mental well-being throughout their life span. Active refers to continuing participation in social, economic, cultural, spiritual and civic affairs, not just being physically active or participating in the workforce (WHO 2002). Active ageing strategies can reduce the incidence of chronic illnesses like VaD.

As the topic of dementia prevention gains prominence certain ethical and practice issues must be considered. Particularly, inequities relative to healthy ageing need to be addressed. We are increasingly becoming aware that inequities experienced throughout the life span critically influence health and well-being in old age (WHO 2002). As the ageing population balloons it is vital that the promotion of healthy ageing, including the prevention of dementias, becomes a key building block in the policies guiding resource distribution. Healthy older adults require fewer resources to maintain their independence. Poverty within all age groups, therefore, must be recognised as a major ethical and practical dilemma requiring intense clinical and research attention.

Although society has always recognised the economic value of education and employment, we are only now beginning to realise the contributions education and employment make to maintaining health and cognitive functioning later in life. Policies creating greater equity in resource distribution amongst all ages must thus be encouraged. As we increasingly realise the ameliorating influence of lifelong learning on dementia, there must be an emphasis at the policy level supporting learning opportunities that include seniors.

Finally, preventive lifestyle practices that can influence the prevention of dementia significantly must be proclaimed to all age groups. In their study of 282 Canadians, 55 years of age and older, Coulson et al (2004) found that although the seniors in their study had a wealth of knowledge about lifestyle behaviours that prevent VaD, they did not necessarily practise them. Strategies going beyond simple education about dementia prevention must be developed to include the encouragement and fostering of healthy lifestyle practices throughout the life span if future health care costs are to be moderated.

Improving healthy lifestyles for older people

Older people have the potential for wellness and health care professionals can help them recognise and achieve healthy lifestyles. Frances, 71, and Sam, 81, have been married for more than 50 years and have twin daughters, both of whom take an active role in their parents' lives. Sam is very determined and active despite having had several seizures and having high bloodpressure. He still drives his car legally. Frances is also very busy in the community and has a strong faith in God.

Sam and Frances recently became concerned that the number of older people over the age of 65 years in their district has grown significantly. Sam and Frances are active themselves, but they frequently comment that too many older people in their neighbourhood have nothing to do.

Sometimes they see an ambulance coming to the rescue of an older person in their neighbourhood. Several of their friends in the neighbourhood, and Sam himself, have high blood pressure. Frances has commented that some of their friends now have vascular dementia.

At a recent community meeting for older people, which Sam and Frances organised, several problems and concerns were identified by the 100 who attended:

- they sit at home and watch too much television because there is nothing else to do;
- they have trouble getting to the grocery store to purchase food and often cannot get fresh vegetables;
- they cannot get to their family physician or other activities because of a lack of transportation in the area;
- they are lonely, but are too frightened to discuss this with their families because they do not want to be a burden to them;
- they feel 'stressed out' and do not know how to relax;
- some felt they had no more goals left to achieve in their life and wished they could just die.

Following the meeting, Sam and Frances spoke to the mayor of the city and received a grant of $50 000 to start the Calder Seniors' Club with the major goal of developing healthy lifestyles for older people.

Activity 5.1

From the above example, identify strengths, potential barriers, strategies and programs that could assist older people in developing the new Calder Seniors' Club to improve their health and well-being.

Conclusion

The prevention of dementia will continue to be a challenge in the foreseeable future. While some dementias may be preventable, others require extensive research to uncover their underlying causes. The issue of preventing or managing hypertension is an important key factor in the prevention of VaD, stroke and heart disease. High-risk lifestyle behaviours that predispose a person to developing dementia can be prevented by individual lifestyle choices and environmental factors. Wholesome lifestyle practices are fundamental to healthy ageing and have a positive influence on cognitive functioning regardless of underlying pathologies.

Another important area that has recently been found to have implications for VaD is the likely use of thrombolytic drugs in the treatment of acute stroke. This may be a double-edged sword. 'Theoretically these will limit brain damage sustained during the stroke, but they may also increase the total number of patients surviving who would otherwise have died without this treatment, perhaps leaving more patients with considerable cognitive impairment' and VaD (Amar & Wilcock 1996, p. 231).

While individuals can change their lifestyle practices to promote healthy lifestyles that prevent VaD, some will continue to make choices that promote illness. Overall, however, people in developed countries have an increased life expectancy. Governments and researchers need to focus on strategies and programs that will enable today's middle-aged cohorts to choose healthy lifestyle behaviours that will lead to their growing old gracefully and fulfilling the definition of active ageing.

6

Work and retirement later in life: Is retirement a relevant concept for the 21st century?

Linda Rosenman

Retirement, the permanent withdrawal from the labour force, and the change in role from 'worker' to 'retiree', has become the passage into, and definitive characteristic of, old age. An expected, and often required, age of retirement has usually been synonymous with the age at which full pension eligibility has been set by the state. This has become the final age by which workers are expected to quit the workforce and as such has become the symbolic age marker of old age.

Retirement has usually been considered as an ageing issue—but, like most ageing issues, retirement is a socially constructed phenomenon. The decision to retire from the workforce is a product of many factors including labour force and employment policies, employer and societal expectations, individual health, social situations, attitudes and expectations, and public policies, particularly those determining pension and welfare programs.

This chapter reviews the social policy, economic and individual issues that shape, and are influenced by, the retirement decisions of millions of individual workers. Similar patterns and trends are apparent in most developed societies, including the major English-speaking countries. Finally, it reviews the issues regarding the future directions of policy since demographic change, and particularly population ageing, is challenging the economic and social viability of a continuation into the 21st century of retirement patterns and expectations established at the end of the 20th century.

The emergence of retirement as a significant life stage

Physical capacity has always been necessary for production, and in earlier societies alternative roles, food and shelter were provided by families and tribes for older people who could not provide labour due to frailty or poor health. Later, however, in many societies the inability to work due to physical incapacity or frailty risked poverty and reliance on charity, often in poorhouses, unless families could provide accommodation, care and support, or a person had been able to make private arrangements that ensured an income regardless of labour force status.

The modern concept of retirement, that is, withdrawal from the workforce at a fixed age, and eligibility for an alternative form of income, appears to date from seventeenth century Europe. In a review of the history of retirement, Encel (1996, p. 7) points out that the diarist Samuel Pepys wrote in 1667 that he:

> would like to retire from his government job and live on his pension. One of Pepys' contemporaries, Daniel Defoe . . . was a very early proponent of the right to retire at a specified age and to be entitled to a pension. He chose 50 as the age [by which people should retire]. The age, 50, was also chosen by another British M.P. . . . who introduced a motion in 1772 calling for pensions to be granted to all old persons who had lived frugal and industrious lives.

> . . . Bureaucratisation of the governmental system . . . provided a model for a new version of the life cycle, based not on biology but on workforce participation, superimposed on the traditional succession of youth, maturity and old age. This linkage soon spread to other sections of the population, especially with the growth of an industrial proletariat which demanded that society should take responsibility for welfare in old age' (Encel 1996, p. 7).

The bureaucratisation of state systems in the nineteenth century led to the bureaucratisation of pensions to support state employees in old age. Concern about poverty amongst the aged generally led to the introduction of state-managed social security for old age in the latter part of the nineteenth century throughout Europe. Australia followed, introducing a national age pension in 1908. In the United States, a national age pension was not introduced until the *Social Security Act* was passed in 1936.

Retirement or age pension programs established in different nations varied in terms of their structure (social insurance or social assistance) and their underlying rationales. They had in common an age at which (male) workers were entitled to apply for a pension, usually 65 or 70. This was high enough to ensure that the majority of workers would die either before, or soon after reaching it and so would be placing very limited, if any, demands on the financial resources of the state. This meant that any period of 'retirement' between leaving income-generating employment and death was relatively brief for the majority of retirees.

The period following World War II shaped the attitudes and expectations of the current generations of mid-life and older people in most developed countries, an era characterised by stable lifelong employment during which industries became highly unionised, with the unions negotiating working hours and the duration of working lives. This included a rigid age categorisation of labour force entry through legislation for minimum ages for employment and wages, and maximum ages for labour force exit. Labour force exit, and a compulsory retirement age, were enshrined in employment contracts. Male employment in heavy industry and manufacturing required physical endurance. The right to retire early recognised the reality of decreasing capacity for heavy physical labour as people aged.

Increasing longevity and improvements in health lengthened the period between the age of pension eligibility and death and led to the emergence of the concept of retirement as a life stage rather than an employment decision. Retirement became identified as a period of leisure that separated paid work from decline and death. In the late 20th century, as longevity increased and retirement ages decreased, the concept of a 'third age' was developed (Moynagh & Worsley 2001). This was conceptualised as a time of active leisure and social re-engagement that commenced with retirement from income-generating employment and for some, but not all, merged into a 'fourth age' of social disengagement, decline in health and activity and the need for care. The parameters of the third age were not bounded by chronological age but rather by work and family life stage and health.

Retirement in western capitalist societies is now being recast to mean more than the point at which a person withdraws from 'an occupation or business to enjoy more leisure'. It is now a life stage and a 'life style', characterised theoretically by unlimited leisure as a result of freedom from the need to earn a living and the reduction in child-rearing responsibilities. The vision of retirement as a lifestyle stage is now an economic and marketing opportunity embraced by a wide range of industries and services, including the finance, housing, travel and entertainment industries. Research and colloquial use still indicates that for many 'retirement' is used synonymously with 'old age', and as such remains an event and a term with negative connotations.

Nevertheless, retirement remains foremost a decision about labour supply and the generation of income through sources other than full-time work. Retirement decisions exist at the intersection of employment and workforce decisions, income security and retirement incomes policies, and personal and family situations.

Labour force, employment policies and retirement decisions

During the last 25 years of the 20th century most economically developed countries experienced even earlier ages of 'retirement' for men. Using Australia as an example, this shift was particularly marked during the decade 1973–82 and interacted with major economic structural changes. Women, whose labour force attachment had been widely viewed as subsidiary to family responsibilities, tended to retire much earlier, often timing permanent withdrawal from the labour force around child bearing and family responsibilities or, if they were employed in later life, around the retirement plans of their (generally older) partners.

Measuring changes in retirement ages is a challenge due to lack of agreement on definitions of retirement. For this reason labour force participation is the most useful indicator. As an example, using figures collected by the Australian Bureau of Statistics for 1968–2001, with those aged over 45 who are neither employed nor looking for employment being assumed to have 'retired', Figures 6.1 and 6.2 show that the age of labour force withdrawal and the proportion of men aged over 45 in employment has been trending downwards over the past 25 years, and that the incidence of non-employment

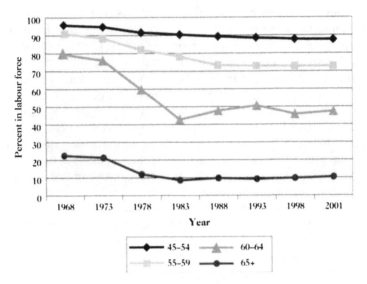

Figure 6.1: Older men: Labour force participation over time by age cohort (Australia)

Source: Australian Bureau of Statistics, *The Labour Force Australia 1987; Historical Summary 1966 to 1984; 1989:24; 1994:19; 2002b:22*

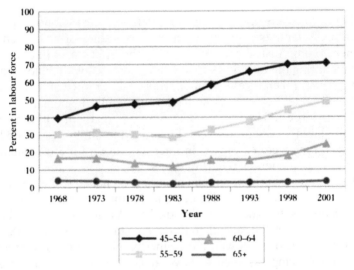

Figure 6.2: Older women: Labour force participation over time by age cohort (Australia)

Source: Australian Bureau of Statistics, *The Labour Force Australia 1987; Historical Summary 1966 to 1984; 1989:24; 1994:19; 2002b:22*

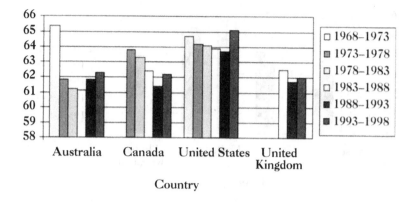

Figure 6.3: Males: Average age of labour force withdrawal

Source: Scherer (2002), *Age of Withdrawal from the Labour Force in OECD Countries*

increases markedly with age. While these trends apply to males who have traditionally remained in full-time employment up until retirement age, women have been showing a slight increase in labour force participation but from a much lower base (see Figure 6.2), and much of this has also been in part-time rather than full-time employment. The general pattern in the United States and Canada, where age discrimination legislation has been enforced for well over a decade, is for the age of withdrawal from the labour force for men to have stabilised, but is now trending back upwards.

Figure 6.3 and Figure 6.4 shows the average age of withdrawal from the labour force over five-year time ranges for men and women in Australia, Canada, the United States and the United Kingdom. This indicates that, while the size of the changes varied across countries, the average age declined for men during the 1970s but subsequently stabilised and began to trend upwards in the late 1990s. Amongst women the patterns are similar but the changes have not been quite so marked. There is also quite a lot of consistency within each country between men and women. Average age of withdrawal is higher for both men and women in the United States and in Canada than in either Australia or the United Kingdom.

These data do not indicate whether or not labour force withdrawal is permanent or voluntary. A considerable amount of 'retirement' is not voluntary. Late-life unemployment and early retirement in

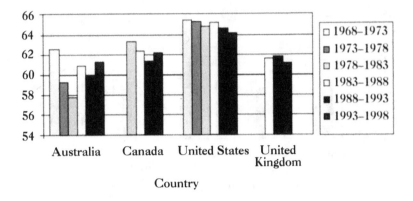

Figure 6.4: Females: Average age of labour force withdrawal

Source: Scherer (2002), *Age of Withdrawal from the Labour Force in OECD Countries*

the developed countries are partly attributable to economic changes which have led to declining work opportunities over the past few decades and which have tended to affect older workers disproportionately. In addition, older workers are influenced by social pressures which encourage them to retire with the expectation that they will make way for younger people.

Over the last 25 years of the 20th century there was a decline in the 'old economy', particularly in the manufacturing and agricultural industries, and a reduction in the size of core public sector employment as part of a move to privatise government operations. The changes led to constant restructuring of the workforce in many industries. Economic cycles and technological change are neither new nor unusual, but a characteristic of this period was the targeting of older and longer serving workers who were offered financial incentives to take early retirement rather than be retrenched. Older men, who were more likely to be working in manufacturing industries, were particularly affected.

Once unemployed, older workers, particularly those with lower levels of education, minorities and migrants from non-English speaking backgrounds and those in non urban areas, were particularly likely to have difficulty in finding new employment (Bittman et al 2001). In response, by the 1990s most countries had expanded access to unemployment benefits and disability pension schemes for older unemployed workers. In Australia, for example, the eligibility criteria for unemployment benefits were relaxed for older people through the introduction of a 'Mature Age Allowance', which limited reporting and job search requirements and expectations regarding re-training, for the unemployed aged over 55. This recognised the economic need and the difficulty of the older, long-term unemployed in finding employment. In the United Kingdom, a special early retirement program allowed a pension for older job leavers if the employer replaced them with an unemployed person. Using disability and unemployment schemes as early retirement programs both reflected and contributed to shifting the acceptable age of labour force exit downwards from 65. In Canada applications for disability benefits under the Canada Pension Plan increased by 78 per cent in the five years from 1988 to 1993.

A large shift to early retirement occurred in the decade between the early 1970s and early 1980s. During that period changes were made to pensions to improve access and benefits for retrenched workers. These changes were seen by some as discriminatory against older workers as they effectively promoted early retirement. Furthermore, the generational shift related to the entry of the World War II veterans (mostly male) into the younger age of eligibility for veterans' benefits meant a downward shift in pension age. In Australia, for example, the availability of the Veterans Pension at age 60 contributed to the dramatic reduction in labour force participation by men aged 60–65 during the mid-1970s.

Older workers are also often the first targeted in attempts to restructure organisations to reduce costs. The reasons for this are multiple. They relate not only to the assumed lower productivity relative to wages of older, more experienced and therefore more highly paid workers, but also to the assumption that they have access to, or are eligible to receive alternative sources of income, namely a state or private pension, or an unemployment benefit. It is also often assumed that their economic needs are less because within chronological and life cycle frameworks they are less likely than younger workers to have dependent children.

Perhaps as important is a quite well-documented systematic discrimination against older workers. This appears to be related to beliefs regarding lower productivity due to assumed lack of adaptability, limited capacity to learn new tasks and new technologies, and blocking the career prospects of the next generation of workers.

Despite numerous studies which show that these beliefs are unfounded and that older workers are as productive, energetic and adaptable as younger workers, evidence persists that workers who lose jobs after the age of 45 find major difficulty in obtaining new employment due to employer preference for young workers (Australian House of Representatives 2000).

Employers also target workers from the age of 55 onwards for early retirement incentives and offers to encourage them out of the workforce, since early retirement is assumed to be less painful than retrenchment. Many older workers are willing to accept financial incentives to retire early since this may accord with their longer term plans, provide the finance to make an employment or lifestyle change, or they wish to go before they are 'pushed'. Nevertheless these contribute to the widespread assumption that older workers are expendable and that beyond the age of 50 their labour force participation is voluntary and their employment optional.

In most developed countries this labour market restructuring slowed down by the mid-1990s and economic growth led to labour shortages, particularly in the growth areas of the new economy—services, finance and information, and communication technology. The 'success' of labour force clearing through early retirement began to be viewed as a policy problem with the recognition of the economic cost of early retirement in terms of high levels of government transfers.

As medical and health improvements are causing significant increases in longevity, concern is now being expressed about the fiscal and social impacts of the potential 20–30 years that people could be spending out of the labour force (Centre for Public Policy 2002). Concomitantly, demographers are raising the possibility of future labour force shortages and the need to delay rather than encourage labour force exit in the future (OECD 2002).

A not inconsiderable body of research into retirement decisions indicates that the decision to leave employment permanently is neither a simple response to economic and social policies, nor is it necessarily a decision to never work again. Quinn et al (1991) document the extent to which retirement decisions have changed in the United States, with 'retirement', at best, meaning leaving a full-time career position for a more flexible level of control over working hours and kinds of work. This includes part-time, casual and contract work.

Table 6.1: Employment status of older Australian workers, 2001

Age/Sex	Full-time	Part-time
Females		
55–59	50.5%	49.5%
60–64	40.9%	59.1%
65+	35.1%	65.1%
Males		
55–59	87.5%	12.5%
60–64	80.5%	19.5%
65+	55%	45%

Source: Australian Institute of Health and Welfare 2002

One of the options to extend working ages and limit early workforce withdrawal is to offer older workers the option of phased retirement, or the ability to reduce from full-time to part-time employment over an extended period prior to complete workforce withdrawal. A characteristic of the Australian economy has been a significant and sustained increase in the rate of part-time employment relative to full-time employment (see Table 6.1). This has been marked amongst all age groups, and includes older workers, particularly older men. Part-time employment at older ages may be an example of phased retirement. Alternatively, it may reflect the difficulty that older people experience in obtaining and retaining full-time continuing employment.

The shift to part-time work later in life is similarly marked in Canada, the United Kingdom and the United States. Amongst men aged 60–64, 15.4 per cent in Canada were part-time workers, a 2.1 per cent increase over the five years 1993–1998, in the United Kingdom 18.5 per cent were working part-time, a 4.1% increase, and in the United States 16.1 per cent, a 0.8 per cent increase over the same period.

To a senior and experienced worker the transition to part-time work can mean a significant drop in status and responsibility. Changing to part-time employment can mean that a worker is viewed as neither serious about their career nor core to the workforce. Furthermore, defined benefit superannuation schemes, which link the retirement benefit to the final years of earnings, are a significant disincentive to people to reduce hours or position if it means a salary reduction. In terms of psychological and financial well-being in retirement it is not surprising that many older workers decide against phased retirement options, even where they could be negotiated with an employer.

Public policies and retirement

The major public policies that directly influence retirement decisions are those relating to income security in older age. The decision to retire from paid work is largely an economic decision about the capacity to live at an acceptable standard on income sources other than employment income. These other sources are predominantly state pensions (government-funded social security) and private pensions (savings through employment-linked superannuation).

Activity 6.1

Identify governmental and employer work-related policies that influence older workers to leave the labour force. What changes would be required to encourage people to continue working?

Retirement incomes policies and retirement decisions

The term 'retirement' is used interchangeably to describe two transitions. The first is the transition in labour force status and the second the shift in income source—from employment-derived to pension-derived income. It is possible for a person to retire but not to draw income from government benefits and in some countries (particularly the United States) it is also possible for the reverse to happen. Nevertheless, fiscal and social policies, especially retirement incomes policies, play a major role in establishing individual and community expectations about whether, when and how people should retire. The United States, United Kingdom, Australia and Canada each have multi-pillar retirement incomes programs, usually comprising a government pension as the first pillar and a tax-subsidised retirement savings program as the second. The third pillar is often employment linked and may or may not be available to everyone. The rate at which employment income is replaced by retirement benefits, and the eligibility criteria for these programs, strongly influence individual worker and employer decisions relating to retirement.

The age of eligibility for the government age pension has been important in setting the upper age by which employers and society expect that people should exit the workforce. In Australia, the age at which people can begin to draw the government pension is 65 for men, and over a 25-year period is increasing for women from the age of 60 to equal that of men by 2016, while in the United Kingdom it will equalise to age 65 over a ten-year period by 2020. In Canada the age is 65 and in the United States it is 67.

The OECD has pointed out that while eligibility ages for national pension schemes are now increasing:

> there are other pathways to withdraw from the labour market at a relatively early age, in particular by using special early retirement schemes, unemployment-related transfer schemes, disability pensions and occupational pensions. While some of these schemes have also been tightened more recently, they still provide important fiscal incentives to retire before the statutory retirement age (OECD 2000, p. 3).

Using Australia as an example, there are a number of other government pensions which have lower eligibility ages than the Age Pension, including schemes which allow people to claim pensions or pension equivalent payments earlier than normal pensionable age. They include the Mature Age Allowance for older unemployed people (over 55), the Veterans Pension which is available at the age of 60 to veterans who have served in the defence forces, and to their spouse after the veteran's death. As concern has grown about the shift to early retirement and the role of government benefits in encouraging older people to leave the workforce early, governments around the world have begun to tighten eligibility ages and criteria for benefits. Unemployment benefits for older unemployed workers and disability pensions have been subject to scrutiny and eligibility criteria tightened. Veterans Pensions are usually maintained but they have become less important as the vast majority of veterans from World War II are now in advanced old age. In the United States it is possible for people to draw an actuarially reduced pension on their Social Security account from the age of 62.

Personal/employer retirement decisions

Saving for retirement through government-mandated, subsidised or tax-advantaged pension/superannuation schemes exists in the United States, United Kingdom, Australia and Canada. Australia was the last to add a private pension pillar with the federal government legislating in 1993 to introduce the Superannuation Guarantee which established a national program for retirement savings. Unlike social insurance programs in the United States, this is not government managed. Government regulations and taxation regimes play an important part in setting the parameters that determine individual and employer plans and expectations about retirement. The minimum age at which people can access their pensions under normal circumstances was set at 55 in Australia but at 60 in Canada. This appears to be the lower limit to expectations regarding a suitable or appropriate retirement age. While reflecting the trend to early retirement such an age provision has the potential to further define retirement age downward. The Australian government has now introduced a phased process by which the age at which superannuation benefits can be claimed will increase from 55 to 60 years by 2025.

Reflecting the recency of introducing employment related pensions, the vast majority of Australians who are age eligible are pension recipients. Overall in 2001, 85 per cent of the age group 65 and over received at least a part pension (Age or Veterans). The proportion was higher at older ages, increasing from 78 per cent amongst those aged 65–74 to 93 per cent among those aged 85 and over. There has been a decline in the extent of dependence upon the Age Pension as the major source of retirement income.

Between 1986 and 1996 the proportion of men aged over 65 whose primary income source was a government benefit fell from 75 per cent to 64.5 per cent, and for women from 73 per cent to 58 per cent. Only 8 per cent reported receiving their main income from superannuation, while 11 per cent reported investment and savings income, and 5 per cent reported employment income, as their main income source (AIHW 2002). In Canada, 10 per cent of the income of men and 2 per cent of that of women aged 65–74 came from work, in comparison with 5 per cent and 1 per cent in the United Kingdom, and 25 per cent and 5 per cent in the United States. Women in all countries were much more likely to have a significant proportion of their income derived from the state pension, and a smaller proportion of their income from employment or from private pensions, than were men (OECD 2002).

The low percentage of people nominating private pensions as their primary income source reflects the relative recency of the introduction of government incentives to encourage or mandate private saving for retirement. It is estimated to take at least 30 years of accumulation for a private pension scheme to mature to the point where it can constitute a major source of retirement income for the majority of older people (Tinnion & Rothman 1999). Nevertheless, the composition of retirement income is changing, with more recent retirees reporting mixtures of superannuation, investment income (including from the investment of superannuation lump sums), together with a part pension.

Planning for income in retirement and managing multiple income sources for, and in, retirement is a growing challenge for older people. Dealing with the complexity of tax, pension and superannuation regulations, and the variability of investment returns, requires a level of financial sophistication that many people do not possess. Research that has been carried out on retirement income expectations suggest that the upcoming generation of people aged over 65 (those currently in their 50s) are likely to have lower expectations regarding both the availability of, and their entitlement to, a government pension in retirement. They also report concern about how they will manage financially in retirement and confusion about the growing complexity of retirement incomes planning (Rix et al 1999; UK Government 2002).

In response to growing concerns in many countries regarding the role played by social security programs in encouraging ever earlier ages of retirement, the OECD began urging its member countries to adopt fiscal and labour market policies that would reverse the trend. A key strategy was to implement the necessary changes to pension policies in order to begin to change both expectations and behaviour about early retirement before the baby-boomer generation enters the ages of early retirement in the early years of the 21st century. The purposes of these policies are to slow and reverse the trends to early retirement by removing the incentives in public policies that encouraged early retirement and, where possible, to encourage continued economic activity in later life (OECD 2002).

A limited number of policy changes have been introduced to encourage people to extend rather than further shorten their working lives. Australia, the United Kingdom and the United States now encourage later drawing of the state pension by allowing a lifetime higher pension to those who delay drawing the pension for a number of years beyond the normal pension age. In most countries it is also permissible to draw at least some pension benefits while continuing to be employed.

There has also been a concerted effort to remove the special treatment for older women under social security programs that had its origins in the social convention of the nineteenth and early to mid-20th centuries that married women should not be in paid employment, particularly in a prosperous society. These provisions included a lower age of eligibility for the Age Pension for women (60) than for men (65), a Wife Pension for the non-aged wife of an Age Pensioner, and a Widows Pension for women whose marriage ended before they were eligible by age for the age pension. These are now being phased out to equalise treatment between men and women in the pension system, although there has been no concomitant attempt to equalise wages and labour force entitlements. Women's earnings remain generally well below those of men, worldwide.

The major area in which change is needed is in the expectation and the encouragement for older people to be able to continue working beyond traditional retirement ages. This requires changes not only to individual worker expectations and plans but also to the attitudes of employers and of society.

Age discrimination policy and retirement decisions

During the 1980s and 1990s legislation against discrimination on the basis of age was passed in many countries, including Australia and the United States, and the United Kingdom is making compulsory retirement ages illegal by 2006. Under the Human Rights Code, Canada prohibits discrimination on the basis of age. Four provinces, however, define age for employment purposes to include only those under the age of 65.

In most cases such legislation has been introduced well after comparable legislation against gender and racial discrimination. Age discrimination legislation has usually been based on research that documented the systemic and widespread discrimination relating to age, one of the most pervasive being a retirement age specified in employment contracts. Research subsequent to the enactment of the laws has tended to indicate that while compliance with overt discrimination, for example, through removal of age of retirement clauses from new employment contracts, has occurred, covert discrimination against older people continues (Sidoti 1997; Australian Human Rights and Equal Opportunity Commission 2000; Gringart & Helmes 2001). This discrimination includes targeting or pressuring older workers to take early retirement, explicit expectations that retirement would occur at a certain age, a refusal to hire people once they are older than 50, and unwillingness to invest in education or training of older workers on the assumption that they will not work long enough for an employer to recoup the training costs.

It seems likely that it will take a long time for attitudinal and behavioural changes to take place regarding the entitlement of older workers to remain in the workforce, or to retire in a mode and at a time of their choosing. Age discrimination is pervasive and widely accepted in society. Expectations and plans about a reasonable point at which people should and can retire are often longstanding, and may take a generation or more to change.

Individual and social factors in retirement decisions

Retirement decisions are effectively labour supply decisions made by individuals within the context of economic and social policies, financial conditions and social expectations. Trends in later life employment and retirement are the result of the individual decisions of thousands of older people. Personal and family factors play a significant, if not a determinative part in retirement decisions as shown by research from a number of countries such as Australia, Canada, the United States and the United Kingdom.

For example, research on retirement decisions of a sample of 640 Australians aged over 50 (Rosenman & Warburton 1997) revealed that retirement timing decisions are complex decisions made within the context of individual family and employment situations, as well as societal expectations concerning both work and retirement. Those who were able to exercise choice and flexibility in their work in later life found it difficult to nominate an age of retirement as they had the potential to continue working beyond any traditional retirement ages, or to cease working at a time of their choosing. The key factor is having the option to modify working hours and responsibilities (for example, seeing only certain kinds of clients) to meet their personal preferences. People who have this capacity were more likely to be self-employed and in professional occupations. Workers employed on a casual or contract basis can also make decisions to vary their labour supply by not seeking or taking further employment. Those who worked part time or casually were more likely to anticipate a later retirement or did not know when they would retire.

Amongst the majority of older Australians their work is part of their identity and thus retirement was seen as a change or loss of identity and associated with lower self-esteem. Other negative perceptions of retirement also caused workers to put off retirement decisions, in particular, its association with old age and death. Some of the younger respondents did not wish to nominate a retirement age as they felt that to do so would identify them as 'old people'. Responses to questions relating to attitudes towards retirement revealed that many of those who did not know when they would retire viewed retirement as a significant phase in their lives in which they anticipated great change. Anxiety about this change and uncertainty about retirement timing was correlated with negativity about retirement. Only 26 per cent of those who could not nominate a retirement age expressed any positive view about retirement, compared with 54 per cent of those who were able to nominate when they would retire. The correlation between negativity about retirement and inability to nominate an age of retirement suggests that many people actually put off making retirement decisions because they fear retirement.

Many acknowledged the association of work with self-identity, which tended to result in viewing retirement as involving a loss of identity and as becoming non-productive. Comments encapsulating this include: 'I looked at others that had given up and realised the hopelessness of not having productive work. I want to carry on ad infinitum.'

The association of retirement with ill health and death was a very real fear for many respondents. As one person told the research team: 'The more you work the younger you feel. The thought of leaving work is like waiting around to die.'

Many said that they did not look forward to retirement as it defined them as entering old age. This was indicated by responses such as: 'I associate retirement with ageing and being unhealthy' and 'It means life is nearly over'.

Such negative images and attitudes to retirement help to explain indecision towards retirement, as for many it is an unwelcome change.

Workers with flexibility and choice about the timing and process of retirement decided to work longer and many preferred to phase into retirement rather than ceasing work completely. Not all workers have the option of working reduced hours with their current employer, or working at a less physically or mentally demanding occupation. Others are induced to retire because the interaction of the Age Pension and superannuation income, and the tax treatment of these combined benefits, can mean a higher income than that earned through heavily taxed employment. Taxation of employment income and the benefit reduction rate on the Age Pension made remaining at work economically unattractive for the majority of low and middle income workers. Resolution of some of these financial barriers to late life employment would allow more workers the option to continue working.

Amongst those who had retired the reasons for leaving the workforce when they did were varied, but it is notable that personal reasons were significant for both women and men, particularly the desire to have more time for themselves and for interests other than work.

The evidence from countries such as the United States, where age discrimination legislation precluding compulsory retirement ages has been in effect for several decades, is that retirement before the age of 65 continues to be common but that both men and women are extending the age of labour force withdrawal. Arguably, however, changes to Social Security that have increased the age at which full benefits can be claimed (to the age of 67) are at least as important in labour force withdrawal decisions as the effects of attitude change due to age discrimination legislation.

Once retired, most people enjoy the flexibility in the use of their time, the time to follow up on interests, to re-establish social and family contacts and the freedom from the routine of going to work. Successful adjustment to retirement is related to planning for retirement, both financially and in terms of being able to establish new interests and a new identity that is not defined by work. Satis-faction with retirement is also correlated with perceptions of having enough money and with good health.

Women's retirement decisions

Almost all of the research on retirement in western societies has focused on men, and has used definitions of retirement that exclude women's employment. This may have been explicable in the past due to the limited labour force participation of older women, but women make up the majority of the older population and are now significant labour force participants. Women's work and retirement decisions are an important component of labour force and retirement incomes policy and planning.

Labour force participation amongst older women has been increasing steadily, although the modal age at retirement for women has remained below that of men. Data on women's retirement need to be treated with some caution, however, for the definition of retirement on which data collections have been based has excluded part-time work (retirement can only be from full-time work). Yet the majority of older women who work do so on a part-time basis (see Table 6.2, p. 124). The extent of part-time work has been increasing over time, particularly amongst women. If full-time and part-time employment are taken into consideration, female labour force participation rates are increasing in all older age cohorts compared with a generally decreasing rate of labour force partici-pation by men.

Research on women's retirement confirms high rates of early retirement amongst most women (Rosenman et al 1996). The majority of older women describe themselves as having retired before the age of 60. In comparison with those who retired at or after age 60, those who retired early:

- had been working in less skilled occupations;
- had lower incomes;
- had been working full time rather than part time;
- were more likely to be married with an employed partner;
- were more likely to be from a non-English speaking back-ground; and
- were less well educated.

Those who worked part time retired later than those who worked full time. Multiple regressions predicting the age of retirement confirmed that family reasons and, specifically, having an employed partner were the best predictors of a woman's decision about retirement age. In general, women who did not have a partner, and those whose partner was not working, were more likely to retire later. A further important predictor of retirement age for women was their socio-economic status as measured by occupation and income. Women in professional occupations and those on higher incomes ended to retire later (Rosenman 1996).

The reasons given for deciding to retire also differed. The main reason given amongst those who retired before 60 was their own health, whereas the modal response for those who retired after 60 was that they reached compulsory retirement age. The second most frequent reason amongst both early and regular retirees was that their partner had decided to retire, which determined their retirement timing. Health, although not proving a good predictor of retirement timing, was one of the most frequently given reasons for retirement reported by all respondents. Being in poor health affects the decision to retire, not the actual age of retirement.

In summary, women who delayed retirement until 60 or older were those with better and presumably more satisfying jobs, and women who were unmarried and presumably needed to work to survive and to save for retirement. Those who worked part time retired later. There are two possible reasons for this: one is that part-time workers have 'more time for themselves' (the reason often given for retiring), as well as possibly not being subject to compulsory retirement. Some part-time workers had also given up full-time for part-time work later in life. Insofar as women are entering more professional and managerial occupations, are becoming better educated and are increasingly likely to be in part-time employment, it is likely that the move towards later retirement will continue amongst women.

There are two other major issues to be canvassed in relationship to women's retirement decisions. First, is the extent to which their retirement decisions are made in a family context, particularly taking into account the retirement decisions of their partners. Although only 16 per cent gave their partner's retirement as the major factor in their own retirement timing decision, amongst those who were married, 29 per cent had retired at the same time as their partners. Of those who retired before the age of 60, more than half reported that their husbands were still in paid employment or had retired after they had. Having an income-earning husband was a major factor in their ability to retire early.

Amongst certain groups, particularly those on lower incomes, pension availability was the other major factor in the decision to retire. In addition to reaching pensionable age themselves, some women retire from paid employment in order to ensure that their husband can establish eligibility for the Age Pension. For women with low paying and often tiring and unpleasant jobs, the need for their husbands to establish pension eligibility can substantially influence their decision on when to retire.

Activity 6.2

Identify policies in relationship to state pensions and private pensions that influence people's decisions about retirement. What changes need to be made to encourage people to work longer? How feasible is it to make such changes? What pressure groups would oppose and who would support change?

Retirement in the 21st century

There seems to be some evidence that the trend towards ever earlier ages of retirement for men has stabilised in most developed countries. Women's retirement ages are moving upwards and their labour force participation at older ages has increased significantly over the past decade. The reasons for very early labour force withdrawal seem to have been linked to the economic and policy environment that encouraged and rewarded early retirement amongst men.

These conditions included economic and industry restructuring that destroyed many traditional blue-collar jobs and reductions in the effective eligibility ages for pension and superannuation benefits. As importantly, however, older workers, and particularly older men's attitudes and expectations, were shaped by social expectations that older workers should retire early in order to enjoy leisure and to create opportunities for younger people. The preference for leisure rather than work increases with prosperity and the last quarter of the

20th century was a period of growing prosperity and increasing expectations for leisure. Earlier ages of retirement for women are understandable in the context of their employment and retirement decisions being made in response to their family needs and their partners' decisions to retire early, and their generally low wages which make the opportunity cost of leisure versus work much lower.

It has become clear that it is no longer viable for most developed countries to support or encourage ever earlier ages for retirement. Reports by the OECD, the World Bank and individual researchers have pointed to the economic and social implications of a continuation of the trends to early retirement observed over the last half century. In developed societies with increasing longevity, particularly a lengthening of the period of healthy old age, people will be spending a significant period of their lives in retirement. The individual and societal impacts of social disengagement caused by long periods of exclusion from the workforce are a major issue. Furthermore, delayed labour force entry due to extended formal education means that the period over which people can save for retirement is decreased significantly if they retire early. The cost to society of supporting people for up to 20 or 30 years of life in retirement through publicly funded pensions is similarly unsustainable.

The major concern is the imminent impact of the retirement of the baby-boomer generation, the demographic bulge resulting from high birth rates during the 25-year period starting in 1946 in most countries. The first members of this cohort turned 55 in 2001. In Australia, for instance, 'the population of 20 to 54 year olds will grow by 4 per cent over the next five years, the age group 55 to 64 will grow by 22 per cent. In 2002 there are 4 people over the age of 55 for every 10 aged 20 to 54; in ten years' time there will be 6 for every 10' (Centre for Public Policy 2002, p. 2).

The OECD has identified that amongst its member countries policies are now shifting in the direction of no longer discouraging employment of older workers. However:

> incentives for an early withdrawal from the labour market are still in place, particularly in continental Europe, where employment of older workers is currently relatively low. Thus, further measures are urgently needed to make pension systems neutral with respect to the age of retirement, to tighten eligibility conditions for unemployment benefits and disability pensions and to remove tax incentives for early receipt of occupational pensions . . . combined

with improving framework conditions for job creation in general and working conditions for older workers in particular. This would help to better adjust the effective retirement age to rising life expectancy and to alleviate the pressure from ageing populations on government budgets and on living standards of both younger and older generations (OECD 2001, p. 17).

The challenge for the future is not only to change policy settings, but also to change the attitudes of employers and of older people. Despite legislation against discrimination by age there is compelling evidence that sustained and systematic discrimination purely on the basis of age exists.

[S]ociety is not prepared to utilize the enormous resource of older adults. Despite the windfall of volunteers, workers, and caregivers, we are only beginning to discuss how to develop and employ this capacity for productive engagement . . . [I]t is clear that older adults face significant barriers and disincentives to their continued or renewed participation in productive roles. While they may wish or even need to engage in productive activities, they are able to do so only with great difficulty . . . [I]nstitutionalised structures of opportunity have failed to keep pace with increases in the capacity of older adults to fill productive roles (Morrow-Howell et al 2001, p. 1).

Conclusion

In a society and culture that is overwhelmingly dominated by youth and physical appearance it is a significant challenge to expect institutions and employers to value and utilise older people constructively. Attitudinal change in the rights and entitlements of older workers is potentially more difficult to achieve than legislative change alone. The demographic reality of the ageing of the baby-boomer generation will force a rethinking of the social institution of retirement, much as its members have caused change in the institutions of, and attitudes towards, education, marriage, parenting and work as they have moved through the life course.

The debate for the 21st century is not simply: 'How can people be encouraged to delay retirement?' It is rather whether or not retirement is any longer a relevant concept. As developed economies move from industrial to post-industrial models of employment, continuous and lifelong employment with a single employer or within a single industry or occupation is being replaced by concepts of multiple careers and portfolio employment. People's employability will increasingly be determined by their capacity to develop their human capital over their entire life span, and their adaptability and capacity to utilise new technologies. Potentially, employment that is rigidly age determined will become irrelevant. Greater flexibility in employment should increase the capacity of everyone to take time from employment when it best suits them in order to further their education, to travel, to parent or provide care to others. As this happens, the boundary between work and leisure at a set age that is formed by retirement should become both unnecessary and irrelevant. The challenge for policy and practice is to introduce the policy settings and the institutional shifts that will enable this to become a reality for all.

7

Housing and older people: Environments, professionals and positive ageing

Catherine Bridge, Hal Kendig

The residential environment has a major influence on older people's capacities to remain independent, to participate in the community and to maintain their sense of meaning in life. Housing and the built environment sustain and support human life, and thus directly and indirectly impact on health, social support, absence of disease, quality of life and well-being. Particularly for older people whose mobility is limited, the home environment encompasses the major activities of everyday life such as eating and preparing food, sleeping, socialising and spending time in meaningful ways.

It is essential that health and other professionals understand how environments influence the lives of older people. This is not necessarily an easy realisation given that the caring professions focus primarily on individuals' difficulties and their related treatment and care. However, in order to improve outcomes in terms of independence and well-being, it is essential to recognise that social and physical environments can play a crucial part in enabling (or disabling) positive ageing for individuals and for the society. As cited in Straton et al (2003), the World Health Organization believes that social and built environments become increasingly important for enabling functional abilities as people grow older (see Figure 7.1).

Figure 7.1 demonstrates that functional capacity has a trajectory that grows during early life, peaking in adulthood and followed by

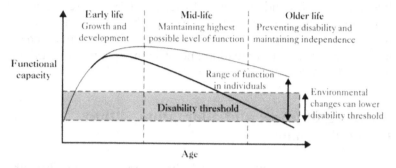

Figure 7.1: Maintaining functional capacity over the lifecourse

Source: WHO 2002, as reproduced in Straton et al (2003)

a decline. However, the rate of decline of functional ability varies between individuals the same age. An abrupt change (bottom curve) implies dramatic functional loss, while on the top curve functional losses are reduced or delayed. Variation, while based on individual physiology and genetics, remains strongly influenced by factors related to the environments in which people live. Consequently, changes in the social and built environment can enable people to remain independent despite the onset of disability. Supportive environments can also facilitate physical activity, making healthy choices easier (Straton et al 2003).

It is widely appreciated that a secure home base enables personalisation, improves life satisfaction, personal meaning and perceptions of control, while reducing stress (Bell et al 2001). The field of environmental gerontology recognises that person–environment relationships are particularly important to support older individuals in ways that minimise dependency and its adverse consequences (Browning & Kendig 2003). *The National Strategy for an Ageing Australia* (Andrews 2002) has charted policy directions for housing and residential environments that are crucial to healthy ageing and quality of life. In Canada and the United Kingdom, the environment has been identified as a primary locus for public and population health initiatives that can improve health and limit escalating health care costs (Dunn 2002; Burridge & Ormandy 1993).

This chapter is comprised of essentially five parts. In the first part, we explore older people's own views on their homes, and related issues concerning older individuals. In the second part, we examine population perspectives underlining the need for new housing strategies and initiatives. In section three, the relationship between housing and health is examined, while in section four the relationship of housing to care is discussed. Lastly, policy challenges are examined in creating and sustaining supportive urban and regional infrastructure.

Meaning of home and adaptation within the environment

In Australia, over 1 million people have reported difficulty with using public transport and steps (ABS 1998). There is an increasing trend towards this environmental vulnerability, given population ageing. As older people do not wish to be socially stigmatised or thought of as being disabled (Clemson et al 1999), they are more likely to consider behavioural changes than environmental modifications. Ageing in place—whether place be defined as formal care, community or home—may result in habituation and gradual adaptation with less awareness of potential risk. Indeed, Rowles (2000, p. 528) defines environmental habituation as the 'process of gradual, often imperceptible, environmental adjustment'. Environments can involve remarkable inventiveness being displayed as older people adjust their use of space in line with changing capacities and interests (Davison et al 1993).

Understanding and valuing people's emotional attachments to physical environments and the objects within them is critical in understanding the individuals themselves and their stance in the world. For instance, a house may be viewed as affording stability, privacy and intimacy in an otherwise hostile universe (Bachelard 1994). Remaining in place from the perspective of older persons preserves familiar and comfortable patterns, including leisure and socialisation patterns, and serves as a locus of meaning (Fogel 1992). However, environments can and do mean different things to different people, and usually evoke emotion, either positive or negative. For environmental interventions to be valued and useful for the individuals who live with them, it is important to explore what they mean to the individuals concerned and to their sense of self.

Deep attachment to home usually begins in childhood; the home can serve as a place of self-expression, a vessel of memories and a place of refuge from the outside world (Marcus 1997). Staying at home in normal housing has been found to be crucial to the sense of identity and independence of frail older people in Australia (Browning & Kendig 2003) and South Africa (Frankental 1979).

Older individuals desire to create and maintain continuity with the world but they may be restricted in their access to it, so emotional nurturance from familiar places becomes increasingly important (Hocking 1997). Failure to explore the significance of objects and home itself to the occupiers is a failure to address the personalisation of space. Personal objects evoke memories of people and places in the past and in so doing make us feel connected and rooted.

The complexities of meaning inherent in understanding housing need are highlighted by research conducted in the United States which found that the majority of older persons do not make special alterations to their homes, nor do they choose housing based on any preconditions for easier living (Filion et al 1992). They also do not spend time planning future alterations to their living environment and, given a choice, opt for living situations identical to their present ones (Wister 1989). What older persons want from their housing can be different to what is perceived as rational by government and other interests (Kendig & Gardner 1997).

Older consumers, families and health care professionals agree that appropriate accommodation can be a critical factor in the reduction of institutionalisation and in promoting integration and inclusion. Older persons consistently report that cared accommodation is a last resort and that they would prefer to live in their own house or apartment, either alone or with a partner, and not to live with others (Cooper 1996; Knapman 1996). While moves to more appropriate housing can be beneficial, re-housing to achieve higher care levels can create 'transition stress' with consequent impact on quality of life and elevated risks to mortality (Bruce 1986).

Harm reduction as a viable approach

The housing occupied by older persons, particularly those on the lowest incomes, can be relatively older and dilapidated. US data indicates that up to 8 per cent (more than 1 million older people) live in homes with serious physical defects (Kendig & Pynoos 1996). Data from the United Kingdom indicates that up to 35 per cent of private dwellings occupied by people with disabilities are unfit (Nocon 1997). Although supporting data is not available, these concerns undoubtedly apply to some proportion of older people in Australia. Quality of housing has become a major concern for enabling delivery of home-based care.

In addition, injury is most commonly associated with housing that is of poor repair or quality (Ambrose 1997), while housing renewal has the potential to decrease accidents and injury with a consequent sevenfold reduction in reported morbidity (Allen 2000). Improving safety and security features in housing increases market potential, as these features appear to be highly valued (Pragnell et al 2000). If home modifications are viewed from a preventative perspective (see Chapter 2), their value becomes obvious in injury prevention and in improving ease of use and efficiency. Improved housing conditions are particularly critical for frail older people (Kochera 2002).

A move to view environments as enablers of independence and as factors important in creating and maintaining quality of life for all is required. This view takes the focus away from the occupants and functional limitations and places the focus on the shortcomings of the design and fabrication of the building instead. An inclusive approach, which is more likely to appeal to 'us', not just 'them', is more likely to be effective in changing attitudes of consumers, suppliers and people within the building industry (Queensland Department of Housing 2001; Vikstrom 2003). Creating and sustaining a viable market can best address factors like resale value and general desirability.

Increasing consumer knowledge

Most of the housing options for older people are available on the private market and older people can require information and support to inform choice and provide protections where necessary. Wylde (1998) makes the point that general knowledge and acceptance of the formal service system are better predictors of use than the demographics of functional capacity. Many potential consumers are unaware of available programs. In Australia as in the United States, there is a general lack of 'help lines' or cross-service information outlining eligibility criteria. In the United States lack of information, not lack of need, has been identified as a critical factor in less than satisfactory home modification and relocation outcomes (Duncan 1998).

Given that health promotion strategies can develop and change lifestyles, and impact on the social, economic and environmental conditions that determine health (WHO 1997), it is of interest that better advertising of housing services has not been more evident. While advertising appears to be an effective way to increase consumer knowledge, to date this has not been a very high priority for service providers who have instead sought to decrease service demand. Nevertheless, mainstream media (publications, radio and television) advertising is needed that touts the beauty, desirability, affordability and other benefits of home modification and adaptable housing construction—which itself is hampered by negative stereotyping of older people within the building industry (Frain & Carr 1996).

Educational efforts need to meet the consumers on their terms in their preferred language. For this to be effective, more research needs to be conducted with consumers about preferences for language, images and packaging. Aspects of aesthetics and appearance must be improved—need is not enough in and of itself to 'sell' products. Home modifications and improvements need to be presented in creative ways, with emphasis on added-value and cost benefits.

A population perspective on environments and housing

As noted by Struyk and Katsura (1988) home modification and relocation are the primary means for altering housing to provide the services required. The ability to adapt or modify a home environment is, however, largely dependent on home ownership and income. Australia, like the United States, has one of the highest rates of home ownership amongst older people in advanced industrial countries (Kendig & Pynoos 1996). Amongst older individuals and couples aged 65 years and over in private households in Australia, nearly 80 per cent are outright home owners, which provides low housing costs—93 per cent paying less than a quarter of their income on housing (AIHW 2002). In the most recent national survey of housing and home modification issues in the United States, 86 per cent of persons over the age of 55 were home owners (Bayer & Harper 2000).

Home ownership remains in many western countries a substantial financial asset that can be used to buy into aged care facilities and/or left as inheritances. While owners face the direct costs of property taxes and maintenance, they are financially advantaged by the tax-free position of owner-occupied housing in terms of use value, property appreciation and eventual inheritance (Kendig & Neutze 1999). Older owners typically are asset rich but income poor, which means that their wealth generally is not available unless they sell their homes and move.

By contrast, most private housing tenants are heavily pressured by high rents as well as low incomes, and neither public nor private tenants have housing assets. The Australian Institute of Health and Welfare (AIHW 2002) reports that approximately 7 per cent of older individuals and couples are private tenants, 6 per cent are public tenants, and another 5 per cent live rent free or have some form of shared equity. Public housing tenants across Australia are advantaged over private rental tenants in that their rental is typically capped. For instance, nearly all public tenants across Australia pay less than 25 per cent of their assessable income in rent as contrasted with private tenants who are not so protected. While owners generally have income well above those of private and public tenants, housing costs for older couples are much lower for outright owners ($38 week) than for those who are renting ($103). Owner occupancy is essential for enabling many older people to have an adequate standard of living while relying on a relatively small government pension.

Home ownership rates are expected to rise as the baby-boomer cohort moves into their retirement years over the coming decades (Kendig & Duckett 2001). However, home ownership rates have been falling for younger cohorts. If this trend continues, there will be a substantial increase in economic inequity in old age. Fewer older people will have the financial benefits of home ownership to offset income reductions after retirement from the paid labour force. Overall, in terms of housing wealth as well as lifetime incomes, it can no longer be assumed that older people are disadvantaged relative to younger people by their cohort of birth.

In 1998, 91 per cent of older people in Australia lived in private households, 6 per cent in health care establishments such as nursing homes, and 3 per cent in other accommodations such as boarding houses. However, amongst the minority of older people with a substantial disability, most resided in some form of long-term care accommodation, including hospitals, nursing homes, hostels, and the care-intensive sections of retirement villages (ABS 1998). Reflecting trends from a number of western countries, including the United States, Canada, Australia and the United Kingdom, widows and never-married older men are more likely to be in residential care than married people of either sex and never-married older women, highlighting the important influence of informal care. Overall, less than half of the people entering old age are projected to ever live in a nursing home or hostel (Mason et al 2001).

Those people who have grown older in urban areas that were designed during the public transport era have relatively good access to buses and trains (Kendig 2000). These older areas tend to have a range of housing types, thus enabling people to move to smaller, less expensive or more easily maintained dwellings without having to move away from familiar neighbourhoods. Increasingly, however, people generally are 'ageing in place' in postwar suburbs with relatively low densities, less variety of housing and poor access to public transport. There are also trends for people who are growing older to move away from rural areas to small towns. An increasing pattern is of coastal retirement migration, in which people cash in on their housing equity in major urban areas and buy into less expensive areas having improved amenity.

Staying in their own homes can be central to older people's identity and sense of independence (Davison et al 1993). Those who choose to move to retirement villages (Gardner 1994), public housing (Brook et al 1998), or coastal retirement areas (Neyland & Kendig 1996), by and large benefit significantly. However, older persons, particularly in Australia, show an overwhelming resistance to entering nursing homes: One recent study reported that most respondents claim they would prefer to die rather than enter a nursing home (Salkeld et al 2000). These intense views are shaped by a fear of dependency as well as of nursing home conditions.

Amongst older people who have substantial disabilities and live in private households, more than half are married and only a third live alone, indicating the importance of informal support in remaining in the community (Bridge et al 2002). Relatively few of this cohort live with an adult child, reflecting older people's wishes to remain independent, their financial capacity to do so, and cultural norms of 'intimacy at a distance'. They have extensive needs for assistance, however, ranging from help with property maintenance (60 per cent), housework (46 per cent), health care (44 per cent), and transportation (42 per cent) to assistance with self-care (29 per cent) and meal preparation (18 per cent). Some 54 per cent of these older people having substantial disabilities report that all their needs are met, 30 per cent that needs are partially met, and 12 per cent that none of their needs are met.

The relationship of housing to health outcomes

Older people's functional performance, community participation and satisfaction with life rely to a certain degree on environmental conditions. Human habitation serves to mediate natural environmental extremes. As such, housing and built environments sustain and support human life, and thus environments directly and indirectly impact on health, social support, absence of disease, quality of life and well-being (Bridge et al 2003). Health can be positively improved by enhanced formal care provision matched to need while maintaining housing choice and personal control, as these are positively correlated to improved quality of life, with decreased acute and cared accommodation costs (Walker et al 1998; Harrison & Heywood 2000).

As previously mentioned, income impacts on the ability to maintain and improve one's accommodation, so it is unsurprising that poor maintenance and dwelling deficiencies are most prevalent amongst older, less well-off sole occupants (Markham & Gilderbloom 1998; Choi 1999). Dwelling characteristics can have adverse impact on life expectancy of frail elders. A Japanese study conducted by Zhao et al (1993), found that the cumulative survival rates of older people with good housing conditions were higher than those with poor housing conditions.

A growing body of evidence indicates that home modification and home ownership improve safety, well-being and mental health (Faulkner & Bennett 2002; Kochera 2002). There is also some evidence that greater accessibility afforded by enhanced dwelling design reduces dependence (Connell & Sanford 2001). On the other hand, policy innovation, such as legislative change to facilitate the creation of 'granny flats', has been less effective than anticipated because dwelling occupancy incentives and design have failed to accommodate older persons with frailty and disability (Chapman 2001). Nevertheless, utilisation of high technology in things like 'smart housing' may also be inappropriate because of issues associated with affordability, learning and cognition (Pragnell et al 2000). In addition, as already mentioned home modification programs are perceived to be difficult to access (Pynoos et al 1998).

Lastly, some qualitative evidence suggests that older persons also perceive that pressure to modify rather than to enhance care might magnify the informal care burden in environments with a concentration of older or disabled persons (MacDonald et al 1994). Indeed, there is some evidence that age segregation may have variable negative impacts on mental health and self-esteem (Percival 2001).

The relationship of housing to care

The complexity of disability, ageing, health, housing and care programs means that funding and management is divided between different sectors of government. The devolvement of program responsibility to non-government and private sector organisations further complicates matters (Kalish 2000). The division of responsibilities, and the piecemeal and historical base for such divisions, underscores the need to consider their joint impact on individuals whose complex needs may require provision across a number of service areas. The division of management and funding responsibilities, together with a narrow focus on accountability for outputs and costs within each of the program areas, does not provide a sound base for provision of integrated accommodation and care.

Further, different states/provinces may have their own acts and legislative frameworks that have major impacts on older persons. For example, in Australia many state governments are trying to fill perceived gaps in national legislation and programs. Crucial areas of state action include disability rights legislation, policy frameworks and property-related tenancy. They also encompass other consumer protection legislation aimed at monitoring quality of dwellings and care accommodation (including regulation of retirement villages). Most states are aiming to overcome some of the policy divides across housing, care, and ageing/disability areas by establishing larger operational departments with a wider range of responsibilities.

Although proper care has traditionally been linked to non-private housing, the fact is that the same level of care can be given in a private dwelling as in a nursing home. That is, provided the in-home care option has appropriate housing design and security. It is housing stability and the qualities of housing design that afford the ongoing provision of quality care by informal caregivers. The provision of both affordable and appropriate accommodation choices and options is a central tenet of international policy and is reflected in recent legislative change. Many if not most countries, including Australia, the United States and the United Kingdom, have anti-discrimination

Acts in place which implicitly preclude discrimination to housing services based on disability. Additionally, in countries like the United States, the *Fair Housing Act* explicitly covers most housing, making it unlawful for a landlord to refuse housing or the installation of reasonable modifications (at the occupier's expense) to accommodate functional impairments. In the United Kingdom, building regulations now require builders to construct new housing to standards that enable disabled people, particularly wheelchair users and those with mobility or ambulant impairments, to visit a house and have access to a ground floor living space and toilet.

Informal care and support networks play a critical role in community service provision, especially in caring for frail older people and older people with disabilities living within the community (see Chapter 8). Unpaid informal caregivers provide the majority of housing support outside cared accommodation settings. Not only are informal carers responsible for maintaining people, often with high levels of functional dependence, within the community, but the absence of an informal carer has been identified as a significant risk factor in contributing to institutionalisation amongst the older population (AIHW 1997).

The growth of models of home-based care relies heavily on the availability of carers to provide the day-to-day support to people who are ill or disabled. As parents and grandparents, older persons are the first line of support for sick adults and orphaned children. For example, in Australia, more than 17 per cent of people aged 50 and over are carers (Wolcott & Glezer 1999). Women are nearly three times more likely than men to be primary carers. In addition, older people are more likely to be carers than younger people, with those aged between 65 and 74 years being twice as likely to be a carer compared with the overall population (ABS 1998). Seventy-five per cent of carers of severely handicapped older people are the spouse of the person requiring care, highlighting the extent to which older people are themselves carers.

The cost of caring is personal (emotional and physical health decline) and financial (cost of care, lost income, and lost opportunities for advancement and promotion), having both immediate and longer term impact (Watson & Mears 1996). The fact that the ability to 'age in place' depends on the availability of informal care is significant because of the economic disadvantage experienced by carers and the increased likelihood that the physical demands of caring will result in acquired disability for the carer. Thus containing residential care cost depends, to some extent, on an improved respite care benefit being provided to carers (Ball 1990). Well-designed home environs can reduce the risk of injury to carers and older persons, as already discussed.

Predictors of transition to formal care include the profoundness of disability-related impairments, particularly neurological disability (Cape & Gibson 1994), in conjunction with social isolation (Bridge et al 2002). Other studies have found area of residence, sex, race and living arrangements significant as predictors of relocation to cared accommodation settings (Dwyer et al 1994). Older persons who are most likely to be doubly disadvantaged are women with disabilities (Currie 1996; Moss 1997).

The secondary data analysis of the 1998 Disability and Carers Survey in Australia provides a population perspective on their circumstances, including those who are not directly known to service systems (Bridge et al 2002). This includes the large numbers of people who, notwithstanding their disabilities, remain largely independent of services, and identifies people who have needs that are not met by the existing services. This same analysis indicates that amongst people with at least moderate levels of disability—that is, having some difficulties with core activities including self-care, mobility, communication—two-thirds reside in some form of care accommodation, including hospitals, nursing homes, hostels, parts of retirement villages, and children's homes. The conclusion is that the primary government response to people with high care needs remains support provision within the restrictive and expensive context of residential care. This is particularly so for older persons, because of the far greater availability and acceptability of residential care for older people.

The trend towards de-institutionalisation and ageing in place demonstrates that community care is becoming the primary and preferred context of care for older people with high care needs. The desire to remain in a familiar environment impacts on older people with disabilities who seek to remain in the community despite high support needs. Ageing in place contrasts quite strongly with the view that transitions are 'normal' and inevitable for older persons with high care needs.

Policy changes that regulate social housing provision, care arrangements and income have all been implicated in negative outcomes for older persons. Large variations in the ways housing and care are coordinated for older persons can impact on outcomes, creating a multiple jeopardy situation (Houben 2001). While a care in the community policy is based on people staying in their own homes, the impact on housing policy is generally poorly considered or factored in. In the United Kingdom, for instance, the impact on housing policy was not considered until eighteen months after the introduction of the *National Health Service and Community Care Act* in 1990 (Conway 1995).

Shortfalls in care have been shown to be most acute in social housing (Malmgren et al 1996) and in rural areas (Karwat 1998). Rural difficulties stem from distance and the ongoing reductions of service infrastructure within smaller townships. On the other hand, shortage of social housing results in more tenants requiring care and support to maintain tenancies (Clapham & Franklin 1995). Additionally, economic incentives that have the opposite effect from that intended, poor linkages and/or policy that increases the complexity of decision making and interdepartmental communication may place care arrangements at risk (Bamford 2001). Changes to benefits may also negatively impact clients' abilities to cover care costs (Houben 2001).

The number and type of housing on offer is also impacting care outcomes negatively. For instance, demographic trend analysis indicates that housing shortfalls will eventuate for severely mentally ill persons whose primary caregivers are ageing (Grosser & Conley 1995). For instance, in New York State, Grosser & Conley (1995) found that up to 1200 adults with severe and persistent mental illness would experience housing disruptions due to the death of ageing caregivers. As a consequence they concluded that additional housing and support were required. Housing location, type and availability impacts informal care availability and community participation. As Felce (1998) states, a decent, homelike and supportive home is necessary but social support and participation is also required to ensure well-being.

Another important implication of recent research is the notion that the level of disability, particularly within social housing, may be a function of lack of physical activity, given that social housing tenants were found to be disproportionally physically inactive (Buchner et al 1997). Lack of physical activity may be a consequence of housing provision that fails to encourage active and healthy behaviours. Factors such as poor street lighting, lack of street seating, high crime rates, lack of accessible public transport and inaccessible public recreation areas may all contribute (Sallis et al 1998). The establishment of pedestrian and biking trails that connect homes with shopping areas, and more attention to hazard and comfort in general infrastructure design, can be used to ameliorate the impact of climate-related disincentives (ice, wind, rain, flooding, etc.).

Community care is enhanced when housing facilitates rather than decreases access to services (Bochel et al 1999). For older persons in particular, remaining in the community with care and support correlates to both better health maintenance and well-being (Faulkner & Bennett 2002). Moreover, there is some evidence that increasing home help services for older and disabled persons correlates to decreased acute hospital costs (Sapey 1995).

Improving quality of housing via renewal and retrofit for people with disabilities can reduce dependency. Special initiatives partnerships can achieve both curative and preventative health gain when core purposes are aligned (Palmer & Molyneux 2000). For example, large scale initiatives between the US Department of Housing and Urban Development and the state of Minnesota, based on Continuum of Care (CoC) regional planning, enable improved access to a logical, interconnected system of housing and social service supports (Schmidt 2002). Indeed, provision of housing tenancy support, socio-emotional support and direct practical support have all been found to improve well-being and self-esteem (Quilgars 2000).

Last but by no means least, the rapid growth of formal home health care services in the United States, Australia and other developed countries (Kalisch 2000), poses unforeseen direct and indirect costs. Another challenge in home care provision remains in improving occupational health and safety performance, as care provision has been directly linked to the creation of injury and disability for carers. In one year, for example, almost half of the total occupational, health and safety claims made in one Australian state related to manual handling by carers (48.5 per cent) (Home Care NSW 2000).

Functional loss equals the need for more supportive housing and care

Disability, housing and care are interdependent and complex and their intersections, particularly in terms of linkages between access, safety and dependency, are often not well understood.

Figure 7.2 illustrates the interrelational nature of accommodation, disability and care policies. Change in one sphere impacts the others, either increasing or decreasing the intersect between spheres and the resultant need, which is a product of all three spheres intersecting. In this way the fit between societal need and governmental policy varies over time. For example, implementation of accommodation policies like reverse mortgages, rental assistance, public housing provision and nursing home admission criteria, determines what accommodation can be obtained.

'Access' to residential accommodation options is the product of the intersect of disability and accommodation. This is because the degree of functional loss and the resultant disability classification typically determine access and eligibility expectations and criteria. Accommodation and care policies are equally interlinked. Nursing home accommodation, for instance, packages personal care with meals, housekeeping and nursing services, under which the safety of care provision rests on national monitoring and accreditation standards. On the other hand, a standard residential dwelling provides no guarantee of on-site support and injury prevention, which remains the responsibility of the occupier.

The intersection of accommodation and care thus raises issues of safety in terms of primary and secondary disability minimisation, and formal and informal carer hazard reduction and risk minimisation. The intersection between disability and care relates to the amount and quality of informal and formal support. The intersection of disability and accommodation raises issues of access to services and implicitly of access to premises. Levels of access, safety and dependency frame need and have implications for disability, housing and care linkages.

The built environment and urban and regional development challenges

Research on the link between older people and urban change is relatively new and is gaining momentum. Both the growth of older populations and urban consolidation are long-term, largely predictable processes (Kendig 2000). For vulnerable older people, the residential environment can have a crucial bearing on independence and well-being. For instance, the ability to independently participate in society, and manage the intrinsic activities of daily

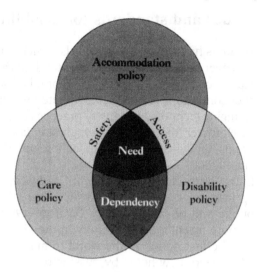

Figure 7.2: The intersection of accommodation, disability and care

living such as banking and shopping, may depend as much on community infrastructure and public transport infrastructure as they do on an individual's functional ability (Malmgren et al 1996).

Building codes provide statements of the minimum technical requirements for the design and construction of buildings and other related structures. The rationale for these is typically driven by human rights and disability discrimination legislation. But the 'where', 'when' and 'what' of building and access falls under the guidance provided by building codes enacted by local legislation in combination with regional planning ordinances. The way or method is guided by national standards and the 'who' by regional controls on licensing of builders and allied trades.

Not surprisingly, in Europe, the United States and Australia, there are significant variations between regions because individual states and countries have statutory responsibility for building regulation within their jurisdiction. Currently, individual governments adopt building codes depending on climatic and regional difference. Consequently, while there are general principles in common there are clinically significant variances in the dimensions deemed to satisfy the provisions. This situation is underscored by a dearth of reliable research into the housing factors relevant to older persons and persons with disabilities.

Building codes and standards for disability

Nearly all countries have disability standards, which unfortunately do not always cover housing infrastructure. Standards are typically written by expert committees set up and supported by government. They are under continuous review, being updated regularly to take account of changing technology, industry practices and community expectations. However, the degree to which standards are implemented depends on whether they are called up in legislation (Bridge & Simoff 2000).

In the United States the *Americans with Disabilities Act* and the Fair Housing laws have worked to provide more adaptable and accessible public and private dwellings (Watson 1990). This has been echoed more recently and forcefully in the United Kingdom which became the first nation in the world to mandate basic disability access in every new home by passing the *Visitable Homes Act* in 1998 (Stewart et al 1999). This Act requires that every new home must have an entrance without steps, a downstairs bathroom, sufficiently wide halls, all doorways passable by wheelchairs, and other elements of universal design.

The Building Code of Australia (BCA), by means of state and territory legislation, requires most new public buildings to have features to enable access and use by people with disabilities, and specifies which classes of buildings, which areas, and how many facilities, should be accessible. However, the scope of the code is limited, covering requirements for new public buildings and works but not existing infrastructure. Building codes tend not to cover areas beyond the building block (streetscapes or parks), nor do they generally cover furniture or fittings, equipment or interiors (Vikstrom 2003).

In most developed countries, local governments have the major responsibility for implementing the provisions of building codes, via building approval and certification processes, generally in accordance with detailed environmental planning instruments covering localities, regions and nations. How effective the system is in practice varies enormously, as many systems have traditionally not considered public access and egress for older persons as a key component in their deliberations (Kendig 2000).

The initial arrangements of building boundaries, roads and public spaces set up patterns of land use far into the future. Urban development, planned and unplanned, has implications that are persistent and often unforeseen at the point of construction, and reflects the cultural preferences, technological realities, and economic imperatives of its time. The critical point here is that only processes that enable better planning for the future, which are inclusive of all within society, are most likely to facilitate positive participatory futures for older persons.

Do I stay or do I go now?

Mary is 69 years old. She and her husband decided to pursue their dream retirement in their late 40s when their oldest daughter went to university, and relocated from the 'rat race' to a coastal farm. Unfortunately, Mary's husband died last year and she has recently been diagnosed with late onset diabetes, and with epilepsy following a drop-fall (a fall that occurs without warning or explanation) which saw her admitted to hospital with a head injury. While Mary has to all intents and purposes recovered well—she is ambulant and has no obvious memory loss—as a result of the incident she has lost both her sense of smell and her confidence. Mary is deeply ambivalent about her housing options. She is fiercely independent but struggles to manage the farm alone and is dependent on being able to continue to drive to maintain her banking, shopping and socialisation activities. While Mary has supportive neighbours she knows she has more limited care and support options locally than in a larger city. However, even if she were to sell her farm in an effort to relocate closer to her remaining family, she cannot now afford a home in the city near her daughter.

Reflecting on Mary's specific dilemma assists in clarifying the general geographic, economic and emotional factors influencing older persons' housing choices. Mary's case illustrates how well-being and quality of life are impacted on by access to housing and care options in the context of changing emotional, physical and safety needs.

Mary may be anxious and ambivalent about taking action but she still has a range of options. The sooner she acts, the greater the potential there will be for her to experience control while achieving a housing outcome enabling her to reduce her risk and capacity demands. Mary's epilepsy and 'drop-falls' can be better managed with improved access to specialists and regular monitoring. However, without access to tel-health facilities this will require Mary to organise and fund regular travel to specialists located in urban or city areas, or may force relocation of her accommodation.

Mary's ability to travel by herself from her farm to her specialist will depend on her ability to both maintain her car and retain her driving licence. Her ability to retain her licence rests on assessment of her functional capacity in combination with prescribed medication. Should Mary be unable to maintain her licence, remaining in her current accommodation setting will be compromised because her rural environment limits access to both services and public transport infrastructure. Lack of transport infrastructure may result in an unwanted reliance on care services for shopping and banking, and will potentially limit her socialisation and care options.

Activity 7.1

Reflecting on the following question will help you to assess the knowledge needed to assist someone like Mary to make more informed housing choices within your local context. What are the environmental positives and constraints that would affect Mary's housing choices in the context of your local housing environment? Consider carefully the:

Social and physical geography impacting on the suitability of older persons' housing:
- Climatic factors including temperature, precipitation, geological stability, etc.
- Design and age of the immediate environs (home, footpaths, roads and shops)

- Access to roads and general physical service infrastructure (water, gas, electricity, etc.)

Care accessibility in light of cultural, social and physical environmental delivery constraints:
- Formal care services available to assist older persons to remain at home, including but not limited to subsidised food, personal care, home care and transport options
- Informal or community assistance available from relatives, neighbours and local cooperatives

Environmental legislation:
- Driving restrictions such as those imposed by legislation relating to age-related testing or those following a significant health concern such as failing eyesight or neurological impairment
- Building codes and standards as they apply to housing construction and retrofit or redesign
- Land use planning as it relates to subdivision, land sale and rezoning

Housing markets:
- Affordability and availability of alternative accommodation options, including but not limited to caravans and mobile homes, 'granny flats', apartments and the like
- Enhanced care and security packaging options within existing local retirement communities, hotels and hostels

Housing environmental maintenance and injury prevention programs:
    Access to individual pre-existing or pre-purchase home safety assessments and or home modification and maintenance intervention services
- Access to helpful technologies, monitoring and security services

Only a multidisciplinary team approach will be able to canvass the full range of social, physical and environmental factors determining optimal housing choices for someone like Mary. However, all health professionals attempting to assist Mary will need to do so within the context of Mary's emotional attachment to her current abode. As previously mentioned, failure to attend to factors of the housing environment that embody emotion and security ignores the importance of the memories, habits and cognitive responses people associate with their home. A careful history of preferred activities in the context of potential barriers and hazards, and the amount and quality of informal and physical supports, are keys to both rapport and to informed decision making. Informed decision making requires detailed and objective observation of intrinsic activities of daily living in the context of the supportiveness of Mary's current environment. For instance, if heating water for cleaning or cooking purposes requires Mary to chop wood, a reliable connection to the local gas or electricity service can fundamentally change the physical demand on her functional capacity. Cognitive demand can also be decreased by automation. For some other activities, factors relating to climate and formal and informal support availability may enable the activity to be minimised, if not eliminated, or alternatively delegated to others. The optimal solution will depend on the economic, physical, legislative and social environmental resources in the context of Mary's functional capacity.

A home assessment report detailing accessibility and potential barriers and hazards in her current home will assist Mary to pay attention to the range of factors likely to impact on her quality of life, both now and in the longer term. This in combination with information about alternative housing options will enable Mary to construct a mental plan that she can use to make informed decisions about what can be done now and what plans may need to be made for a quality future. Mary's housing options will be constrained by her functional capacity, economic resources and current housing in the context of local housing, care and disability policies, as these are what shape financial, care and housing packaging options (in other words, access to and eligibility for home modification and maintenance services, aged care facilities, etc.).

Conclusion

The built environment is an essential foundation for promoting positive experiences in old age. The home and neighbourhood are the primary areas in which older people live their daily lives. Continuity of residential experience can provide an intense sense of meaning and identity for people whose life positions may be threatened by life changes such as shrinking social worlds, reduced income, frailty, or loss of a partner. For vulnerable older persons, a supportive residential environment can make the critical difference in enabling continued independence and well-being and maintaining healthy ways of living. Owner occupancy is the main source of economic security amongst older people while those who are tenants face high housing costs and limited security in use of their homes.

Understanding person–environment relationships provides outstanding opportunities to improve living experiences for all people but especially for those who are vulnerable. While health professions focus primarily on treatment and rehabilitation, good outcomes also can be achieved through environmental interventions. For example, a person who has experienced a stroke may require rehabilitation to use a chair, but the function of sitting can also be facilitated by the design and provision of more user-friendly chairs. Similarly, while people without cars can be transported to shops, they can be more independent if shops are located within easy walking range.

The challenges facing older people in regard to housing in the 21st century centre on affordability, accessibility and adaptability. Firstly, affordability varies depending on savings, interest rates, loans, subsidies and land value. In many developed countries the baby-boomer generation is relatively well off, with a large percentage owning their own homes, this capital providing them with a degree of control and choice regarding housing options. However, the same is not true for younger generations, with the ability to invest in housing rapidly moving out of reach for the pre-retirement cohort, who will reach their later years mid-century. Greater urbanisation and consolidation pressures, particularly in the more sought-after coastal areas, largely determine affordability. Housing is likely to remain cheaper in rural areas, but here range and choice are limited and services, particularly health and care services, remain limited and expensive.

Secondly, accessibility rests on innovation in assistive technologies and renewal of urban and rural infrastructure. Creating more accessible residential environments requires long-term forward planning to reap maximum benefits and cost-effectiveness. Local planning varies between states and countries, but has great potential for enhancing access. Successful implementation of standards and legislative requirements depends on understanding of those requirements and commitment to enforcement, through many layers of people and processes.

Lastly, adaptability outcomes depend on design and technological innovation in combination with regulation of residential housing. The long-term livability of housing environments can be greatly enhanced in the future by designs that anticipate and are responsive to the diverse needs of people over their entire life course. However, our ability to achieve this vision is presently limited by lack of comprehensive ergonomic information on the diverse anthropometric data regarding strength vision and light sensitivity of older people required to maintain function across a range of meaningful daily activities. Lack of performance standards for design and technology intended to overcome functional limitations associated with ageing limits the impact of anticipated regulatory reform and innovation within the housing sector.

In summary, the environmental approach to supporting older people can be pursued usefully in many ways. Assessment for community care services in clients' homes can consider their individual capacities and explore possible interventions specifically in terms of the demands and supports of their local environments. Interventions can include aids and home modifications as alternatives or complements to the provision of services. On a larger scale, building regulations and land use regulations can ensure basic supports in the environment that may be essential for vulnerable people and a convenience for everyone. Comprehensive public and private actions can support the independence and well-being of older people through self and informal care, care services and environmental interventions.

8

The challenge of caregiving

Neena L. Chappell, Glenda Parmenter

Caregiving has been, and remains, the mainstay of support for older people. This chapter provides an overview of gerontological research in this area, beginning with studies conducted in the 1970s and 1980s. Early research in the field established the importance of social support and caregiving in the lives of older people, debunking myths about their loneliness and social isolation from family and friends. Since that time, research has demonstrated the importance of social support for the health and well-being of older people both on a day-to-day basis and during times of stress (Cohen and Syme 1985; Chappell 1992). It has also revealed the predominance of caregiving from family and friends as the primary care system as we age, unveiling both its extensiveness and the sources and types of assistance that are provided.

Despite the popularity of this area amongst gerontological researchers, there is much that we do not know. This chapter discusses current issues in the caregiving area, including the misnomer of the concept of the 'generation in the middle'; the emphasis on burden and stress within the caregiving experience; the lack of attention to satisfactions and, relatedly, an understanding of the experience from the caregiver's point of view (research on the meanings of respite is provided as an illustrative example). The implications of health system reform for family caregivers are then generally discussed. Finally, attention turns to the primarily western domination within caregiving research, drawing on studies of Chinese older persons to indicate the importance of cultural values and the need for more research to help us understand cultural differences and similarities in this area.

A brief history of caregiving

Throughout time, family and friends have cared for one another when the health of one declines. This remains true today. The concept of social support began receiving attention in the gerontological literature in the 1970s, amidst common beliefs that in western society older individuals tended to be socially isolated and lonely, abandoned or neglected by their families and institutionalised if possible. Modern western society's individualism and materialism, it was believed, valued only those who remained productive within the labour force. The fact that most older people are retired, combined with ageist attitudes, would mean relative isolation in old age.

Early research identified the multi-dimensionality of the concept, without consensus on its precise meaning. Lopata (1975), for example, referred to the informal network as the primary support system involving the giving and receiving of objects, services, and social and emotional supports deemed by the receiver and giver as important. Cobb (1976) defined support as including one or more of emotional support, information that leads the person to believe he or she is esteemed or valued, and the feeling that the individual belongs to a network of communication and mutual obligation. Three typical components include Cohen and Syme's (1985) notion of emotional function, information that may or may not lead to confirmation or heightening of self-esteem, and tangible support such as assistance with activities of daily living. House and Kahn (1985) refer to social networks, social support and social integration. Social support refers here only to the functional content of social relationships such as the three components identified by Cohen and Syme (emotional concern, instrumentality and information).

Social support has been used to refer to all relationships, implying that social interaction is necessarily positive. Any number of terms may refer to a similar idea: social network, group affiliation, interpersonal interaction, social integration, social support, emotional support, information, feeling of belonging, tangible support, to name only a few. Most of the research has focused on emotional concern and instrumentality, as well as the social network, usually focusing on size and/or composition. Emotional aspects often distinguish between companionship and confidantes. Instrumental assistance typically refers to assistance with activities of daily living—basic, instrumental or both.

The nature of social networks has been influenced by changes to the structure of the family, particularly in the industrialised, western world, which occurred in the mid-20th century. These changes were documented in a large study (Phillipson et al 2001) that compared the structure and function of modern British families with those described some 50 years earlier by Sheldon (1948) and Townsend (1957). In the intervening period the most notable change to the structure of the family was the decline of the multi-generational household in which older persons and their adult children lived together. This decline had increased dramatically since the 1960s, with older persons increasingly more likely to live with a spouse only or to live alone. Accompanying this was a decrease in the general proximity of family members as children moved away from their parents to find employment or as their ability to undertake a greater range of employment opportunities at more distant locations increased, particularly for women. Despite this decline in the extended family and the increased geographical distance between family members, the study found that the family remained the principle source of support for its older members.

Research in the 1970s and early 1980s documented the variety and extent of social interaction during old age, debunking common assumptions that the nuclear family abandoned its older members. These assumptions were documented as generally false; the vast majority of older people are embedded in extensive social networks (Antonucci 1985; Chappell 1992; Chappell et al 2003). A study of social isolation amongst older people in Wales (Wenger et al 1996), for example, found that for those older people identified as isolated and lonely, the critical factors were living alone, having a very small social network, belonging to a lower social class and being in poorer health. Those people who experience a decline in the amount and variety of social interaction in old age tend to be those who are 'old-old', in poor health and with fewer economic resources.

Much of this research focused on marriage during the later years, a status which tends to characterise those who are young-old, with higher incomes, better mental and physical health, assured companionship and larger social networks (Verbrugge 1979). The research demonstrated that married men typically name their wives as their confidantes whereas married women name their husbands plus children or friends; married men name their wives as their best friends while women name their offspring or female age peers (Strain & Chappell 1982, 1985). Married men's exclusive emotional reliance on their wives led to much concern that they are at risk, especially when they become widowed. Men are much less likely to become widowed than women, but when they do they are likely to remarry. For women, on the other hand, widowhood has become a normal life stage wherein they typically have many peers in the same situation.

Amongst older people today, the divorced and never married constitute but a small proportion—something that will change as the baby-boomer generation ages. Lifelong singlehood, it would appear, promotes self-reliance (Johnson & Catalano 1981). As the prevalence of a greater diversity of relationships increases as the baby-boomer generation ages, more gerontological research will focus attention here. The sibling relationship received some attention in these early days, revealing itself as especially important to the never married, the childless, the divorced and the widowed (Cicirelli 1982, 1985). More recent research supports these earlier findings. Campbell et al (1999), for example, examined the role of siblings in the lives of 678 older Americans. They found that in general, siblings are more likely to provide instrumental and emotional support but companionship was more commonly provided by spouse and friends. However, amongst single and widowed women and the childless, sibling ties were found to be particularly important. They concluded that for the childless this is not the substitution of the parent–child relationship but the result of a lifelong closeness. Those without children have the opportunity to invest more time and energy into relationships with their siblings.

Next to spouses, children have received more research attention than other relationships. The majority of older people have at least one child living and tend to both live near at least one child and have weekly contact with their children (Rosenthal 1987; Chappell 1989). More interaction takes place between older parents and their children than with any other kin. As early as 1963, Rosenmayr and Kockeis coined the phrase 'intimacy at a distance' to describe the general preference of older people in the west not to live with their children, but to maintain close ties. Ties with children are maintained even when there is geographic distance. The relationship with children is especially important for women, who consider it more important and more satisfying than do men. The mother–daughter tie is one of the closest.

Although less attention has been focused on grandchildren, early research suggested that a gendered interaction reflected the socialisation of the times—grandfathers emphasised task-oriented involvements with grandchildren, while grandmothers tended to be involved in interpersonal dynamics emphasising the quality of the relationship. Same-gender ties tend to be more prevalent amongst these generations and the grandmother–granddaughter tie is reported to be the closest (Hagestad 1985). By old age one has accumulated a large number of social relationships simply by having been around for so many years. There are, therefore, a large number of relationships from which to draw and to form friendships (Matthews 1986), and their importance has been noted for emotional support, affection and quick integration (Lee 1985).

Early research in the area of social support, then, focused on social interaction but assumed its supportiveness. In other words, if a relationship could be documented, it was assumed to be supportive. This research on the extent and type of social supports in the lives of older people continues today, but the 1980s saw a major shift in focus. Gerontologists began to ask the extent to which this interaction was indeed supportive and to examine the relationship between social support and well-being.

Much of the research in this area assessed the direct affects view that social support is important in meeting needs that require fulfilment on a more or less daily basis, regardless of whether the individual is experiencing stress. Simply being a member of a group or receiving support from others is beneficial, but it is mediated through one's perception, that is, subjective support. Generally research confirms this view. Several reviews in the mid-1980s concluded that the direct affects view was correct although the aspect of social interaction that is the most crucial in this relationship is not always consistent. Cohen and Syme's (1985) review concluded that it is the degree to which an individual is integrated within their social network that is the most important element. House and Kahn's (1985) review, however, concluded that of all the measures of social support, network size is the most consistently related to health and well-being.

The buffer hypothesis argued that social support is important for quality of life during crises or stressful events. Here, social support is seen as mediating the effect of stressful experiences; it protects us against the harmful effects of stress. Again, the bulk of research in this area confirms this postulate although findings are not always consistent. Kessler and McLeod (1985) argue that emotional support is the most important type of social support. Antonucci (1990) argues that the quality of social support shows a stronger relationship than quantity for both men and women but the impact is greater for women. Cohen and Syme (1985) conclude that there is more evidence demonstrating a link between social support and mental health, and between social support and mortality, than there is for a link between social support and physical illness.

Despite its popularity as a subject for research, the area is nevertheless plagued with conceptual and empirical inconsistency as well as the confounding of concepts and causality. For example, measures of stress and social networks are confounded. Widowhood, retirement and relocation all include losses, discontinuation or disruptions to social ties and are considered stressful life events. In addition, social interaction can be both positive and negative, although the negative effects receive considerably less attention. Rook and Pietromonaco (1987) are an exception; they reveal four types of detrimental functions of close relationships including ineffective help, excessive help, unwarranted help and unpleasant help. Wortman and Conway (1985) provide poignant examples in healthy persons' efforts to cheer up individuals with cancer. The recipients of this 'support' consider it to be unhelpful, with such unrelenting optimism seen as disturbing and unauthentic. In addition, although conceptually social support is seen as having beneficial effects, we do not know the extent to which causality works in the other direction. That is, individuals with greater well-being may well attract more social support. Within this literature, furthermore, there is also confusion between caregiving and the broader concept of social support. We turn now to this discussion.

A special type of social support

Caregiving, also known as caring, in this context refers to support provided to older people because their health has deteriorated and they can no longer function independently. The defining characteristic of this support is the provision of assistance. Despite governmental and media attention to the cost of the formal health care system as the population ages, care and assistance from the informal network of family and friends has been the mainstay of care for older people throughout history. 'Informal care' refers to unpaid assistance from family and friends. Although there is some objection to the term 'informal' on the grounds that there is nothing informal about the care that is provided, a distinction does need to be made between family and friends who provide care without remuneration and health care personnel who are paid.

Indeed, in a review of all of the scientifically rigorous studies that had been conducted up to the late 1980s in industrialised countries of the west, Kane (1990) reported that approximately 75 per cent of care to old people came from the informal network, primarily families, irrespective of whether the country had a universal medicare system. The formal health care system provided only about 25 per cent of care. These caregivers tended to be spouses if there was one, or a child, especially a daughter. Families today continue to provide this care despite trends (such as more women working for pay, increase in divorce rates, greater acceptance of differences and geographic mobility) that were supposed to test this commitment. Families overwhelmingly continue to provide care and there is no evidence of this changing (Brody & Schoonover 1986; Chappell 1992). In the face of increasing demands, caregivers forfeit their own leisure time, they give up having coffee with friends, weekly dance lessons, family boating trips, etc.

A confusion arises from the fact that informal caregiving is a type of social support and, as noted in the preceding section, social support is viewed and has received confirmation as good for one's health. However, one typically receives informal assistance when one's health decreases. Given the wide array of measures of social support, it perhaps is not surprising that inconsistency is found in the literature both in how the relationship between assistance and other types of social support are related to one's health and in how they are related to one another. For example, Roberts et al (1994) found that women who experience mobility limitations receive significantly more emotional and instrumental support (assistance) than men. That is, emotional and instrumental support would seem to be related to one another positively. However, McColl and Friedland (1994) found that physical impairment was related with fewer family contacts, fewer friendship contacts, a reduction in both belonging and tangible support, and a tendency to provide less material assistance to others. That is, declining health is related to less social support.

Seeman et al (1996) found that greater frequency of instrumental forms of support (assistance) was a predictor of increased risk of activities of daily living (ADL) disability for men. Hayes et al (1997) similarly found that those who received assistance were more likely to experience functional declines. Seeman et al (1996) also found no significant protective effect of emotional support in delaying ADL disability. Looking at the opposite causal direction, Kemper (1992), Choi and Wodarski (1996) and Boaz and Hu (1997) found the most reliable predictors of the amount of help received with the number of ADL disabilities to be the extent of the network of helpers and their living arrangements. That is, there is no consensus on either the causal direction of assistance or its relationship with broader/other social support dimensions. Using cross-sectional data, some authors see functional disability as a predictor of the receipt of support, while others see the receipt of assistance as predictive of physical health. In some instances assistance is seen as a predictor of another type of social support. For this area to advance there must be a clear distinction. While more research is needed in order to understand the relationships it would appear logical that physical decline leads to assistance, and that assistance would not lead to physical decline except in cases where caregiving is promoting undesirable dependency.

Some of the confusion in this area could be clarified by distinguishing between support received because of a physical limitation or a long-term health problem and support received for other reasons (an agreed-upon division of labour, love, etc.). Canadian data are illustrative. Keating et al (1999), drawing on the 1996 national General Social Survey, distinguish between three groups of older people receiving assistance: those with long-term health problems, those experiencing a temporary difficult time, and those who receive assistance because of the way things are done within the family. They report almost 80 per cent of those aged 65 years or less, and 73 per cent of those aged 65 and over, living in the community are receiving assistance. However, only 3 per cent of those receiving assistance who are 65 years or less do so because of a long-term health problem or a physical disability, whereas the figure for those 65 and over is 22 per cent. Only 4 per cent altogether receive assistance because of a temporarily difficult time such as a short-term illness or minor injury. According to the survey, just over one-quarter of older Canadians receive no assistance. This probably includes those who are independent and do not require assistance as well as those requiring but not receiving any assistance. Amongst those receiving assistance for long-term health problems there are higher proportions of women than men, of the unmarried than the married, of the older rather than the younger, and those in poor health. Overwhelmingly they receive assistance with household tasks (fully 93 per cent). That is, most older people receiving care do so for the instrumental activities of daily living, not for the basic activities of daily living. If we did not refer to 'assistance' for those without physical or mental decline (those without need), it would go a long way in avoiding the present confusion.

A similar picture emerges for Australia. The Australian government's policy on aged care has led to a trend away from institutionalised care and a consequent increase in community-based care. This has meant that a significant proportion of the burden of the care of older persons has been shifted back to families (ABS 2001). In 1998 there were 2.5 million carers in Australia and one in five of these were identified as a primary carer. The majority of these carers (75 per cent) provided care to a member of their own family who lived in the same household (ABS 2001).

In Australia the likelihood of being a carer increases with age and is also influenced by gender. Women are more likely to be carers when they reach the 55–64 years age group, but for men this is delayed until they are at least 74 years old (ABS 2000). Daughters are more strongly represented in the 35–64 years age group of primary carers and are more likely to be performing a number of roles simultaneously, such as participating in the paid labour force (49 per cent) and caring for children under 18 years of age (33 per cent) (Murphy et al 1997). As many of the carers are relatively older there is also a degree of infirmity amongst this population. Some carers have similar disabilities to those they are caring for; in fact, 28 700 Australian carers have been identified as having profound to severe core activity restrictions (ABS 2000).

The Australian literature has also identified the positive aspects of caring such as increased closeness with the care-recipient and a feeling of satisfaction with the caring role (Murphy et al 1997; Wells & Kendig 1997), with the caregiving experience involving both positive and negative aspects. However, the negative effects that caring has on the carer's life continue to be emphasised. These negative effects include a decreased participation in the labour force with a consequent decrease in income, and free time for leisure activities (ABS 2000). The effect of caring on the carer's relationships with her network has also been studied; the results show an enhanced or unchanged relationship in the majority of cases (77 per cent) and a deterioration of the relationship in the remainder (ABS 2001).

The issue of 'assistance' extends to help received by the caregiver. Most of the focus in research in western societies is on the primary caregiver. Tennstedt et al (1989) note that spouse caregivers are the least likely to receive assistance from others with their caregiving tasks, but that child caregivers and friends who are primary caregivers usually have secondary caregivers involved with them. When a child is the primary caregiver, it is usually a daughter; sons and sons-in-law as well as grandchildren living with her often assist. Friends are more often secondary rather than primary caregivers (Chappell & Penning 1996). Amongst siblings who are caregivers one tends to be the primary caregiver with others as secondary caregivers (Brody et al 1989). Veilleux (1991) reports that secondary caregivers help alleviate the burden for primary caregivers, but Pruchno (1990) reports that secondary caregivers do not reduce the burden of primary caregivers. Chappell and Penning (1996) report that 7 per cent of caregivers self-identify as 'sharing equally' rather than as primary or secondary caregivers. However, those sharing equally are more similar to secondary than to primary caregivers other than in labelling themselves this way.

Because women tend to marry men a few years older than themselves and have a longer life expectancy than their husbands, they are available to provide assistance when their husband's health deteriorates prior to death. Older couples tend to cope by redistributing domestic chores, but there is less of a change when the husband's health deteriorates and the wife is a caregiver since the wife's traditional tasks include cooking, cleaning, and attending to the husband's needs. Spouses more than any other category of caregiver provide care during periods of greater illness and disability and continue to do so even as their own health declines (Hess & Soldo 1985; Chappell 1992). Once the woman is widowed it is her children, a daughter if there is one, who provide care as her health deteriorates. Children are the next most frequent caregivers after spouses. Sons and daughters tend to provide differential gender-based care with daughters providing more hands-on emotional care and sons providing more supervision and money if and when needed. If, however, a daughter is not available either because there is none or she is geographically distant, sons do provide the needed care (Horowitz 1981).

The childless are a group for whom the provision of care in later life is potentially a problem. They include those who married but had no children (or who have no surviving children) and those who did not marry and remained childless. This group of older people make up a significant proportion of the population and their care arrangements are of some interest. A study of the support received by 1156 older people living in the north-west of England (Wenger et al 2000) found that one-fifth were childless and that single men and married women were most adversely affected by the lack of children. They concluded that for women the investment in a marriage may be at the cost of forming other relationships that might replace the support normally provided by children.

The role of friends and neighbours in providing care for an older person has received less attention in the research literature. These people often form relationships with the older person through being conveniently located and able to provide frequent interaction and rapid assistance when necessary. Studies of the types of support offered by the friends and neighbours of older English people (Nocon & Pearson 2000) and older Americans (Barker 2002) found that these carers assumed the position of 'quasi-kin' and many went to great lengths to provide care. They undertook the role of carer in cases where the older person had no living or available children or received inadequate support and care from their nearby children. They provided help to people with whom they were already acquainted and their involvement as carers gradually developed from a few small tasks to more time-consuming and complex ones. They sometimes provided care in lieu of formal services that the older person had rejected as less flexible and less able to meet their individual needs.

There is some evidence to suggest that the friendship networks of people in advanced old age are different from those formed and maintained at earlier stages of life. A British study (Jerrome & Wenger 1999) which drew data from the Bangor Longitudinal Study of Ageing examined the influences on the friendship networks of this older age group over a period of sixteen years. Changing circumstances brought about by the death or infirmity of friends influenced these older people to relocate to be nearer to family or to seek accommodation in aged care housing. In such circumstances older people tended to form new friendships with younger people who functioned as surrogate family. The opportunity to form new friendships with people in their own age group existed but due to the constraints of later life, such as declining health and mobility, their new friendships were influenced by more pragmatic motivations and often depended on proximity and opportunity.

Caregiving is also influenced by its cultural context, which determines which family members undertake caregiving and at what point and to what extent formal services are utilised. Research in Japan (Yamamoto & Wallhagen 1998) found that despite the increasing westernisation of Japanese society the burden of caring for elderly parents continues to follow traditional norms and to fall to daughters-in-law and, to a lesser extent, to daughters. These women are obliged to undertake such care and, as the use of formal caregiving services is stigmatised in Japan, they are required to negotiate with other family members if they feel the need for such help. The success of such negotiation depends upon three factors: whether or not such services were available, the strength of the carer's authority within the family and whether the family (and the carer herself) feel that the carer's burden is sufficient to justify the use of formal services. Such justification requires the carer to have reached the very limit of her physical and emotional resources. The level of the caregiver's authority within the family is a strong determinant of the chances of receiving formal support. Such authority rests upon the carer's position within the family and the daughter-in-law, whose authority position is usually lowest but who is also more likely to assume the role of carer, is least able to speak on her own behalf and to have her opinions respected. This research highlights the need for health professionals to be alert to the range of influences that may operate to determine the likelihood that a family will seek support for caregivers. The seeking of such support will not depend solely on the level of burden experienced but will rely on the interplay of a number of complex factors which will vary from family to family. While this research was undertaken to examine the circumstances of a particular culture it serves to point out the possible influences on the decisions regarding carer support which operate to a greater or lesser extent in all families regardless of their cultural background.

Despite the abundance of research on informal caregiving, its popularity has not waned. Indeed new issues continue to arise and its complexity, while recognised, is still not well understood. We turn now to a discussion of some of the current issues in the caregiving area.

Current research issues

The number and types of issues that arise in this area are countless. Here several are discussed, including the concept of the 'sandwich generation', 'caregiver burden', 'caregiver coping' and 'respite care'. The next section goes on to discuss current policy concerns.

The terms 'sandwich generation', 'hidden victims', and 'the generation in the middle' have received popular media attention for some time now. They refer to middle-aged children, primarily daughters, who have multiple demands including having to care for aging parents, still raising their children and working in paid labour. Despite the popularity of the notion, however, it is not middle-aged adults with children who are providing extensive help to their parents—it is children, who no longer have their own children living at home, doing most of this caregiving (Rosenthal et al 1996; Penning 1998). The terms therefore are misnomers. 'Serial caregiving' is a more accurate term, because most women raise their children, then give care to their parents, then provide care to their husbands, in succession rather than simultaneously.

A major focus in the caregiving literature is unquestioningly on the stress and burden of caregivers. Burden, referred to by a variety of terms including stress effects, caregiving consequences, caregiving impact, stress and strain, refers to any negative consequences for mental, physical, psychological or emotional health, social involvement and/or financial difficulties. Tebb (1995) refers to it as the inability to be resilient. Burden includes both objective (such as changes in daily routine, employment and health) and subjective (including emotional reactions such as low morale, anxiety and depression) components, with the subjective usually regarded as the most important.

Most of the literature on caregiver burden has focused on caregivers to those who suffer from Alzheimer's disease or other dementias. Caring for dementia sufferers is considered more burdensome than caring for those who are physically frail (Zarit &

Zarit 1983; George & Gwyther 1986). In addition, behavioural manifestations of dementia are more problematic than the condition per se and not all stages of the disease are as problematic as others (Chappell & Penning 1996). Amongst behavioural problems, those that are most problematic are those that restrict or confine the caregiving time and space and those requiring personal bodily contact (Montgomery et al 1985). The negative impact of caregiving has been well documented using a variety of outcomes such as depression (Parks & Pilisuk 1991), guilt, worry/anxiety, loneliness (Barusch 1988), emotional stress and strain (Fast & Da Pont 1997), lower physical functioning, lower social functioning, or worse general health (Hughes et al 1999).

A British study on caring examined the relationship between the history and quality of the marital relationship and levels of adjustment amongst the older carers of psychiatrically impaired spouses (Murray & Livingston 1998). The findings of this study show that those carers with better health and adaptation to caring were those who were able to recognise the continuity in the connection and intimacy they had with their spouse before he/she was affected by a mental illness. Conversely, those spouse carers who 'look back on marriages that have been low in intimacy and reciprocity, derive no satisfaction from caregiving and are themselves at risk of mental illness' (Murray & Livingston 1998, p. 669). The former group is less likely to seek formal assistance with the care of their spouse than the latter. Those with a history of a happy relationship resent the intrusion of outside people and wish to provide the care for their spouse themselves. Those from a relationship with an unhappy history feel trapped by the demands of their spouse and seek outside help to reduce their burden. Therefore, consideration should be given to the nature and history of the relationship between the carer and spouse when support services are being planned or offered. The type and extent of services may depend on the nature of the caring relationship. The health of the carer should also be kept in mind, with more extensive intervention being required by carers who have a history of a less happy relationship with their dependent spouse.

While family members provide the majority of the informal care to older persons within private residences, caregiving is not relinquished when the care-recipient enters a nursing home. Rather, family and friends modify their caregiving roles to encompass predominantly social and emotional support, while nursing home staff take over the more instrumental aspects of care (Naleppa 1996). Recent Australian research on visiting in rural nursing homes (Parmenter 2003) has identified those members of the residents' social networks who undertake a continued involvement in the residents' care through frequent visiting. Analysing a sample of 876 family and friends, the study found that the majority (68.9 per cent) of visitors were female, with this gender bias holding across both the age and relationship (spouse, child, grandchild, sibling, friends) categories of the visitor. Frequent visitors were from the older age groups (71.6 per cent being aged between 40 and 74 years) and were the spouses and children of these residents. There was a relative absence of younger visitors, and grandchildren comprised only 11.9 per cent of the total sample of visitors.

The continued caregiving role within the nursing home was found to be a predominantly social one with only a minority of family members providing instrumental care. The overwhelming majority (86.6 per cent) of visitors had come to the nursing home to provide the resident with companionship, although other more instrumental activities were also undertaken. These included bringing supplies such as clothes, toiletries, etc. for the resident (15.9 per cent), bringing food (9.8 per cent), helping the resident with meals (9.4 per cent), and taking the resident out for a walk (9 per cent). These relatively low levels of instrumental care may reflect the degree of infirmity amongst this population of residents, with the more demanding, physical aspects of care becoming the responsibility of the nursing home staff. However, it may also represent a degree of uncertainty amongst visitors regarding the roles that they may perform within such institutions. This is confirmed by the qualitative data gathered in this research project, which showed that many of the family members felt uncomfortable within the unfamiliar nursing home environment and uncertain of how to behave toward frail and demented residents. This uncertainty may restrict the range of caregiving tasks that visitors undertake. It may also make visiting particularly difficult for those family members who derived personal satisfaction and an enhanced closeness in their relationship with the resident from their former community-based caregiving role. Such difficulty may result in a feeling of discomfort and be reflected in a decreased duration of visit to nursing home residents. An interesting finding was that the duration of visit to residents was predicted by the level of community involvement within the nursing home, such as volunteer groups, support groups and fund-raising activity. Its association with longer duration of visit may further reflect the importance of the degree of comfort that visitors feel and the level of connection that the nursing home provides with the broader community. That is, visitors who feel more familiar with the nursing home and more at ease within it may stay for longer periods.

The focus on stress and burden, together with a lack of focus on the positive or more satisfying aspects of caregiving, suggests that caregiving is only or primarily a negative experience. When asked, however, caregivers provide a number of reasons for giving care including love, affection, reciprocity and commitment (Horowitz 1985). A province-wide Canadian study (Chappell & Litkenhaus 1995) reports that almost all (93.4 per cent) caregivers can list rewards to caregiving including, for example, seeing the care-receiver happy and watching them improve, the closeness of the relationship, and being able to help. Fully one-third say that the caregiving relationship is the closest relationship they have ever had with anyone in their lives and 40 per cent say that it is as close as any other relationship. Keating et al (1999) report that over three-quarters say they are giving back what has been given to them (87.7 per cent) and that it strengthens their relationship with their care-receiver (88.7 per cent).

Furthermore, when examining the actual prevalence figures of burden amongst caregivers, the vast majority do not emerge as overburdened and unable to cope. In the British Columbia study just noted, while two-thirds say that they find caregiving stressful, two-thirds of this group say that the burden is intermittent and only 9.2 per cent say it is extreme. Over 90 per cent say that they are coping well. Keating et al (1999) report nationally that only 18.2 per cent say they felt burdened in helping others. Schulz and Williamson (1991) report depressive symptomatology as stable amongst most caregivers, with most able to meet their demands without becoming dysfunctional. That is, most caregivers are not at risk of burnout, at risk of giving up caregiving, or at risk of becoming a major user of the health care system. This is despite the fact that the heavy focus in the caregiving literature on stress and burden suggests the opposite. The research linking personality characteristics to better coping and less burden suggests that caregivers higher on hardiness, sense of coherence and personal resiliency are likely to report less burden and better overall well-being, to use formal services less, and to be in better health (Braithwaite 1998; Mockler et al 1998).

Relatedly, we know little about the experience of caregiving. This is exemplified in the research on respite (referring to a pause in/or temporary cessation of caregiving tasks and an interval of rest). In practice and in research it is primarily referred to as a service or a group of services that provide periods of relief to caregivers (Feinberg & Kelly 1995). Services that explicitly target the caregiver rather than the care-recipient, for example, often include sitter attendants who come to the house and look after the care-recipient while the caregiver leaves the house to do shopping, etc.; day care or day hospital programs where the care-recipient is taken for a few hours; and respite beds in a facility where the care-receiver stays for days or weeks. Chappell et al (2001) have argued that researchers and service providers have gone astray in conceptualising respite as a service, that it is rather an outcome, something (relief, a break) the caregiver experiences.

Using in-depth qualitative interviews, and confirmation in a random sample of 250 caregivers in Victoria, Canada, Chappell et al (2001) derived a typology of what respite means to caregivers themselves. The resulting six meanings were different from what researchers and service providers assume, over half encompassing meanings that researchers and service providers had not referred to. 'Stolen moments' was the most prevalent category (48.1 per cent), referring to brief periods away from the actual tasks of caregiving, involving activities or situations that temporarily take the caregiver away from caregiver tasks but maintaining the daily caregiver routine. It includes all manner of activities, such as taking the dog for a walk, taking a bath, cooking, having a haircut, grocery shopping—activities that are done in the time 'stolen' from caregiving and generally referring to activities that must be done anyway. They provide a break from actual caregiving tasks. This research illustrates that it is time for researchers to turn increased attention to the experiences as lived by caregivers themselves. We turn to this topic next.

Caregiving and health reform

The 1990s saw the industrialised world focus on reform of their health care systems with an emergent vision that recognised family caregivers and embraced stronger community care. The new vision called for a broad definition of health that included, but went far beyond, a biomedical model, an emphasis away from hospital and institutional care toward care in the community, a focus on health promotion and disease prevention, and an embrace of informal caregivers in community care (Chappell 2001; Mahtre & Deber 1992). This widely accepted vision thus recognised caregivers but did not distinguish between informal/family care and community care. This lack of distinction has proved problematic because, if it is assumed that family care is equivalent to community care, it means an even greater demand on informal caregivers. Community care, on the other hand, calls for resources in order to build community infrastructure. That infrastructure includes the social components, such as homemaking services for ill and disabled persons in their own homes, transportation to and from appointments, and community support groups, as well as formal educational and recreational systems. It calls for an infrastructure that will facilitate community development.

While there has been much restructuring, particularly since the mid-1990s, there has been virtually no attention directed towards health promotion and disease prevention or to building the formal community support system. Indeed, recent evidence (for example, from Canada) suggests the opposite—community support is turning into intensive post-acute care and a medical support system while traditional support for the long-term chronic care so needed by older people is being dismantled (McDaniel & Chappell 1999; Chappell 2001). Research by Penning et al (1998) reveals increased dollars to home care have resulted in fewer people receiving more hours of service and in greater need as measured by level of care. There is a redirection of home care services from clients who are less needy and therefore may have the greatest potential for prevention. This interpretation is supported by evidence that surgeries are increasingly being performed on an out-patient basis, to the point where some hospitals are performing 80 per cent of their surgeries on this basis (Deber et al 1998). This is similar to the experience with diagnostic related groups in the United States when they became the funding formulae for acute care hospitals. Earlier discharges from hospital and increased demand for intensive post-acute home care resulted in a restriction of social services available through home care (Estes & Wood 1986).

The recently released Kirby and Romanow Reports on Canada's health care system both recommend the government begin with a national post-acute home care program—which will reinforce home care as a type of medical support program. And yet, recent Canadian evidence demonstrates that home care can be a cost effective substitute for long-term institutional care. Hollander and Tessaro (2001) compared four health units that differentially implemented cuts to 'homemaking only' services. Regions making these cuts paid for more services for the individuals who were cut three years later, through their greater use of hospital beds, increased use of homemaker services in the second and third years after the cuts, and increased rates of admission to nursing homes, than regions not cutting the service. It is important to note that the greater overall costs did not emerge immediately. In addition, a higher proportion of those who were cut from the service died.

Restructuring and privatisation of services has also had an impact on the residential aged care industry contributing to the rise of larger, more cost-effective facilities located in urban centres. This trend away from smaller facilities has had a particular impact on older persons living in rural areas. In a study of rural nursing homes, Joseph and Chalmers (1996) found that a combination of factors has led to the decline of services for the elderly in rural New Zealand. These factors, the increased cost of care in metropolitan nursing homes and the decline of rural community-based services, leave older people who elect to 'stay on' in the rural area with a dramatic decline in available and affordable supports and services. These older people are faced with declining community and domiciliary support and loss of access to local residential aged care facilities. A further exacerbation of this problem is the decline of the population and the economic base in rural areas and the out-migration of younger members of the community (Keeling 2001) which contributes to a generally older age profile of these communities. Such rural older people are isolated in small, relatively poor communities which lack the resources to support them in their own homes and forces those who cannot afford to move to a metropolitan nursing home to live in less than ideal circumstances. Those who remain in their service-poor rural locations into their infirm years are therefore disadvantaged in terms of care services. This raises the question of how small rural communities will care for their aged as the elderly population expands and the services to rural communities decline.

Hollander and Chappell (2002), analysing costs to government of home care clients compared with long-term residential care clients for several years at the same level of care, reveal that costs for home care clients are 40 per cent to 70 per cent of the costs of facility care depending on the level of care (lower levels of care have a greater differential). The costs of home care are in the transitions, that is, those who change their type or level of care cost considerably more than clients who remain within their level of care even though transition individuals still cost less than facility clients. In a separate study, Chappell et al (2003) compared overall societal costs, including costs to families as well as to governments, in two Canadian cities. Again they report home care cost less than long-term residential care even when costs of informal caregiving are set at replacement wage value. Other research (Allan & Penning 2001) shows that in the 1990s, as hospital outpatient surgeries were increasing, hospital lengths of stay were decreasing and home care was shifting to a medical support system for intensive post-acute care following hospital discharge, the utilisation of costly physician services, especially specialist services, was increasing.

At the present time the forces of the globalisation of American-style capitalism appear to be resulting in a dismantling of the welfare state, at least in the area of health care services. Health reform, for example in Canada and Australia, suggests fewer services delivered less comprehensively—a retrenchment to the biomedical model of health as opposed to the broad vision of health care as proposed in the many visions for a new health care system launched in the early 1990s.

Cultural differences

Gerontological research on social support and caregiving has been conducted primarily in the United States, although other western countries, including Australia and Canada and a variety of European countries (notably the United Kingdom), have also been researching this area for some time. A minority of this research examines caregiving amongst subcultures within the host country (older Chinese people in Canada, older Korean people in the United States, etc.). Recently there has been increased interest in national comparisons to explore cultural differences as well as a growth in the attention to the area within other countries such as China. We shall explore this area of cultural differences in caregiving briefly here with reference to Chinese seniors living in China.

Asian cultures, and China in particular, have long been noted as culturally different from western societies. Chinese culture is known for filial piety, respect and care for older people, and familism (Streib 1987; Chen et al 1996), notions that are being questioned in present-day China, most noticeably in the Chinese (rather than English) research literature. Liu (1994), for example, argues that it is no longer adequate to point to the traditional role of the family as caring for older people, that expectations and conditions have seen profound change in China as elsewhere. Similarly, Xia and Ma (1995) note that cultural values have been changing. Empirical studies are inconsistent. McKinnon et al (2001) report that even older people living with their children feel distant from them, yet Gui (2001) reports that, in Shanghai, older people overwhelmingly want their children and grandchildren to live with them, provide care and pay for their care. Zhu et al (1994) report that in Beijing it is the old-old and those who are widowed who are more likely to live alone. Xia and Ma (1995) reveal from a 1987 national survey that only 6.9 per cent of older people were cared for by their children, and 5.3 per cent by their spouse. Ikels (1990), more than a decade ago, argued that it was a housing shortage rather than traditional values of co-residence that kept the generations living together.

Recent research (Chappell 2003) comparing older people in Shanghai and non-Chinese older people in Canada, suggests some interesting similarities and differences in caregiving across cultures. Those data suggest that some common stereotypes concerning caregiving in China, with its historical emphasis on collectivist values including filial piety, and materialistic western culture, may no longer be true. There were important differences in living situations—older people in Shanghai have much less formal education than those in Canada, are much more likely to rent than own their dwelling, are much more likely to live in an abode where they have no independent room to call their own and are considerably less well off financially. And the Chinese elderly in Shanghai (this is also true of Chinese elderly living in Canada), are much more likely to receive financial assistance from kin, especially children, than is true of non-Chinese Canadian elderly. In Shanghai, older people are in worse health, and receive fewer formal services.

In terms of social support, whether for an emergency, as confidantes or for companionship, Shanghai Chinese tend to choose their sons, rather than a spouse or daughter as in the west. However, when examining the correlates of life satisfaction, social support and health emerge as the major predictors, as they do in the many studies conducted in the west. Those with more social support and in better health report higher life satisfaction. Importantly, the form the social support takes differs; sons are more important in China, consistent with cultural values that prefer sons. Similarly, amongst caregivers, their situations differ. In Shanghai, caregivers spend considerably more hours per day at this task yet are less likely to have work interruptions. However, they are not necessarily more burdened as a result. In examining the correlates of burden, it is the deteriorated health conditions of the care-receiver that is significant, as has been the case in many western studies. In other words, the data suggest tremendous differences in living situations in the two countries but also reveal that when it comes to subjective quality of life, whether in terms of life satisfaction for older people or burden for caregivers, there are universal predictors. The forms that these predictors take, whether the type of social support or the particular health problems, vary between cultures.

The area of cross-cultural differences in social support and caregiving is only now receiving more attention in some non-western countries. As this research accumulates, we will learn more about similarities and differences.

Activity 8.2

This chapter has raised a number of issues related to the provision of care for the elderly. The following are some questions for you to consider in relation to this topic.

- Write down a list of people you believe will care for you in old age should this become necessary. If there is more than one person on your list, how will these people divide the tasks of care between them? Which people will perform which tasks? Are there aspects of care you would like performed by some and not by others? Why?

- Who will you be responsible to care for in their old age? Do you expect that such care will be required? What aspects of care do you anticipate will be most rewarding and which do you think will be most burdensome? Will there be anyone available and willing to assist you with this care? What formal care services are available to assist you? What are your feelings about the use of formal care services and residential aged care facilities?

Conclusion

The area of social support and caregiving has a long history within gerontology, for good reason—it is tremendously important for us as we age. The state in modern industrialised societies has never totally replaced private arrangements, and those private arrangements have been assumed, by and large, by the nuclear family. However, the extent to which informal caregivers are now recognised and applauded is new, and it is the cornerstone of the new vision of health care around the world.

Much knowledge has been gained, but there is much yet to be learned, from caregivers themselves. One thing that appears clear is that the importance of social support and caregiving does not diminish over time or across cultures. People caring for people, fortunately, seems to be characteristically human. The challenge is to learn how to best support people helping others. We are therefore directed to new questions for study in our search for greater understanding of the meaning and experience of caregiving and how we can best ensure that we care for one another throughout the life span.

9

Delivery of care for older people

Lyndall Spencer

It is widely acknowledged today that the provision of services to older persons represents a significant financial impost on societies in the developed world. The World Health Organization (WHO 2000) indicates that countries such as Canada, Australia, the United States and Japan are striving to meet the triple challenges of assuring quality of care, guaranteeing equity of access to services for potential users while, at the same time, attempting to be cost effective and use their nations' taxpayer-funded resources to best possible effect.

A related issue concerns the rise in the number of older people as a proportion of the whole population. In Australia, for example, the *National Strategy for an Ageing Australia* (Bishop 1999a,b) indicated that the ageing of the population has accelerated in the past two decades and is projected to rise further over the next 30 years. In addition, the greatest increase is occurring in the very old, those aged 85 years and over (Kinnear 2001). While this does not necessarily signify a problem, Mason et al (2001) indicate that the probability of entering an aged care home after turning 65 is 0.42 for women and 0.24 for men. Further, Liu (1998) commented that almost all women over 90 years and many extremely old men will do so. Thus aged care policy makers, managers of residential facilities and members of the wider community need to be prepared for future increases in service demand with a concomitant rise in associated costs. This challenge is also being faced elsewhere. Statistics Canada (2002), for example, highlights that amongst all the developed countries Canada, along with Japan, has the most rapidly ageing population with an increase not only in relative and absolute numbers of those aged 65 years and over, but particularly in the oldest segment of the population. Between 1991 and 2000, the Canadian population aged over 80 years increased by 41 per cent to 930 000 and by 2011 this cohort will have passed an estimated 1.3 million people. As noted by Tirrito (2003) in his book, *Aging in the New Millennium*, the United Nations predicts that by 2050 the number of people aged 85 and over will experience a sixfold increase and the number of people aged 100 and over, a sixteenfold increase. By the year 2030 one in four persons in the developed world will be aged 65 or older. In Florida, USA today 19 per cent of the population are seniors. Japan will hit this mark in 2005 as will Germany in 2006.

A short history of aged care service delivery

In many developed countries, until the early 20th century older persons came to public attention only if they were recipients of care in institutions for the destitute. This highlighted two issues that the community was obliged to address: income support and accommodation and shelter for those too old and frail to meet their needs independently. In 1909 the Australian government became one of the first to legislate for the provision of aged and invalid pensions, and in so doing attempted to tackle the matter of income support for the aged. A variety of services came into being to meet their shelter and care needs.

Residential care

During the four decades that succeeded the 1909 legislation, charitable organisations throughout Australia established cottage-type housing facilities, serving communal meals, for older citizens with limited means (Kendig & McCullam 1990). In 1954 the *Aged Persons Homes Act* was passed to provide matching government funds directly to voluntary organisations to accommodate older couples and allocated a capital subsidy to approved not-for-profit organisations to support self-contained and hostel-type services. In 1966 the capital subsidy was incorporated into the provision of nursing home and hostel beds, subject to limitations on the proportions in each service area. Nursing home beds occupied by the voluntary sector could now attract both capital and recurrent funding. In 1969 recurrent subsidies were also made available to hostel residents with substantial disabilities.

The *Nursing Homes' Assistance Act 1974* provided an alternative method of financing not-for-profit homes via a subsidy equal to the home's operating deficit. As Gibson (1998) identified, this resulted in a large (47 per cent) increase in not-for-profit nursing homes between 1975 and 1980, compared with a more modest (7 per cent) increase in private-for-profit establishments in the same period.

The for-profit sector had been a component of the industry more or less since its inception, largely as an extension of the private hospital and convalescence homes established in the 1950s, available for long-term patients needing nursing care who belonged to a private health insurance fund. Private-for-profit providers were also eligible to receive recurrent subsidy for residents in their care. In 1974 the *Aged Persons Homes Act* was retitled the *Aged or Disabled Persons Homes Act* and expanded its provisions to include services for handicapped adults of all ages.

The 1980s saw the development of the *Aged Care Reform Strategy* following a series of investigations into nursing home and community based services. In 1986 the health of older people was declared a national priority under the *Health for All Australians* policy developed by the (then) Better Health Commission. During the following year the Australian government implemented new recurrent funding strategies and in-service training for nursing home staff. It also established the Users Rights Advocacy Service and the Charter of Residents Rights and Responsibilities (Rolands et al 1989). From 1 July 1987 nursing homes began a gradual transition to a uniform national funding level for infrastructure costs, known as the standard aggregated module (SAM). Deficit funding of homes was revoked from this date and outcome standards were implemented.

One other change to emerge by 1987 was the inception of criteria for eligibility to enter residential care. Prior to this, entry into nursing homes had been determined largely by general medical practitioners and government medical officers, in collaboration with managerial teams in each sector of the industry. This resulted in a process that lacked both rigour and consistency. In 1985, a pilot system was developed whereby a team of professional aged care practitioners, known ultimately as Aged Care Assessment

Teams (ACATs), determined eligibility for entry into nursing homes. These teams incorporated representatives from many of the disciplines associated with the provision of services for the aged including doctors, nurses, social workers and therapists of various kinds. They were established to conduct physical and psychosocial assessments of potential residents to ascertain their need for care and the level of care needed. By 1987 national guidelines for admission had been established. While each state developed its own processes, in all circumstances eligibility was determined by the individual scores on a nationally consistent set of dependency items. The process of eligibility assessment expanded progressively in the 1990s to include entry into hostels. Further, psychogeriatric units established within the ACAT structure in 1994 enabled the assessment process to take into account the challenges of older people with cognitive impairment.

The numbers of beds necessary to accommodate dependent older people was a matter for community debate more or less since the establishment of subsidies and was the subject of regular revisions (Gregory 1993, 1994; Gibson & Liu 1995). By 1993 the national residential care planning ratios were 52.5 hostel places, 40 nursing home places and 7.5 Community Aged Care Packages (CACP) per 1000 people aged 70 years and over. They were amended in 1995 to 50 hostel places 40 nursing homes places and 10 CACPs.

The current principles that govern the Australian aged care sector emerged in the 1990s. Paramount amongst them is the *National Strategy for an Ageing Australia* (Bishop 1999b), which incorporated an assortment of legislation and regulations including the *Aged Care Act 1997*, the Standards for Aged Care Facilities (Department of Health and Family Services 1997b) and the Residential Care Guidelines (Department of Health and Family Services 1997a). Their historical foundation was, in part, the framework that emerged in June 1987 through the publication of a groundbreaking report entitled *Living in a Nursing Home: Outcome Standards for Australian Nursing Homes*. This heralded the beginning of monitoring the performance of Australian nursing homes, and the quality of the care they provided for their residents.

In 1997 a new policy direction was introduced that incorporated five strategic positions with which the industry was obliged to comply by 1 January 2001, or cease to receive subsidies for the care it delivered. The five reforms depicted in the *Aged Care Act 1997* included a mandatory system of accreditation for care provided in nursing homes and hostels, and certification for all the buildings and grounds in which this care is delivered. In addition, prudential arrangements were incorporated to protect resident accommodation bonds, concessional resident ratios for financially disadvantaged older people were determined, and a protocol was put into place to familiarise residents with their rights and responsibilities.

Community care

Community-based care has also claimed high levels of funds over the decades. Until 1985 when the Home and Community Care (HACC) program was introduced, services in the community were provided through four separate programs under several pieces of legislation. These comprised the *Nursing Home Subsidy Act* (1957), the *States Grants (Home Care) Act* (1969), the *States Grants (Paramedical Services) Act* (1969) and the *Delivered Meals Subsidy Act* of 1970.

In its seminal 1994 report on the HACC program, *Home But Not Alone*, the House of Representatives Standing Committee on Community Affairs indicated that HACC operates as a partnership between participants in community care, including governments, service providers, consumers and their carers. The Commonwealth is responsible for financial assistance to the States and Territories for the provision of community care, plus monitoring HACC funding expenditure and maintenance of national data base systems. The States and Territories are responsible for the day-to-day management of the program. A range of providers including local government, community organisations and religious and other not-for-profit organisations provide service delivery. The exact structure and relationship varies between states.

Another community-based service available to frail older people in need of hostel-level care was introduced in 1992, the Community Aged Care Packages (CACPs) scheme. Eligibility to receive these services is also determined by ACAT assessment and assistance may take one of several forms. These include: clinical care, support for activities of daily living and some domestic duties. Early in the 21st century a further service based on high care levels of need was also introduced. Entitled the Extended Aged Care at Home (EACH) program, this service is considered to be a pilot study providing help in private residences for people who would normally require nursing home levels of assistance. Its future remains unknown.

In 2002, of the people aged 70 years and over in the population, about 7.9 per cent were in residential care, 0.7 per cent received Community Aged Care Packages (CACP) and 12.2 per cent received HACC services (Department of Health and Ageing, 2002, p. 7). There are about 4000 Home and Community Care funded services providing resources to approximately 300 000 people at any given time or about 470 000 people per year with about a 5 per cent monthly turnover.

During the same period the United States was also addressing issues of income support and the provision of care and accommodation for its older people, according to the Centers for Medicare and Medicaid Services (2003). In 1965 the *Social Security Act* established both Medicare and Medicaid. Medicare was a responsibility of the Social Security Administration (SSA), while federal assistance to the state Medicaid programs was administered by the Social and Rehabilitation Service (SRS). SSA and SRS were agencies in the Department of Health Education and Welfare (HEW). In 1977 the Health Care Financing Administration (HCFA) was created under HEW to coordinate Medicare and Medicaid effectively. In 1980 HEW was divided into the Department of Education and the Department of Health and Human Services, and in 2001 HCFA was renamed the Centers for Medicare and Medicaid Services (CMS). The present CMS is the federal agency that administers the Medicare program that provides coverage to approximately 40 million Americans (2003). It is the national health insurance program for people aged 65 years or older, together with some who are younger than 65 but with disabilities, and all people with end-stage renal disease regardless of age.

In the United Kingdom, the social security benefit system offers financial assistance for elderly people to complement the health and social services provided by the National Health Service and local authorities. Around 11 million Britons were in receipt of one or other of these benefits in 1998, 78 per cent of whom receive a retirement pension (Office of National Statistics UK 2004).

Models of service delivery

In common with many developed countries, within the Australian context there are two principal modes of aged care service delivery: in the community and within residential facilities. In each, a variety of models prevails. As most government funds are directed towards residential care these services will be addressed first.

Residential services

Three models of service delivery apply in residential settings across the nation—one of which is self-funded and the other two dependent to a greater or lesser degree on federal government subsidies. The first comprises a range of independent living arrangements attached in one way or another to communities of retirees and auspiced by commercial proprietors, not-for-profit organisations or local governments. Residences may include stand-alone cottage-type dwellings or, more usually, semi-detached villa-type apartments, units or town houses. Older people who choose to live in these centres purchase a title to the property in a manner not dissimilar to any other real estate purchase. They receive the security of tenure associated with ownership of conventional real estate, within certain prescribed constraints. They share common property such as landscaped gardens, outdoor facilities like barbecues or sporting equipment and pay a maintenance fee, usually quarterly, to support the upkeep of these resources. Ultimately this property may become a component in its owner's estate should he or she die while in residence.

As with all property owned jointly, residents in these units are obliged to comply with any occupancy rules such as the permissibility or otherwise of pets, numbers, frequencies and times of guests, and similar regulations. The precise nature of the rules varies from facility to facility, but each organisation that sponsors accommodation of this type must provide a handbook or other documentation detailing the rights and responsibilities of owners who join the community prior to any purchase being completed. Incorporated in this document are any conditions which would apply should it be necessary to reconsider the occupancy status of residents, including conditions of purchase or repurchase if the owner is obliged to vacate the premises for reasons such as the non-payment of maintenance fees. In a small number of cases it may be possible to rent accommodation in villages of this type, although it is much more usual for occupants to purchase the property. There are no limitations or eligibility criteria connected with entry to this type of accommodation other than having the purchase/rental price, funds to meet any additional services and being willing to comply with the 'house rules'.

Other forms of independent living include rental in the general market, serviced apartments and boarding houses. The latter two rarely offer value-added services, but may have house rules of their own with which seniors must agree to comply. Fees are usually at commercial rates for the area in which the facility is located, and security of tenure is seldom an option other than traditional lease arrangements in the private rental sector, with service providers free to terminate the arrangement in common with other landlords.

Of greater consequence to taxpayers are the models of residential service delivery that incorporate some level of therapeutic intervention for which specialised staff must be employed to ensure its delivery. Traditionally these models have been segregated into services which provide low levels of care and which were known as hostels, and services that delivered high levels of care entitled nursing homes.

With the advent of the *Aged Care Act 1997*, accommodation services were incorporated into a single delivery mode entitled a residential aged care facility. They are governed by a philosophical approach to service provision described as 'ageing in place', where possible suppliers aspire to ensure that residents are able to remain in their location of origin but receive increasing levels of services as they become more frail. The formal difference between a hostel and a nursing home may have disappeared from legislation, but in practice the wider community continues to make the colloquial distinction, perhaps in part because many facilities designed as hostels are ill equipped to deliver the more intensive level of services required by high care residents as they age.

Funding associated with the provision of residential care is drawn from several sources. In addition to government subsidies, residents are obliged to make a contribution. For people whose only income is the Aged Pension, it is usual to contribute 85 per cent of their pension to meet the cost of their care. For those who have other income such as superannuation, money from investments or other sources, additional daily charges apply according to an established means-tested standard. In addition, amongst those entering hostel level establishments a proportion of those with income in addition to the pension will be required to pay a means-tested admission fee previously called an entry bond. The exact amount for the entry fee is determined by the service provider, who is obliged to ensure that residents retain a specified minimum amount in assets.

A further residential care model available to older people and their carers is that of residential respite care. Individuals may receive up to nine weeks of service in a residential setting. This permits older people who normally dwell in the community to receive supported accommodation, thereby enabling them (and/or their carers) to have a break from each other. Not all facilities maintain respite beds, and some require an ACAT assessment to determine the potential resident's eligibility for the service. However, it is a useful option for those in need of a reprieve from the challenges of living in the community.

Ribbe et al (1997) conducted a comparison between nursing homes in ten nations to illustrate demographic differences and recent trends in the provision and models of care in long-term settings. Seven European countries participated—Denmark, France, Iceland, Italy, The Netherlands, Sweden and Switzerland—as did the United Kingdom, the United States and Japan. Taxpayers in all participating nations to a greater or lesser degree subsidise the care given to their seniors in nursing homes. Between 2 per cent and 5 per cent of older people in the participating countries reside in nursing homes, a figure comparable with Australia. Interestingly, Iceland, the 'youngest country' in this study, had the highest rate of institutional living, but no relationship appeared to exist between the ageing status of the country and the number of nursing home beds. Characteristics which were seen to be significant included differences in the organisation of long-term services, in the amount of responsibility assumed in the care for elderly people by each sector, and the availability of long-term beds.

Community-based services

In addition to the provision of residential care for seniors, Australia supports several models of service delivery into their own homes. Mention has been made previously of the Community Aged Care Packages model and the pilot Extended Aged Care at Home (EACH) program. Other types of services include delivered meals via the Meals on Wheels program. While subsidised, it also attracts a user-pays contribution from the majority of its clients. Referral to this service is usually through the client's general practitioner or a community nurse familiar with the client's circumstances. Domiciliary nursing is available for older people with significant clinical need, such as being recently discharged from an acute care facility. Home help is a service often provided by state or local government in which housekeeping and/or other home maintenance needs can be met. A modest fee may be attached to the provision of home help but it is usually based on the cost of materials alone, with labour either provided by volunteers or subsidised by government.

The preeminent model of community-based service delivery is that of the Home and Community Care (HACC) program. Designed to focus on the psychosocial rather than clinical care needs of older people and disabled younger adults, HACC offers a range of services. These may include assistance with the activities of daily living, leisure interests, entertainment and transport, amongst others. HACC programs are offered in purpose-built day centres as well as senior citizen facilities and private homes, depending on the client's needs. In some instances all HACC fees are met by one of the three tiers of government. In other circumstances clients are requested to make a financial contribution towards the cost of the service they receive, usually calculated according to their means.

Respite is also available in the community. Older people may be entitled to receive several hours a week or month in a day respite centre, thereby freeing their family carer to undertake private activities or simply be relived of the responsibility for caring. Respite centres almost always maintain their own transport, usually in the form of a bus, which enables them to collect and return clients to their homes, thus relieving them and their carers of the challenges associated with the use of public transport. Respite centres and many senior citizen centres provide a hot midday meal for clients at a modest fee. Older people or their carers may be referred to community respite by local health care workers, clergy, or other industry gatekeepers.

Another model of service delivery in the community is founded in the voluntary sector. Organisations such as the Alzheimer's Association, National Seniors and the Carers Association draw on the strength and experience of their members to meet shared needs. In some instances these organisations receive subsidies from one or other of the tiers of government, while others are self-funding. The nature of the services they provide varies widely, from practical help to education, entertainment, legal and financial advice, amongst others.

The American Health Care Association (2003) points out that, in the United States, under the traditional system for the delivery of home and community based care, the states contract with home care agencies to provide home care workers, direct services and monitoring of the quality of care delivered to clients. With the rise of the Independent Living Movement in the 1970s clients began to reject the agency-directed model in favour of a more consumer-directed model where the client could choose the type and relative amount of services to be received. Although consumer choice of services has implications for the quality of care received by the client, as research by Doty et al (1998) indicates, most consumers prefer to have choice and are generally more satisfied with services when they have control over the type and provider of those services. Further, as Glickman et al (1997) indicate, consumer-directed care is not for everyone, particularly clients with cognitive difficulties, and those who may be unaccustomed or uncomfortable with hiring, paying or firing personal assistants.

In the United Kingdom, major developments in domiciliary care did not come until World War II, and by the 1970s over half of all home care cases were related to people aged 65 years and older. The General Household Survey of 2001–02 (Office of Statistics UK 2004a, b) found that 2 per cent of those aged 65–69 years had used the District Nurse, Home Health Visitor or some other personal social service in the month before the interview. Amongst those aged 85 and over the figure was 19 per cent.

Defining quality of life and quality of care

As demand for residential and community care proliferates, the need to ensure adequate standards and quality in each setting becomes more urgent. In the opinion of Bartlett and Burnip (1998), the challenges faced by service providers in achieving acceptable standards, taking into consideration quality of life and quality of care, have not been adequately explored.

Quality of life

It is widely acknowledged that 'quality of life' is an imprecise concept which is difficult to define (Bowling 1997; Byrne and MacLean 1997; Ball et al 2000). While there have been many attempts, a consensus of opinion has yet to be achieved. McDowell and Newell (1996, p. 32) described 'quality of life' as an intuitively familiar term, suggesting that everyone believes that they know what it means while, in reality, the meaning differs from person to person. This disparity has resulted in the development of many scales that purport to measure 'quality of life', an outcome not without its limitations. As McDowell and Newell (1996, p. 492) note: 'This embarrassment of riches . . . militates against understanding and acceptance of these types of measures for clinical research and clinical practice.' The literature (Fletcher et al 1992; Steward et al 1996) reveals that definitions of quality of life include both objective and subjective components. Courtney et al (2003) identified three broad categories: those which focus on objective indices, such as economic circumstances, housing and functional status; those which measure purely subjective aspects, such as morale, happiness and life satisfaction; and those which contain both objective and subjective components, such as the health-related quality of life measures. Courtney et al (2003) speculate that health-related quality of life measures have proliferated over the last two decades in part as a consequence of an increasing interest in health outcomes beyond simple survival rates. This is of particular interest within the aged care context, given the increasing life spans of people within developed and developing nations, and an associated increased risk of disabilities or chronic conditions which have the potential to compromise the quality of life. Frytak (2000), however, cautions against the concept of health-related quality of life, suggesting that the focus on health inherent in such definitions narrows and limits the concept.

According to Stewart et al (1996), one of the other challenges for quality of life research with older people is that the cohort represents an extremely heterogeneous population. Within the 65 years and over group, people range from those who are healthy and functioning independently in the community to those who are frail, in very poor health and in need of supported accommodation and care. However, the researchers do acknowledge that mean scores on health indicators tend to decline with age.

Frytak (2000) suggested that broader concepts of quality of life are necessary for older people and that the psychosocial domain becomes particularly important, especially in the context of declining physical health. Kane (2000) found that older people often score more highly than younger adults in psychosocial aspects of well-being, as well as for subjective impressions of quality of life, despite poorer physical health. It has also been found, however, that expectations of quality of life amongst seniors decline with increasing age. Kane (2000, p. 526) further cautions, 'the well are prone to discounting the value of a disabled life, but many people with disabilities seem to cling to their lives all the same'.

Quality of care

Donabedian (1966) made the simple point that the definition of good quality care can be almost anything one wishes it to be. Mooney (2000) expressed similar views three decades later. For example, principal amongst Australian notions of quality of aged care are those set out in the *National Strategy for an Ageing Australia* (Bishop 1999a). By implication this document suggests that the provision of care includes the nurturing of and attention to older persons by other members of the community. It also encompasses attributes such as sensitivity to their needs, forethought to ensure these needs are met and the protection of their interests. The American Health Care Association (2003) echoes these sentiments in terms of quality of care in the community, while Philips et al (1997) demonstrate how quality might be measured in nursing home settings with reference to four international sites in Denmark, Iceland, Italy and the United States.

It was noted in the discussion on quality of life that the health status of the individual has profound implications for their perceptions of their own well-being. Insofar as those aged 65 years and over are able to meet their own physical and psychosocial daily requirements, their perceived care needs do not differ significantly from those of younger age groups. This finding does not apply amongst those with compromised health, especially those who live in residential care, as Guse and Masesar (1999) indicate. In this chapter, consideration of quality of care for older people will focus primarily on the provision of services to meet the health and daily living needs of those unable to accomplish these goals independently.

Balancing costs with quality of life and quality of care

The need to balance the costs of service delivery with quality of life and quality of care for service consumers has preoccupied aged care policy makers for at least a decade. As Withers (1994) pointed out in his foreword to an Economic Planning Advisory Council report: 'Pessimists point to what they see as unsustainable demands on public social expenditures from an ageing population structure, while optimists point to the constructive and increased roles they see the aged as playing in our society.'

The Department of Health and Ageing repeated the message in 2002 when it stated that the purpose of Australia's aged and community care program is to support healthy ageing for older Australians and quality, cost-effective care for frail older people and support for their carers. Furthermore, it established a Quality Outcomes Branch within the overall department responsible for a range of quality improvement mechanisms for the aged care program including compliance functions and managing a number of key funding and accountability issues.

Anticipated changes in the demographic structure described earlier will add to pressures on government to develop aged care policies and programs that are effective and affordable. It could be argued that the policy agenda for the aged, particularly in the past, has been over-medicalised and that this has been a fundamental contributor to the high cost of services. With the introduction of the HACC program and CACP, services that focus on 'care in the community' rather than 'cure in institutions', Australians may look forward to a time when the cost of caring for frail aged in residential facilities, if not the community, may be more contained.

One issue that must be addressed in the debate between cost containment and quality of life and/or care concerns hidden costs. While the cost to government of looking after an aged person in residential care is high, and care in the community involves fewer public outlays (Department of Health and Ageing 2002), there are substantial private costs associated with providing care at home to be considered.

The role of the informal caregiver, such as spouse or child, is a fundamental issue that needs to be factored into any cost-benefit analysis (see Chapter 8). If family carers elect to remain in the workforce, the challenges of fulfilling obligations to employers as well as caring for loved ones not infrequently results in the diminution of carer health or well-being with its associated claims on Medicare and the health care sector. Carers who abandon careers to attend to the needs of loved ones have the potential to become claimants on the state as recipients of carer or unemployment benefits. Demand on respite services may also expand as carer and care-recipient seek to obtain relief from exposure to each other for short periods. Individual care-recipients are also more likely to be obliged to meet fees for services, such as the use of a physiotherapist or other therapists, privately. In residential facilities, the federal government allocates subsidies for therapeutic services such as these.

A range of solutions to the cost of care problems has been suggested over the past decade. Clare and Tulpulé (1994) debated the merits of universal insurance for long-stay care. They also addressed the possibility of increasing migration rates to overcome the diminution in Australia's fertility rate, thereby expanding the workforce and providing increased sources of taxation revenue. To the present, policy makers have adopted neither option.

Campbell and Ikegami (2000) note that, in Japan, mandatory long-term care insurance for seniors was introduced in that country on 1 April 2000 with a view to cost containment amongst other goals. Long-term care insurance covers both institutional and community-based care provision and every person aged 40 years and over pays premiums. Everyone aged 65 and over is eligible for benefits, based strictly on physical disability in six categories of need. Benefits take the form of service provision with no cash allowance for family care and are generally valued at 90 per cent of need. Consumers can use whatever services and providers they prefer including the use of for-profit companies.

Gender issues are important in the debate, throughout western countries, over costs and quality outcomes (Gibson 1998). The bulk of government-provided aged pensions plus care subsidies in residential facilities are received by females. This reflects both their longer average life expectancy and their traditionally lower involvement in the paid workforce and superannuation schemes of the past. Changes to superannuation arrangements which facilitate female membership over broken periods of employment for reasons such as child bearing, combined with increased participation rates by females in the paid workforce, may help redress the imbalance in the future.

Another strategy for aged care service cost containment, which simultaneously enhances quality of life, is to target the relatively high incidence of risky behaviours amongst young males. Health promotion activities to minimise alcohol and substance abuse, high-speed driving and similar potentially dangerous behaviours may achieve positive long-term savings for men to enable them to reach retirement age in greater numbers for minimal government outlays.

An additional issue which has implications for both expenditure and quality outcomes and therefore should be included in the debate concerns the labour required to meet care needs. Gibson (1998) has identified that the majority of both professional and informal care providers (as well as care-recipients) are female (see also Chapter 8). Further, family care providers have been women traditionally, as are the vast majority of volunteer caregivers. The same is true for professional care providers, irrespective of whether they are nurses, social workers or other welfare officers.

However, it would be unwise for policy makers to rely on this source of labour into the future. Female participation rates in the paid workforce in most western countries have more than doubled in recent decades, which leaves many fewer individuals to provide care for family members, labour in voluntary organisations such as the Alzheimer's Association and so on. Further, the difficulty of recruiting workers of either gender into the caring professions such as nursing has been widely documented (McCallum 2002), with little evidence of change apparent in the foreseeable future.

Measuring quality

Quality of life

A wide range of measurement tools has been developed to determine quality of life, possibly due to both the absence of a cohesive definition and the subjective nature of the concept (Arnold 1991; McDowell & Newell 1996). Further, Frytak (2000) suggested that the 'gold standard' for health-related quality of life measures should include physical, psychological and social health as well as global perceptions of health and well-being. In addition, as already discussed, health status and physical functioning in health-related quality of life instruments often have such a strong emphasis that any resident in a nursing home, for example, would appear to have very limited quality of life if measured by these instruments alone.

A further challenge associated with the measurement of quality of life concerns differences in perceptions between older people themselves, their families and friends, and the clinicians applying the measurement tool. Consequently, there is some debate in the quality of life literature over whether reports from independent representatives should be used. Frytak (2000) and

Stewart et al (1996) advocated against such a practice, stating that only in the most extreme cases should it be considered, given the highly subjective nature of quality of life. Byrne and MacLean (1997) agreed, finding that when nurses assisted residents with responses to a quality of life questionnaire, the ratings tended to be higher than when residents responded independently. Paradoxically, when other staff or family members assisted residents, their ratings tended to be lower than resident-only responses. Hence, measures should be as client-centred as possible, in the view of Arnold (1991), and self-report tools should be preferred over observational tools, except in cases of significant cognitive or communication impairments. When obtaining consumer feedback from clients of home-based community care services, the majority of whom were older people, Cooper and Jenkins (1998) found that self-report tools and client-centred instruments more accurately represented their clients' views.

The ambiguity associated with measuring quality of life does not apply to the same degree with measuring quality of care, although there is also a wide range of instruments available to attempt this process. Again using Australia as an example, prior to the implementation of the conditions of the *Aged Care Act* in 1997 a variety of quality systems were available for voluntary implementation. None of them had a specific focus on the provision and measurement of quality care for seniors, although each could be modified or reconfigured for application in aged care services.

Measuring quality of care in residential settings

Currently within the Australian industry there are two instruments that contribute to measuring quality in all residential facilities that receive government subsidies. While not necessarily designed with that purpose exclusively in mind, each is driven by a philosophy of continuous quality improvement and each addresses the quality of clinical and psychosocial aspects of care for residents.

The care delivered by the residential sector of the industry is governed by a set of four Accreditation Standards with a combined set of 44 outcomes with which providers must comply. They consider all manner of attributes, from management practices to sleep patterns, skin care and aspects of the environmental setting. These are addressed in more detail in the section below on Accreditation and Best Practice.

The second instrument used in all residential facilities is the Resident Classification Scale (RCS). Designed primarily as a funding tool, the RCS focuses on 20 aspects of service and care that are provided at one of eight levels. Those in receipt of Level 1 care are individuals in need of greatest support, who receive the highest levels of subsidy and are accommodated in what was previously termed a nursing home. Those nominated as eligible for Level 8 care do not receive any subsidies for their care. They are perceived to have retained considerable degrees of independence and traditionally would have been accommodated in hostels.

The 20 aspects of care addressed by the RCS (Department of Health & Family Services 1998) include communication skills, mobility, meals and drinks, personal hygiene, bladder and bowel management, understanding and undertaking living activities, problem wandering or intrusive behaviour, verbal disruption and noise, physical aggression, emotional dependence, danger to self or others, other [problematic] behaviour, the social and human needs of the care-recipient and the social and human needs of family and friends, medication, technical and complex nursing procedures, therapy and other services. Each is graded into one of four categories from A, in which a person is able to manage independently of staff, through B and C to D, in which they require assistance from at least one and usually two members of staff to accommodate their needs. Points are awarded for each item. It is extremely rare for a resident to have D levels of need in all 20 categories of care and an RCS score is calculated by adding the totals from the assessment of each of the 20 categories. For a resident to attain a Level 1 ranking they must accumulate 81.01 points or higher; anyone who attains a Level 8 rank has achieved a total of 10.5 or fewer points. Eligibility to receive high (nursing home level) care implies care needs at Level 4 or higher.

It was suggested earlier that, in the Australian context, continuous quality improvement is the approach adopted to ensure residential aged care facilities meet quality of care standards (Department of Health & Family Services 1997; Department of Health & Aged Care 1999; Department of Health & Ageing 2002). Other nations focus on 'indicators' of quality to achieve quality standards (Zimmerman et al 1995; Fitzgerald et al 1996; Anderson et al 1998; 1999). Several researchers at the Center for Health Systems Research and Analysis at the University of Wisconsin

(CHSRA 2000) have also focused on this means to measure quality of care.

CHSRA researchers (<www.chsra.wisc.edu>) distinguish between quality indicators and quality measures. Quality indicators are perceived as pointers indicating potential problem areas that need further investigation. They represent the starting point for a process of evaluating the quality of care through careful investigation. In their view a true measure of quality identifies an aspect of care where there is definitely a problem and describes the extent of the problem. Quality measures are their own endpoints and no further investigations are needed in order to make judgements about the quality of care.

Measuring quality of care in residential settings— North America

The Nursing Home Reform Act of 1987 provided an opportunity to ensure good clinical practice by creating a regulatory framework that recognised the importance of comprehensive assessment as the foundation for planning and delivering care to US nursing home residents. A Resident Assessment Instrument was developed in association with a minimum data set (MDS-RAI) in 1988–89 under a US Health Care Financing Administration contract with a consortium of researchers from the Research Triangle Institute, Hebrew Rehabilitation Center for Aged, Brown University and the University of Michigan (<www.interrai.org>). The 1987 Act mandated that the instrument be introduced into all US nursing homes and it was subsequently adopted voluntarily by nursing home proprietors in several Canadian cities and provinces. Following its initial implementation in 1990–91 the tool has been revised on several occasions and nation-specific variations have subsequently been applied in Canada and several European and Asian countries. The current version RAI 2.0 addresses 18 domains of care: socio demographics, prior customary routine, cognition, communication and hearing, vision, mood and behaviour, psychosocial well-being, physical functioning, continence, disease diagnoses, health conditions, oral and nutritional status, oral and dental status, skin condition, activities, medications, special treatments and discharge potential. It is the subject of further evaluation with the view to produce a new generation in 2004.

Quality care measurement in community programs

In Australia there is no single instrument that measures the quality of the care that older people in the community receive or that providers deliver. Those in receipt of Community Aged Care Packages are reviewed in a manner similar to recipients in low-level residential facilities like hostels. The quality of care delivered to individuals in receipt of other community-based services, such as the Home and Community Care program or Meals on Wheels, is not determined by any uniform standard at present, although the matter is debated periodically. In 1991 guidelines for seven National Service Standards were agreed and published for the Home and Community Care program. These were further broken down into 27 'consumer outcomes' but function only as guidelines and, unlike the accreditation standards for residential facilities, do not as yet include a monitoring or measurement function. Each service provider is free to apply his or her own criteria for measuring the quality of the care or service they deliver. As Gibson (1998, p. 111) states:

> Given the range and degree of fragmentation of home based care services in Australia and the involvement of several levels of government, as well as the private-for-profit and not-for-profit sectors in the funding and provision of such services, the difficulties in agreeing on and implementing such a system are indeed formidable.

International instruments to measure quality of care in all service settings

Within the international context one suite of instruments has been the subject of multi-national acceptance and application following extensive testing for reliability and validity in a variety of care settings and locations. These instruments have been designed by InterRAI (<www.interrai.org>). Over the past fifteen years, this international collaborative of approximately 50 clinicians and scientists from 23 countries has focused on the development of data sets for health delivery with an emphasis on older persons and chronic disease management. The original tool, the Resident Assessment Instrument-Minimum Data Set for residential care (RAI-MDS) has been expanded to tools for home care (interRAI-HC), acute care (interRAI-AC), post-acute care (interRAI-PAC), palliative care (interRAI-PC), mental health, in all age groups (interRAI-MH) and community mental health (interRAI-CMH). This suite of assessment instruments permits an older person to be tracked through the systems of care, and his or her health and care status to be measured and reviewed on a regular basis in almost all settings in which care might be delivered. In all instruments, the following core indicators are assessed: cognition, communication and vision, mood, psychosocial well-being, physical functioning, continence, disease diagnoses, health conditions, oral and nutritional status, skin condition, medications, legal responsibilities and/or directives, together with a range of demographic details. In addition to the core items each instrument addresses aspects of the client's life and environment of particular relevance to the setting in which it will be applied.

Accreditation and best practice

Accreditation of the aged care industry is not a universally practised phenomenon, although many governments do aspire to deliver best practice standards of care, as the World Health Organization attests (WHO 2000). One country in which accreditation does apply is Australia and a discussion of its practices will serve to highlight protocols which might be utilised elsewhere to ensure the best possible care. Since 1 January 2001 all residential services have been assessed against four standards: management systems, staffing and organisational development, health and personal care, resident lifestyle and physical environment and safety systems. Between them the standards contain 44 expected outcomes. There is no formal process of accreditation for community-based services.

The accreditation process commenced in September 1999 when registered aged care quality assessors started auditing more than 3000 residential aged care facilities under the scheme that came into law with the *Aged Care Act 1997*. The Standards and Accreditation Agency (2001, p.1) indicates that, by the end of 2000, all facilities that received federal subsidies had been assessed and 93 per cent were awarded three years' accreditation. In May 2002 the first of these services were required to submit applications for a further period of accreditation, and all will be obliged to do so approximately six months in advance of when their current period expires.

Few elements of the accreditation process changed between Accreditation Mark 1 and Mark 2. The legislation did not change, nor did the Accreditation Standards (Department of Health and

Family Services 1997) or the Accreditation Grant Principles (Department of Health and Aged Care 1999) that set out the matters for the accreditation decision. The philosophical approach founded on continuous improvement also remained unaltered, albeit with an increased focus on responsiveness to residents' needs.

Many of the processes associated with achieving accreditation will also remain the same. For example, services will be required to submit a self-assessment—previously described as a desk assessment. They will also be subject to a site visit by a team of Aged Care Standards and Accreditation Agency auditors at a date close to the expiry date of their current accredited period. An exit report at the conclusion of the site visit will be provided by the auditors at the time of the inspection, but the audit team does not make the final determination about the outcome. The Standards Agency Decision Maker has that responsibility, to be supplied to the service within fourteen days of the visit.

One of the most significant areas to change between the two accreditation cycles is in the ratings for the accomplishment of the accreditation outcomes. Accreditation Mark 2 ratings will vary significantly from its predecessor in which each of the 44 expected outcomes of the four standards could have attained one of four grades: 'commendable', 'satisfactory', 'unacceptable' and 'critical' for the level of service provided by the facility. In the second version, each expected outcome will be rated as either: 'compliant', 'non compliant', or 'non compliant with serious risk'. Being compliant with the Standards means being compliant with each of the 44 expected outcomes, having systems in place to achieve the expected outcomes consistently and being able to demonstrate that achievement. Services must use the criteria and considerations contained in the Standards for Aged Care Facilities (DH&FS 1997) and Residential Care Guidelines (DH&FS 1998) to guide them. There are no separate ratings at the Standard level in the new round of assessments.

A new system of recognition of higher-level services has been devised and it will apply to the service as a whole and not to individual standards. One of two awards can be made: 'accreditation with merit' or 'commendable'. A service must apply for the higher award separately to but simultaneously with its application for re-accreditation. Essential to being eligible to receive the higher award, the service must have mature continuous improvement systems in place which have been in operation for either two years, for 'accreditation with merit' or three years for a 'commendable' service. Further, high order services must demonstrate leadership, the use of data and measurement and effective and sustainable continuous improvement and innovation. Any service applying for a 'commendable' award must also exhibit outcomes at benchmarking standard to achieve the higher award. Benchmarking will constitute Australian best practice in the delivery of residential aged care services into the foreseeable future.

Another area of change concerns the accreditation period. Previously services were awarded accreditation for three years if they achieved a 'satisfactory' grade for the majority of their outcomes. If auditors considered there was any doubt, or serious problems had to be rectified, a shorter period of usually one year could have been awarded. With the new ratings system, services that achieve a 'commendable' rating may be awarded up to four years' accreditation. Lesser periods may be awarded, depending on circumstances.

Activity 9.1

Select a model of service in which you have been responsible for the delivery of services to older people in your district. It may be a community-based program or one offered in a residential setting. With the aid of the data collection system used in that service, calculate the cost of delivering care to that service for a 12-month period and prepare a written report for the service's management team. As you conduct your investigation, identify one or more areas in which savings can be made without compromising the quality of the care the service provides. Include these suggestions in the form of recommendations for service improvement, with evidence to justify your suggestions, in the report. Examples of information collection tools which can guide your data collection processes include instruments such as the RAI-MDS Version 2.0 for Nursing Home Resident Assessment and Care Screening, mandated for use throughout the United States, and used voluntarily in many Canadian provinces and English local authorities. Other examples are the Resident Classification Scale and the Aged Care Assessment Team Minimum Data Set used in Australia.

Your analysis may focus on a single service or facility within your district, or you may view the program in its entirety as it applies to a whole district, state or even country, in which case your report should be prepared for the relevant senior bureaucrat or politician.

You will need to address issues pertaining to your client group as individuals in terms of numbers, degrees of frailty, use of specialist therapies, length of stay within the service, rehabilitation potential and the financial resources of people to meet any fees for service. (The proportion of clients who are recipients of social security support such as aged pensions compared with those who are self-funded retirees may impact on the range of options your service is able to offer and so must be taken into account.)

You will also need to consider issues pertaining to staffing the service, including numbers of licensed and non-licensed staff, the hours they must be employed, the availability and accessibility of specialists needed to meet client needs and casual personnel to cover contingencies such as the winter influenza season. Other matters to consider include the environment in which the service is provided. Calculations will need to take into account capital works for the year, building maintenance, client transportation and external funding sources, because it is extremely unlikely that client fees and government subsidies will be sufficient to meet all the service's financial requirements.

Conclusion

A variety of issues remain to be addressed by aged care researchers, policy makers and care providers alike. Two in particular warrant immediate attention. The first concerns the diminution in the supply of a qualified workforce available to provide care for older people in both residential and community settings. In common with many other subspecialities within the nursing profession, there is a paucity of gerontic nurses offering themselves for service in this area. As a direct consequence the existing aged care workforce is ageing. In combination with high turnover rates, a result of burnout due to the heavy nature of the work and the modest remuneration compared with other nursing subspecialities, the failure to attract new recruits to the sector bodes poorly for the immediate future.

O'Conner (1999) found that the mean age for registered nurses in this speciality was 45.6 years. The same investigation estimated that by 2008 (1999, pp. 31–2) in New South Wales alone there would be a projected shortfall of 418 qualified aged care nurses and 2466 unqualified aged care nurses to meet anticipated demand. As the report highlights (1999, p. 34) 'the significance in these results is that as requirements increase, workforce supply will not increase adequately, either for qualified or unqualified aged care nurses'. The study proposed a twofold solution: an increase in the number of funded positions in both the public and private sectors together with an increase effort to minimise the workforce wastage rate.

The second issue of urgent concern is the provision of care for non-mainstream older citizens. In the aftermath of World War II, the Australian population was expanded by an influx of European-born settlers escaping the vicissitudes of the compromised economies of their homelands and the privations of postwar lifestyles. Many of these new settlers were young men and women in their 20s and 30s. In the early years of the 21st century they have reached or surpassed retirement age. Non-English speaking older persons present unique care challenges, such as the communication difficulties posed by those who never learned to speak English or who have forgotten the English skills they once had with the onset of cognitive impairments which accompany illnesses such as dementia. Older Australian Aboriginal persons may also fall into the category of non-English speakers. The definition of 'older person' may warrant revision when focusing on the needs of Aboriginal Australians, whose average life span is considerably shorter than Australians of non-indigenous descent.

Policy makers have attempted to address some of these issues as evidenced in, for example, Expected Outcome 3.8 of Aged Care Standard 3 (1999) which states 'Individual interests, customs, beliefs and cultural and ethnic backgrounds are valued and fostered'. However, the specific needs of individuals from non-mainstream cultures have rarely been described, let alone offered solutions. Because they are likely to make up almost a quarter of the over retirement age population for the first two or more decades of the 21st century, it is essential that these challenges be included in any investigation of the cost of care.

10

Vehicles to promote positive ageing: Natural therapies, counselling, music and the creative arts

Judy Harris, Terrence Hays, Jeffrey Kottler, Victor Minichiello, Ina Olohan, Peter Wright

The new millennium sees people living longer than ever. Demographers tell us that in the developed countries today's young adults can expect to live past 80. Biologists inform us that increasingly older people will live healthier lives. They predict a 'compression of morbidity' that will result in older persons experiencing long, healthy and active lives with short periods of severe disability or debilitating illness before death (Fries 1984). The buzz-word in the gerontology field these days is 'active life expectancy'. Kart (1997, p. 105) defines this concept as 'the period of life free of limitations in activities of daily living'. People are asking the question, 'How many years can we expect to enjoy?'

Not surprisingly, the emphasis of many health programs and policies, and increasingly more so in the future, is on longevity and quality of life. Scientists argue that certain lifestyle habits improve the quality of life and may prolong life (National Institute of Aging 1993). A study on centenarians found them to have a positive outlook and sense of optimism (Poon et al 1992), highlighting the importance of mind and body connections. As Tirrito (2003, p. 83) notes, health is linked to life satisfaction and well-being and 'people who have good health are happier, have a better sense of well-being, have friends, and tend to be satisfied with life'. This message is increasingly being appreciated by consumers. More and more people are recognising that lifestyle offers one of the greatest paybacks in terms of improving health and quality of life (see Chapter 2).

Older consumers are more receptive than ever to the benefits of healthy living, as they search for less invasive solutions and smarter health choices than those offered by pills or short consultations with general practitioners. Studies show that the use of complementary therapies and counselling services is high amongst the baby boomers, the current cohort of middle-aged persons (Astin 2003). Governments and medical insurance companies are also beginning to acknowledge the health and economic advantages of a lifestyle approach. Health professionals now in training are learning not to be mindless slaves to the biomedical model but to pay close attention to the social context of health. They have come to appreciate how much can be gained by using compassion, sensitivity and holistic lifestyle interventions. Even back in 1973 Michel Foucault remarked that the days of western medicine discounting other forms of experience and expression in its claim for mastery over disease were fading. Other forms of 'healing' are emerging in the new millennium and attracting acceptance and popularity.

This chapter discusses some of the interventions (the natural therapies and counselling) and lifestyle choices (music and arts) not usually found in gerontology textbooks, but increasingly used by older persons to achieve a positive approach to life (Brett 2002; Tirrito 2003). We begin by describing various types of natural therapies and their benefits. Next we illustrate the utility of the wellness promotion approach offered by counselling and outline some specific techniques that can be used to foster personal initiative and choice amongst older clients. Finally, we discuss how music and the creative arts, through playback theatre, can enhance quality of life by promoting connection with people and community.

Activity 10.1

Go to <http://www.livingto100.com>
What is your life expectancy? Consider the factors that impact on your life expectancy.

The natural therapies

The increasing popularity of natural therapies is one of several indicators of the changing health care market. The provider–patient relationship is shifting from the traditionally held view of a willing, passive and dependent patient to an activist health consumer who demands and seeks out timely, diverse and accurate health information (Jacobs et al 2003). Integrating natural therapies with biomedicine creates the opportunity for expanding the scope of health care beyond the domain of pharmacy and surgery, and of improving the quality of life in addition to prolonging it.

Natural therapies are characterised as much by their underlying philosophies as by their distinctive treatment protocols (Zollman & Vickers 1999), and have the common goals of improving vitality and balancing energy, as well as assisting the eliminative functioning of the skin, lungs, kidneys and digestive system (Jacka 1989). Natural therapy modalities may be grouped into biochemical therapies such as the botanical medicines, including traditional Western, Chinese and Native American herbal practices; manual therapies such as massage and chiropractic; and energy-based modalities, including acupuncture. Many modalities do not fit conveniently into a single category, as they incorporate one or more of the biochemical-manual energy principles; examples include aromatherapy, reflexology, shiatsu and homoeopathy. Ayurveda, Traditional Chinese Medicine and naturopathy are examples of integrated healing systems incorporating more than one modality (Kuhn 1999).

The use of natural therapies dates back many centuries. Ayurveda, the holistic system of medicine indigenous to India, has been widely practised there for more than 5000 years, and incorporates fasting, herbal medicines, yoga and massage (Lad 1985). Traditional Chinese Medicine, which utilises a combination of acupuncture, herbal medicine and diet, has a 2300-year history. Its underlying philosophy is the protection of human life by preserving the conditions under which it thrives, by the cultivation of wellness as well as the correction of ill health (Beinfield & Korngold 1991). Naturopathy grew out of alternative healing systems of the eighteenth and nineteenth centuries, but traces its philosophical roots to the Hippocratic school of medicine *circa* 400 BC. Naturopathic practice integrates diet, herbal medicine and massage therapies, emphasising the maintenance of health and prevention of disease by seeking the underlying cause of disease, rather than treating and suppressing its symptoms (Murray & Pizzorno 1990).

As well as these integrated healing systems, the natural therapy modalities most commonly utilised singly in western countries include acupuncture, massage and botanical medicines (Astin et al 2000; Morling 2001). Increasingly, these are the modalities utilised in the management of a number of conditions affecting older people (Vickers 2000).

Acupuncture

Acupuncture focuses on the regulation of the balance and circulation of energy, achieved by the insertion and manipulation of fine needles at specific points on the body's meridians, or channels of energy flow (Kenyon 1987). In the United States, acupuncture practised by non-physician practitioners has expanded within the larger context of the holistic health movement, emerging concurrently with increasing dissatisfaction with the bureaucracy and iatrogenic effects of biomedicine (Baer et al 1998). Acupuncture offers a relatively safe and inexpensive form of therapy that appears to provide relief from a wide variety of chronic ailments, and has significant application in management of chronic pain in older people.

Massage therapy

Massage therapy involves the manual application of general or regional sequences of movements to the soft tissue of the body surface to achieve mechanical, reflex, physiological, psychological or psychoneural effects (Andrade & Clifford 2001). A treatment modality with a 4000-year history, massage therapy disappeared from the US medical scene approximately at the time of the pharmaceutical revolution of the 1940s, and came thereafter to be regarded as an 'alternative therapy' (Field 1998). Massage therapy is currently one of the most widely practised and utilised natural therapy modalities (Morling 2001).

Botanical medicine

The use of plants for healing purposes is as old as human history, and forms the origin of many modern pharmaceuticals. Western botanical medicine emphasises the pharmacological effects of plant extracts, generally administered in a non-purified form through ingestion, on the functioning of individual body systems (Vickers & Zollman 1999). Aromatherapy, which may be considered a specialised form of botanical medicine and often incorporates the added dimension of massage or other forms of touch, utilises plant-derived volatile oils principally in external application, to regulate both physiological and emotional well-being (Fischer-Rizzi 1990).

Who uses natural therapies, and why?

Natural therapies are currently used by a substantial proportion of the general population (Harris & Rees 2000), and their use is growing rapidly as consumers drive the demand for more cost-effective and personalised health care (Josephek 2000).

The largest group using natural therapies are professional women aged over 35 years (Hall & Giles-Corti 2000). However, between 35 per cent and 60 per cent of all adults surveyed in a number of western countries reported using some form of natural therapy (Astin et al 2000), with older people comprising a significant population of those users (Luskin et al 2003). Recent surveys in America targeted at people aged 65 years and over indicate that in this age group, 30 per cent of Americans overall, 41 per cent of California residents and 58 per cent of those attending one of two New York City medical clinics had used at least one type of natural therapy within the previous year (Astin et al 2000; Foster et al 2000; Cherniack et al 2001).

Concurrent with an increase in patients seeking natural therapy treatment is the increase in natural therapy practitioners. For example, the number of natural therapy practitioners represented in Australia by the Australian Traditional-Medicine Society approached 10 000 at the beginning of 2003, compared with just 4300 at the end of 1995 (Fawcett 1995, 2003). In Western Australia, 90 per cent of general medical practitioners had each been approached by over 30 patients seeking advice on natural therapies in the nine months prior to the survey, while around half of the practitioners surveyed had undertaken postgraduate study in one or more natural therapies, predominantly acupuncture, meditation, herbal medicine and hypnosis (Hall & Giles-Corti 2000). In addition, over 60 per cent of medical schools in the United States report offering elective courses in natural therapy, or including these topics in required courses (Wetzel et al 1998). US nurses increasingly incorporate natural therapy techniques, such as massage and aromatherapy, into their practice (Buckle 2001), and there is a growing emphasis on the incorporation of natural therapies in the nursing care of older people (Brett 2002).

People in most western countries use natural therapy not so much as a result of being dissatisfied with conventional medicine, but largely because they find these therapies to be more congruent with their own values, beliefs and philosophical orientations toward health care (Astin 1998). Users of natural therapy differentiate between the socially legitimised and widely accessible but disempowering and mechanistic attributes of conventional medicine, and the holistic and empowering but relatively less accessible and less legitimate nature of natural therapy (Barrett et al 2000). Patients claim that natural therapy does a better job than conventional medicine of meeting their emotional needs and respecting their religious and cultural beliefs (Boozang 1998). They value the emphasis on treating the whole person, and believe natural therapy enables them to take a more active part in maintaining their own health (Vincent & Furnham 1996).

Natural therapies have a proven efficacy in the management of a number of conditions predominantly affecting older people, and can provide cost-effective treatment relatively free of side effects (Luskin et al 2003). In addition, natural therapies appeal to people on an emotional and philosophical level, and may help to promote the perception of being more in control of individual health and treatment. Natural therapies also provide reassurance through human touch, adding a caring dimension which may otherwise be perceived as lacking (Brett 2002). All of these elements contribute to an increased quality of life for older people.

Natural therapies and older people

Natural therapies are gaining increasing medical acceptance as research shows their effectiveness in managing specific conditions, many of which predominantly affect older people. Natural therapies are increasingly utilised in the treatment of chronic conditions in particular, characteristically the painful, debilitating and often incurable conditions such as arthritis and cancer which are prevalent in older people (Arcury et al 2000). Treatment modalities such as acupuncture, massage and botanical medicines appear most effective in the treatment of pain, anxiety and depression (Vickers 2000).

Pain

Chronic pain, most often resulting from arthritis and cancer, is common amongst older people. Left untreated, pain can lead to depression, social isolation, sleep problems and difficulty in performing daily activities (Young 2000). Pharmaceuticals alone often are not sufficient for the treatment of chronic pain and its attendant symptoms, and natural therapies such as acupuncture and massage are increasingly utilised to increase patient comfort and decrease medication requirements (Pinkowish 2001).

Pain is the major complaint of the estimated 1 million people in the United States who use acupuncture each year, and acupuncture is now available as a treatment option in most pain clinics in countries such as Australia, Canada, the United States and Hong Kong, for example (Ezzo et al 2000). Acupuncture holds the promise of being able to treat certain patients with chronic disease or otherwise difficult-to-treat conditions, and to achieve palliation with virtually no side effects. Results of randomised controlled trials have found acupuncture to be safe, practical and effective in the treatment of chronic and post-surgical pain, and post-operative nausea (Ernst 2001a). This is particularly significant, as debilitating post-operative nausea occurs in 60–70 per cent of patients, with standard anti-emetics being frequently ineffective and accompanied by severe side effects (Leake & Broderick 1998). Acupuncture is a particularly appropriate alternative for older people who cannot tolerate typical medical interventions.

Natural therapies, including acupuncture and aromatherapy, are utilised by a significant proportion of cancer patients (Yates et al 1993; Ernst 2001b). Used more frequently as a supplement to, rather than a substitute for, conventional care [for many cancer patients] natural therapies fulfil an important psychological need (Downer et al 1994). Such support is increasingly regarded as an integral part of good cancer medicine.

Osteoarthritis is a major cause of pain and disability in Western populations. It is estimated that treatment of arthritis-associated pain constitutes around half of the workload of traditional acupuncturists (Walker-Bone et al 2000). Natural therapies, such as acupuncture, show potential in providing relief from the chronic pain associated with osteoarthritis (Zashin 2000). Massage therapy is also an effective treatment for this and other types of chronic musculoskeletal pain (Young 2000; Pinkowish 2001).

Sleeplessness, anxiety and depression

Sleep patterns change as a person ages, sometimes with troublesome effects (Maher 2001). Botanical medicines such as valerian (*Valeriana officinalis*) are attractive alternative medications to many people with sleep disorders, who may be unable or unwilling to use conventional pharmaceuticals (Gyllenhaal et al 2000). Valerian has been shown to decrease sleep onset time and to promote deeper sleep. Some of the plant-derived essential oils used in aromatherapy, such as lavender (*Lavandula officinalis*), are calming or sedative in effect (Kayne 1998) and may also be utilised to help promote sleep.

Massage and aromatherapy applied pre-operatively have been shown to reduce anxiety associated with surgical procedures (van der Rit 1993; Norred 2000), as well as the anxiety associated with chronic back pain and breast cancer (Field 1998). The reassurance provided by these tactile therapies helps to offset the often impersonal and frightening atmosphere of a hospital, and they are increasingly being incorporated into perioperative nursing practice.

Chronic pain and cancer are often associated with depression. Massage therapy improved mood, lowered depression scores and resulted in increased serotonin and dopamine levels in sufferers of chronic back pain, as well as reportedly improving mood and body image awareness, and decreasing depression in patients with stage I or II breast cancer (Field 1998).

Botanical medicine may also be used to treat depression. Extracts of St John's Wort (*Hypericum perforatum*) have been proven in double-blind clinical trials to be more effective than placebo for the treatment of mild to moderately severe depressive disorders (Linde et al 1996). It has been shown to be therapeutically equivalent to imipramine and to be better tolerated by patients (Woelk 2000). St John's Wort is approved for medical use in Germany for the treatment of depression, and is the best-selling antidepressant in that country (Ness et al 1999). However, because interactions between St John's Wort and common concurrently prescribed pharmaceuticals are understood to be both extensive, and not yet fully documented (Moore et al 2000), care needs to be exercised with its use by older people.

Dementia

Alzheimer's disease is the most common cause of dementia in older people (Khosh 2001). Natural therapy treatments, including botanical medicine and aromatherapy, may be used to ameliorate the symptoms of Alzheimer's disease and improve the quality of life of people in the later stages of cognitive decline (Free & Chambers 2001; Rauckhorst 2001). Over half of primary caregivers surveyed had administered at least one natural therapy treatment to the individuals with Alzheimer's disease under their care (Coleman et al 1995).

The botanical medicine ginkgo (*Gingko biloba*) contains compounds which have antioxidant, neuroprotective and cholinergic activites relevant to Alzheimer's disease mechanisms. The therapeutic efficacy of ginkgo extracts in Alzheimer's disease in placebo-controlled clinical trials is similar to currently prescribed drugs such as Tacrine or Donezepil. However, it differs significantly from these in producing minimal side effects (Perry et al 1999).

The administration of ten minutes' gentle massage to the hands significantly reduced agitation in long-term care nursing home residents with moderate to severe dementia (Remington 2002). Such measures, which are low cost and suitable for application by lay caregivers following minimal training, may contribute significantly to improved quality of life in older people with dementia.

Activity 10.2

Interview an older person who uses natural therapies regularly. Find out why this person uses natural therapies and what benefits it provides to him or her.

Counselling older clients

In many ways, counselling the older person is not significantly different to counselling any other population. Older individuals have needs similar to anyone else—they want to lead meaningful, productive lives; they want to be understood and valued; they want to be involved in significant, intimate relationships with others. The work of the counsellor is to help individuals to recognise and meet their needs through the gaining of insight and skills, and also to assist them to deal with the unique challenges they will face. Older people deal with a number of health and personal challenges that are unique to their stage in life, including existential issues related to mortality, loneliness and the creation of meaning from their life's work. These are areas in which counselling can often provide support, guidance, companionship and constructive input. For example, older people are far more likely than the general population to be struggling with multiple loss issues. This includes the loss of lifelong friends and loved ones and, while the majority of older people live highly functional lives, some will also experience the loss of their optimal physical and cognitive functioning at some stage. They may struggle with a number of presenting concerns that also lend themselves to work in counselling, including retirement with its accompanying redefinition of productivity, loss of status and decision making, loneliness, decreased financial support and finding meaning in their life (Bright 1996; Gross & Capuzzi 2001).

As Richards (2001, p. 12) points out, these are challenges which, as we grow older, 'we either meet and engage or seek to avoid'. The counsellor can help the client to engage with these tasks and challenges of later life through a variety of therapeutic modalities, as well as through engagement in an authentic caring relationship that emphasises personal initiative and choice in decision making. The perspective taken here is one of wellness promotion rather than the medical model of illness prevention. We suggest methods that will assist older people to enjoy and maintain healthy lives, to retain their sense of vitality, to encourage connection to community and social supports, and to address a holistic view that emphasises physical, emotional and spiritual dimensions.

What health professionals need to know

The health professional must be knowledgeable about the various life issues which affect the older person, as well as the particular developmental and transition issues that impact on them. As shown in Table 10.1 this includes knowledge of physical illnesses, their treatments and prognoses, and the emotional consequences of illnesses and their treatments.

Table 10.1: Knowledge areas in counselling the older person for health professionals

- Cognitive functioning including strengths and weaknesses
- Incidence and manifestations of substance and prescription drug abuse
- Developmental stage theories related to emotional, physical and spiritual evolution
- Family issues surrounding needed support
- Sexual issues related to older persons
- Death and loss issues and their treatment
- Constructions of meaning for later maturity
- Coping strategies for dealing with declining health and dependency
- Cognitive strategies for adjusting to life changes
- Spiritual and social support in the later years
- Negative stereotyping and ageism
- Transference and countertransference issues

Health professionals need to be aware of the specific emotional/ spiritual/ interpersonal challenges faced by older clients. For example, there are risks of misdiagnosis and over-medication with older people, especially when health professionals fail to recognise underlying psychological/emotional issues at the heart of presenting complaints (Slater 1995). A patient might be diagnosed with, and treated for depression, when an adequate background check or familiarity with the client's story might reveal a loss issue which has gone unrecognised and unprocessed. Intervention through grief counselling may not only preclude the need for medication but also assist in the process of rebuilding the client's engagement with life and rebuilding social and family support systems. Alternatively, the patient might be reporting symptoms which they attribute to memory failure or physical illness or 'growing old', when a diagnosis and treatment for depression is necessary. The health professional will therefore need to be aware of various support services and make appropriate referrals.

Just as often, it may simply be necessary to provide some degree of human compassion and caring within the context of a short-term counselling relationship. The goals of such a consultation are modest: demonstrating empathy and compassion; encouraging the patient to tell his or her story; attending actively to the narrative, clarifying and reflecting when appropriate; responding to communicate deeper level understanding; and when indicated (and often it is not), helping the older person move to taking some small constructive action.

The health professional's job, in consultation with the patient and other medical staff, will be to distinguish between functional limitations and psychological factors (such as pain due to anxiety and pain due to physical injury) and to provide any advice on appropriate interventions. Let us consider the following example. Sam did not respond to the assortment of medical interventions directed his way; if anything, he became steadily worse even though his doctors and nurses could find no organic cause for his problems. The secondary gains from his illness were intrinsically rewarding in a number of ways: he enjoyed the attention from others; he felt powerful in that he managed to stymie professionals who were supposedly so smart and talented; he felt stuck and so was excused from investing the time and energy needed to engage more fully with life; and he manipulated family members by instilling in them a sense of guilt. Before successful intervention would be possible, the health professional would first need to understand and respond to these underlying psychological 'pay offs' (Kottler 2000).

The health professional will also need to ascertain the client's ability to participate in the helping process, taking into account any difficulties with pain, memory, cognitive processing or sensory impairment. Developmental issues that include loss of sight and hearing, and systemic issues, which include historical, family, social and cultural considerations, are also important to take into account to promote effective communication and suitable choice of therapeutic interventions. Candace, for example, complained constantly about chronic pain associated with a degenerative neurological condition—but what the health professional had not taken the time to understand about her condition was that it was mediated by both her family and cultural context. It would have taken little extra time to discover that amongst her extended family and ethnicity, talking about what is wrong with one's body and life are a usual means of communication. When professionals ask the question, 'What is wrong?' they are going to hear a litany of complaints. On the other hand, older patients could also be asked, 'In addition to those things that bother you, what else can you tell me about what is going right in your life and that you are quite satisfied with?' This counselling strategy, sometimes called 'accentuating the positive', or 'discovering unique outcomes', helps people to balance problems with things that are actually going quite well (O'Hanlon & Beadle 1999).

Helping skills

An important role for the health professional is to establish a caring and supportive relationship with the older patient. The primary task is to build rapport and trust in order to facilitate some degree of commitment and engagement in the process; without this alliance, helping efforts often prove to be useless. Being fully present to the patient (Pt) demands a combination of skills and qualities from the health professional (Hp) that includes kindness, acceptance and attentive listening. Here is an example.

Pt: '. . . so I can't get this idea out of my head. It's . . .'

Hp: 'You're really disturbed by these thoughts and they frighten you.' [*reflection of feeling*]

Pt: 'Yeah, I guess so. I never used to have this sort of problem before. When I was a younger man, about your age . . . I told you about the time when I worked in the mill . . .'

Hp: 'Yes, you did. But we were talking about those thoughts that scare you.' [*redirecting the conversation*]. 'Tell me more about that.' [*probing*]

Pt: 'I've just been having these thoughts more and more. I don't sleep so good any more. And I can't seem to concentrate on things for very long. My daughter, she tells me . . .'

Hp: 'You were saying that your sleep is disrupted, that you have difficulties concentrating, and that family members are starting to notice.' [*summarising, focusing*]

Pt: 'It just ain't easy, if you know what I mean. It's not like it was before. It's . . . I don't know . . . It's just all so hard. Sometimes I wonder if it's worth it.'

Hp: 'You feel so discouraged, and even depressed, that you wonder if life is worth continuing.' [*reflection of content*]

Pt: (Nods.)

Hp: 'What about the things that are going well for you?' [*accentuating the positive; open-ended question*]

In this five-minute conversation, the health professional learns quite a lot just by listening and responding attentively and compassionately, keeping the patient on track, reflecting back what is heard and understood, and asking a few open-ended questions (those that are expansive) that help the patient to explore deeper. In a remarkably brief period of time, these counselling skills are used to build a more intimate, trusting relationship. The patient leaves feeling that he was heard and understood.

Countering negative attributions and ageism

The skills outlined above indicate an attitude of respect and client-centredness which helps to mitigate against the situation of disempowerment and denigration experienced by many older people. Not only is it common for older citizens in western societies to experience a multitude of losses and reduction in personal contacts, income and choices, they can also be subject to ageism, condescension and negative stereotyping (see Chapter 1; Bright 1996; Berk 2001). Negative stereotyping of the older person by self or others as impaired or incapable can diminish their feelings of independence and their self-esteem, leading them to overestimate the decrease in their own capacities and to a negative expectation of their abilities. It is a cycle that can lead to debilitation and dependence in the older person as well as withdrawal from the world, instead of continued productive and creative contributions to society (Lassey & Lassey 2001).

On the other hand, the older person may need to re-appraise and modify what it means to be competent and able at their stage of life so that they have a realistic expectation of themselves against which to measure their self-esteem (Sprenkel 1999). Realistic and positive expectations from both the older person and from the health professional will go a long way towards the health professional selecting the most appropriate and least intrusive remedial steps needed at a given time and towards the older person retaining a high level of agency and coping ability. The older person can be encouraged to value their own life experience and to recall and draw on coping mechanisms they have developed throughout a lifetime. Health professionals can be encouraged to examine their own myths and stereotypes regarding ageing and to seek appropriate education and supervision to prevent these interfering with the therapeutic process. The shift away from the focus on ageing per se to the person and the situation will also reduce unneeded control by health professionals and allow space for the older person to be what Sprenkle (1999, p. 224) describes as 'a true partner in their health care'.

A further barrier to constructive help for the older client may be the emergence of transference and countertransference issues (Knight 1996). For example, as the health professional can often be younger than the patient, there are particular patterns to be aware of, such as the older person being seen as a parent or grand-parent to be protected or even despised, or the helper being identified with an emotionally significant other from the older person's life. The younger health professional also needs to be clear about their own attitudes toward pain, disability and death, and to be clear about any fears, anxieties or avoidance around these issues if they are to be able to work constructively with people who are dealing with these challenges and transitions in later life (Richards 2001).

Life review

Life review, originally conceptualised by Butler (1963), has been widely discussed as a useful way to help older people to think about and understand developmental transitions and experiences and to reconstruct their identity and self-concept. Reminiscence may be a natural developmental task of the older person, but negative outcomes can result if this activity veers towards rumi-nation, which can result in depression and despair. Research has shown that ruminative self-attention is strongly predictive of a negative perception of the past, low self-concept clarity, lack of meaning and purpose in life, and negative death attitudes (Anderson 2002).

Conversely, life review as a form of guided reminiscence pro-vides a supportive vehicle for the client to look at their life story and to reconstruct a self-concept that will be helpful and life en-hancing. For the health professional, using the skill of life review may mean taking time to listen to the patient as they recall life events and treating them as a whole person with an identity sep-arate from their sick role. This orientation takes the health professional beyond the conventional medical model, which emphasises symptom relief and the pre-eminent importance of medical expertise, to therapeutic caring and a more holistic view of health care. There are many ways that life review can be conducted, both formally and informally, as shown in the following example.

Rose—a study in grieving

Rose, an older patient, was soon due to return home from a stay in hospital. She appeared to receive the news of her discharge with great disappointment and withdrew into herself, talking of past times when her husband was alive. She protested that she was sick and could not possibly manage on her own at home. It was clear that Rose was at risk of becoming severely depressed. The health professional charged with her physical rehabilitation took advantage of the therapy periods to ask Rose about her life, her husband, and how she had been coping since his death. Rose reminiscenced with fondness about her life with her husband, but she also explained how she had kept contact with her friends and had a full and active life which included playing bridge and attending the theatre. Through these narratives Rose was allowed an opportunity to grieve, and eventually to began to reconnect with her present life. She began to take an interest in her recovery and to remember her plans to join the 'active retirement' group in her suburb and perhaps travel abroad with them next year. The process of life review helped her to re-engage with her sense of herself and to accept the future and her role in it.

Therapeutic caring in action

Therapeutic caring has been described as 'working with' rather then 'doing to' the patient (Disley & McCormack 2002). This promotes a more respectful and equal relationship with the patient and accounts for individual variation in the experience of illness. It is an approach which also views the patient not as an object but as a resourceful and reflective person who can be active in their own journey of healing. An example is given in Activity 10.3.

The power of the story to make human life meaningful to the engaged listener cannot be underestimated in the healing and helping process (Engel et al 2002). As Atkins et al (2003, p. 16) write, 'The recognition of the self by another, the experience of

Activity 10.3

At the age of 86, Dora suffered a fall, followed by a minor stroke which seriously impaired her sense of balance and left her unable to walk independently. She also experienced difficulty with concentration and short-term memory. Dora was treated in hospital and then admitted to a convalescent home while adaptations were being made to her home environment. What difference might it make if the health professionals involved in Dora's care took time to ask about her life, as well as taking care of her medical needs? They would learn that Dora was a nurse in her younger days and worked in a busy outer London hospital from 1939 to 1945, when England was at war with Germany. She experienced the war, bombing and rationing at first hand and mixed professionally and socially with health care professionals. She later became a hospital matron and supervised many trainee nurses. Could this information be used to encourage Dora to be active in her recovery rather than a passive recipient of medical care? How might her convalescence be enhanced if her carers know her story?

connection with each other's stories at a soul level is profoundly healing and transformative for both client and therapist'. Getting to know the patient means the health professional must be prepared to participate in a reciprocal relationship where the humanness of both participants is encountered. This authentic engagement in relationship may require an investment of time and, in these times of managed care and staff shortages, this expenditure of time may even be discouraged by health care institutions. However, as many health professionals would already know, genuine engagement with the patient/client can also be conveyed in the moment with a look or touch of compassion. The reciprocal nature of the relationship can perhaps bring about benefits for staff as well as patients, where the 'expansion of spirit' for both is facilitated (Hudson 2002).

Spiritual perspective

While there is widespread recognition that biopsychosocial care is important in promoting health and well-being, consideration of complete personhood must also take into account the spiritual dimension. The spiritual dimension may be overtly visible in the display of the patient's religious practices or may be hinted at in meanings the patient attaches to things, people or events (Coulson & Ronaldson 1997). The helper may need to listen and watch for subtle clues as to these meanings. Promoting spirituality not only taps into the patient's life meanings but also can provide the patient with coping strategies and in this way can become an active inner resource in the healing process. For example, James, an elderly Christian man, widower, used the rituals of his religion to create a 'sacred space' where he could find some relief from grief and some comfort from his belief in an afterlife. Involvement in his congregation also kept him in touch with his social support network and linked into church and community services. He was able to remain independently in his own home into his final years.

There is much written about the vital relationship between spirituality and health and susceptibility to illness, interpreting spirituality in its broadest sense of meaning of life, inner peace and hope for the future (Gaskins & Forte 1995; Ross 1995; Coulson & Ronaldson 1997). Even in a hospital or other care setting the health professional can play a vital role in helping the older person to create around themselves surroundings that reflect their sense of identity and the continuity of their lives. It may be helpful for the health professional to look at the medical setting from the patient's point of view, and from this perspective, try to develop an understanding of how the patient may see this environment. In this way, the health professional may come to understand that the patient is living in a contracted environment, a space designed for health management rather than for individual diversity and spirituality. Such insight into the subjective world of the patient/client may lead to finding ways to adapt and transform the environment to cater more to individual needs and to focus on the whole person, not only on the illness and care needs. Ways of doing this are numerous and might include encouraging the patient/client to display familiar possessions such as photographs and gifts relating to their lives (Cram & Patton 1993). Opportunity for choice is seen as an important contributor to a sense of well-being and satisfaction in older people (Lassey & Lassey 2001).

The balancing of individual, institutional and care needs is a paradoxical theme in work with older individuals. On the one hand, such patients/clients may have become accustomed to settling into particular habits and patterns that have been developed over the course of a lifetime; on the other hand, adaptability and flexibility increase the likelihood of greater adjustment to a different environment. To facilitate this adjustment, health professionals must themselves be flexible, creative and adaptable in order to mediate between diverse patient needs and the resources and options available. Achieving a satisfactory life in later years will be dependent on a range of social, economic, psychological and health issues, both intrinsic and extrinsic to the client. Notwithstanding societal and individual patient/client variables, the health professional is well placed to facilitate interactions and interventions that can contribute to well-being and an optimal quality of life for older people.

Activity 10.4

Interview an older person who uses counselling services. Find out how counselling has helped this person deal with his or her life.

Music and well-being

The literature shows that the role of music in people's lives is varied and has meaning with regard to daily well-being (Hays et al 2002). For example, people may use music as a form of recreation, as life-long learning and education, for social contact, and as a form of emotional expression, self-therapy and spiritual expression. According to Campbell (1995), we are just beginning to realise the deep and profound scientific, medical, psychological and spiritual questions involved in the power of music. These include, for example, the use of music as an anaesthetic, for synchronising brain waves, modifying behaviour and stimulating physical responses (Campbell 1995; Clair 1996; Juslin & Slobada 2001).

Not surprisingly, music has been found to elicit responses that range from cognitive and emotional through to physical responses (Bright 1995). Tame (1984, p. 14) explains this phenomenon in his book, *The Secret Power of Music*, by stating:

> whenever we are within audible range of music, its influence is playing upon us constantly such as speeding or slowing, regularising or irregularising our heartbeat, relaxing or jarring the nerves, affecting the blood pressure, the digestion and the rate of respiration. Its effect upon the emotions and desires of man is believed to be vast, and the extent of its influence over even the purely intellectual, mental processes is only beginning to be suspected by researchers.

Today music is widely used in areas of medicine that include labour and delivery, neonatal care, intensive care units, cardiac care units, paediatric cardiac catheterisation, pre-operative and post-operative care, coma units, surgery, dentistry, neurology, psychiatry, gerontology, rehabilitation, oncology, and pain and stress management (Harvey 1995).

Music can help reduce stress and tension and facilitate a sense of relaxation. Ortiz (1997) further states that music can function as an interpreter by translating pain waves into healthy sound energy. For this reason, music can play, for example, an important role in clinical practices where people can be made to feel more comfortable and less anxious when attending consultations. It is now widely recognised that music therapists have an important role to play in supporting the health needs of older persons (Guzzetta 1995).

Bunt (1996) describes how music can help people attain health and well-being by suggesting that music:

- articulates a feeling through a musical gesture
- suspends time
- provides a transcendental experience
- releases a wide range of emotions
- resolves what is hurting and painful
- provides an insight into one's self and/or others
- links significant events in our lives, [and]
- evokes memories of the emotional context of past events and times.

Music can also be an important medium to gain a better understanding of people's subjective experiences. It is a powerful symbol that allows people to assign meaning to experiences (Juslin & Slobada 2001; Hays 2002).

The utility of music

Hanser (1985, p. 283) states that 'one of the foundations of the use of music in therapy, education and society is its appeal to so many people, regardless of functioning level, age, or ability'. For older people, music can provide a way of exploring new creative directions and re-living past experiences. It is an activity that the healthy, the impaired, the talented and the interested can enjoy. Since the 1960s, the importance of music as a therapeutic tool in aged care has been well researched and documented (Jonas 1991; Sacks 1992). Music has two main roles in the lives of older people. Firstly, it can have an evocative effect on emotions, memories and past connections in an older person's life, and secondly, it provides opportunities for people to enjoy shared interests and activities (Bright 1993, 1997). It is for these reasons that Bright (1997) argues that music can be justifiably regarded as a branch of preventive medicine.

In psycho-geriatric work, music has been found to provide motivation for patients to take an active role in becoming well, or facilitating the withdrawn individual who may lack interest and self-expression to become animated. An example of this is Miss D in Sack's (1973) book, *Awakenings*. It is especially so for people suffering from dementia because music can stimulate memory. Through music people recall special associations and/or meanings of particular times or emotions in their life such as their childhood, courting days, parenting, relationships, joy, loss or, in some cases, grief (Bright 1997). Research documents how participation in group musical activities can help older people take a more functional role in life. For example, Clair (1994, 1996) found that planned recorded music and participation in music activities had a beneficial effect on the behaviour of older patients who lived in residential care and suffered from dementia. Music helped these people to be less aggressive, engage in less verbal and physical reaction to hallucination, experience reduced frequency in incontinency, develop greater interest in group activities and improve their attention to personal appearance.

In a study that researched the meaning and function of music in the lives of older people, Hays (2002) describes the diversity of the experience and how music has emotional, social, intellectual and spiritual meaning and roles in their lives. The findings revealed that music provides people with ways of understanding and developing their self-identity, connecting with important life events and other people, maintaining well-being, experiencing and expressing spirituality, and enhancing cognitive and physical functioning. The results also showed that music contributed to quality of life and positive ageing for many older people. The participants reported that music provided them with ways to maintain positive self-esteem, feel competent and independent, and avoid feelings of isolation and loneliness. Music not only offered meaning in the participants' lives, but was used to achieve various functions such as maintaining well-being, connecting with others, with beauty and life experience. The following extract by one of the participants provides an insight into the importance and meaning of music:

> Music oftentimes besides the intellectual pursuit, can be an extension of how I feel. Reflective music, interesting, if I happen to be . . . if I'm doing something on the computer and I have to type out some ideas, I like music in the background. I usually like music that's fairly robust, vigorous, because it seems to excite what I call the words that must flow out of my thoughts because when I do anything, my hands are the extension of my mind. To that extent, music in a sense complements the thought processes and the physical processes of putting down in writing my own thoughts. So music does have that emotional effect . . . and just getting immense pleasure just out of listening I think to beautiful music. It does add that one extra dimension to life. Because without music, I would find it extremely hard to be excited about a lot of things. Music does help to give that spurt and that energy to all of my undertakings.

The following extract from a participant in the Hays study demonstrates why music is important for people.

> Music to me is fairly well a reflection of how I feel. Oh yes, you can get a great smile, it really does make you feel better. And to me, you can take all the tablets you like under the sun, you can go and see all the psychiatrists, all the doctors and you can think and read,

but music pulls you out . . . I've had a couple of illnesses, particularly bypass surgery and music was one of the first things they gave me when I came out [of recovery] because I was inclined to be a bit edgy because all of a sudden I realised that that it could give me a lot more that would help me in my recovery. Ever since then I have had music on all the time and when it gets to the exciting part turn it up and conduct the orchestra. I probably sing atrociously out of tune but feel so much better for it, particularly if I'm a bit down, I've got the flu or something like that. Oh no, music can give you so much pleasure. It adds so much to your life. It's the best way to keep healthy.

Music can provide older people with alternative solutions to everyday problems or stress. For example, a person presenting with a condition that might at first be diagnosed as early stage dementia may in fact be the result of loss, loneliness or mild depression in their life. Such a person may not necessarily need a prescription but rather social connection with other people to share experiences. By being engaged in music activities a person may feel less isolated and be more stimulated, thus leading them to feel less anxious, inwardly focused or prone to depression (Bright 1997; Kirkwood 2001).

Activity 10.5

How do you use music in your life? Consider the function it serves.

Playback theatre and ageing

Playback theatre is one of the recent developments in the field of applied theatre—that is, the application of drama and theatre to health, education and community cultural development—that holds potential for promoting positive ageing amongst the wider community and for older people themselves. Developed by Jonathan Fox, Jo Salas and members of the original Playback Theatre Company in upstate New York in 1975, playback theatre is a form of non-scripted theatre that is now practised in over 30 countries worldwide.

In playback theatre members of the audience tell stories from their lives and actors and a musician spontaneously (re)present those stories using movement, sound and words. A 'conductor' who acts as a bridge between the teller, the actors and the audience facilitates this process. Recent research by Wright (2002) indicates that playback theatre has the potential for education (learning), therapy (healing) and community building, and can be seen more broadly as a part of the developing understanding of how the creative arts can contribute to health and well-being.

Playback theatre can make a number of contributions to positive ageing. First, the social-aesthetic nature of the form lends itself to inquiry into the experiences of older people. For example, playback theatre links cognitive, affective and embodied ways of knowing, thereby encouraging the emergence of nuances and subtleties in people's stories that might otherwise remain hidden. Hence, this form of inquiry has the potential to reveal a wide range of issues—including quality of life, connection with community, identity, and self-expression—that will impact on older people in the 21st century.

Second, the experience of playback theatre is grounded in the stories of those who participate, thereby validating and affirming their lived experience by giving meaning, providing affirmation, and (re)building identity. One participant in the Wright (2002) study described it this way:

> What I find with the playback is that they are touching something that is more of the essence of who we are, or what we do. Or what we feel or we express, or what happens to us or whatever in the same way as a dream in a way can be more real than the experience of real life. So when you go in there and you find that they're acting out scenes or moments or stories or feelings that are thrown to them by members of the audience, and you see it being brought to life. You can see, I feel anyway, that there's something very strong creatively happening at that moment and you think: 'Yes, yes, that's what it's all about and that's what it feels like' or 'now I know what that person was feeling'.

Third, playback theatre builds community through constructing bonds between those present as they bear witness and relate to the stories of others. For example, when a story is played back by the actors and musician in an aesthetic way, the story of an individual becomes everyone's story. This means that issues become access-ible and participants can identify with them. In the words of another participant:

> [W]hile I watched the face of the people presenting, you know offering their story, I was watching their reaction to the performers and seeing where there were connections and where there weren't. In all deliveries there was understanding and experience which went beyond what was there before. The sharing, the openness, is comforting. It helps to be able to share something with people you didn't know five minutes ago even if that something can be a deep and serious experience in your own life. This can be a break-through.

Fourth, playback theatre also provides opportunities for personal, social and instrumental learning where there is learning about the self, the self in relation to others and spontaneity. For example, when participants see themselves enacted they often see aspects of self revealed that they might not have been aware of. One partici-pant described it this way:

> [I]t's educational to sit down and hear other people's experiences. It's education for the self, to see how you appear in other people's eyes . . . [and] it's educational for the audience in terms of expand-ing their understanding of other people.

Playback theatre is a resource for health professionals in that it is a social-aesthetic experience where there exists a 'dialectical com-munication between the . . . actor and [the] audience . . . [with the potential to] continually construct and reconstruct subjectivities, societies, and selves' (Haynes 2001, p. 1). Essentially, playback theatre reveals what it means to be human with potential for per-sonal and social growth, and connection with others. This is reflected in a participant in the Wright study who described her playback theatre experience this way:

> [H]umanness was a key thing that came through, that we are all human. The story about that man is not dissimilar to the story about me. That woman and what is happening to her could

happen to anybody. I didn't realise one woman was going through that while she was just sitting there two seats away from me. It is an opening up of awareness.

Playback theatre is available in many large and some small centres and various companies offer both commissioned and public performances. Workshops for a variety of purposes are also offered. Information about playback theatre, including an online newsletter, is available at <http://www.playbacknet.org/iptn/index.htm>.

Conclusion

As the population ages, a challenge facing governments is assisting older people to live independently and healthily, with access to good quality health and services. The emphasis on the promotion of independence and well-being for older people is consistent with a 'care rather than cure' approach to health, and is one of the driving forces behind the emergence of integrative health. In such a model the individual, rather than the disease, is placed at the centre of the healing process (Diamond 2001).

One can expect that common sense and good business will dictate that tomorrow's health care industries will focus on managing wellness and good health. Within this context, emerging fields, such as the natural therapies and counselling, and the use of music and other forms of art and expression, might force us to challenge assumptions about the dependent, disengaging and fatalistic ageing person that can only be looked after by the tools of high tech medicine. While this chapter has discussed some of the recently acknowledged forms of successful interventions that may assist older people to achieve positive outcomes in their lives, the 'gerontological imagination' of the future, if we may borrow a term used in sociology, is to search for other forms of interventions that promote good health in later life.

11

Gerontechnology: Optimising relationships between ageing people and changing technology

James L. Fozard

'Gerontechnology' is a composite of two words: 'gerontology', the scientific study of ageing, and 'technology', research on and development of technically based products and environments. Concerned with the biological, psychological, social and medical aspects of ageing, gerontechnology is 'the study of technology and ageing for the benefit of a preferred living and working environment and of adapted medical care of the elderly' (Graafmans et al 1994, p. 12). As a theory or world view of ageing, gerontechnology is a transactional view of the dynamics of person/environment relationships that occur with secular changes in the built environment and the changes within and between the generations of ageing people who create and use the environment.

This chapter has four parts. The first defines the areas of application and impact of gerontechnology. The second addresses the proper role of ageing and older people in the guidance of technology development, and argues that the consumer should participate in the planning phases of development and distribution as well as the evaluation of technology-based products, services and environments. The third describes the major publications about gerontechnology, and provides an overview of current and recent research. The fourth relates gerontechnology to other views about health and ageing and to some other ecological views of person/

environment relations concerned with health promotion, as described in Chapter 2.

Areas of application

Gerontechnology concerns the development, dispersal and distribution of technology as targeted toward ageing and older people. It is an integrative discipline constructed from the applications of engineering, biological and social sciences. There are five domains or areas of application of gerontechnnology: health and self-esteem; housing and daily living; mobility and transport; communication and governance; and work and leisure. These human activities increasingly utilise significant technological support in their execution in urban, man-made environments that are the common living environments in the emerging knowledge-based society of the industrial world (van Bronswijk et al 2003):

- *Health and self-esteem*—technology supporting physical, cognitive and emotional functioning as well as the treatment and prevention of disease. 'Self-esteem' refers to the use of technology in the maintenance of individual independence.
- *Housing and daily living*—technology that supports independence, convenience and safety of everyday activities.
- *Mobility and transport*—technology supporting personal mobility and the use of cars and public transport.
- *Communication and governance*—communication technology that maintains and expands social contacts and enhances the governance or remote monitoring of the health and functional status of older persons.
- *Work and leisure*—technology that helps older persons to continue work and to enhance opportunities for educational, recreational and artistic activities.

Throughout history technical aids have been utilised where the strength and skill of humans did not suffice to deal with the demands of specific environment. Today, the complexity of the interactions between changing technology and longer life is continuing to increase. 'The life history aspect of ageing and technology interaction has been accorded little attention in theoretical discussion thus far, and the nature of its treatment in empirical studies has been more practical than theoretical' (Mollenkopf & Fozard, 2004).

Gerontechnology shares basic concepts of other ecological accounts of person–environment relationships, particularly as related to health and health promotion. Frankish (2001) identifies several qualities of a healthful environment that affect human ageing including sustainability (energy use, renewable resource consumption), viability (air and water quality, contaminants) and livability (housing, density, transportation). He points out that there is little research on how an ageing population affects environmental resources or how physical environments serve as a context for values and definitions of well-being of older adults. The gerontechnology view of sustainability is: 'In the planning and managing process of urban environments, a number of sustainabilities are involved: economic sustainability, social sustainability, sustainable health and sustainable development. Gerontechnology especially addresses the last three mentioned' (van Bronswijk et al 2003, p. 170).

Activity 11.1

A central concept of gerontechnology is to directly involve the user in the design, dispersal and distribution of technological products, services and environments. Picking one or two examples, for example, home control and alarm systems or a communication device, apply this concept to product development, dispersal and distribution. Consider the issues of market size, demand, proprietary interests, costs and profits, advertising and training of consumers.

Classification of impacts or uses of gerontechnology

There are four main uses or domains of application of gerontechnology—their relative importance in the five application domains varies.

Prevention and engagement

This refers to the use of technology to delay or prevent age-associated physiological and behavioural changes that restrict human functioning. It concerns accidents in and around the home and environmental factors contributing to allergies, depression and other modifiable conditions. 'More so than in some other domains, the technological environment ranks higher than technological products in themselves. This approach asks for rather immediate investments for long-term societal results' (van Bronswijk et al 2003, p. 171). Prevention thus represents a public health use of technology that is most relevant to lifestyle factors that affect physical strength, mobility, and cognitive and perceptual functioning. Most applications of technology for prevention would be classified as primary prevention in the public health literature (see Chapter 2).

Compensation and assistance

This refers to the use of technology that compensates for age-associated losses in strength and perceptual-motor functioning. Applications range from simple, 'one size fits all' mobility aids to robotic and programmable equipment and products that adapt to the needs of individual users. This is the most frequent use in all domains of application, but especially so in health, mobility and communication. 'In the short run, these impacts may lead to sizeable reductions in societal costs of care' (van Bronswijk et al 2003, p. 171). Most applications of technology for compensation would be classified as secondary prevention in the public health literature (see Chapter 2).

Care support and organisation

This refers to the use of technology by caregivers—often elderly themselves—of older persons who suffer physical or behavioural disabilities. Technological support of caregiving activities includes devices that lift and move physically disabled persons, machines that administer and monitor the use of medications, and equipment that provides information about physiological functioning. Such products are used increasingly by non-professionals, such as family caregivers. The ergonomics of such equipment becomes increasingly important as the range of users increases. Aid to caregivers usually falls under the public health rubrics of tertiary or secondary prevention.

Enhancement and satisfaction

This refers to the innovative uses of technology; for example, virtual-reality, self-adapting equipment to expand the range and depth of human activities with respect to comfort, vitality and productivity. It is most relevant to applications of work, self-fulfilment (artistic activities, education) and communication. 'In the case of communication and governance, consider journals, radio, television, Internet, the cellular phone, or automatic translating devices as well as forms of citizenship making a more intensive use of the experience of older persons to enhance societal cohesion' (van Bronswijk et al 2003, p. 171). This area represents the most opportunities for new research and development. Enhancement emphasises the expanding of human activities rather than compensating for defined limitations, so it does not fit readily into the public health notions of primary, secondary and tertiary prevention.

Gerontechnology broadens the scope of development of specific technology on ageing. The goals of prevention and enhancement are not usually considered in research on medical rehabilitation or care. For example, it has been proposed to use digital hearing aid technology to determine the long-term effects of noise on age-associated hearing loss as well as to reduce its effects (Fozard 2001). The unique applications of technology in artistic activities described by Bouma and Herrington (2000) derive directly from the use of enhancement described above. The idea of using smart or self-adaptive technology in the control devices for technology-based products is being considered as a way to simplify user interfaces by customisation of the controls to the unique preferences and needs of individual users.

Dynamics of the interaction between ageing people and changing technology

Technology's opportunities and consumer needs

A central goal of gerontechnology is to achieve an optimal balance between the preferences, interests and needs of consumers of technology (consumer pull, in short) and the rapid developments of scientific engineering knowledge that provide the bases for developing and marketing new technological products and services (technology push) (Bouma 1992). Technology push may result in the development and marketing of technology-inspired products that contain novel combinations of functions, for example, cellular telephones that may also be used for playing games or as a camera. The dynamics of consumer pull and technology push can change in complex ways over time, frequently affecting persons of different ages in different ways—the first experience of using a menu-driven control device for a new electronic game for a child is very different from that of an older adult who may have lived most of his or her life without the product or, in the case of an existing product, with an earlier configuration of displays and controls for interacting with it, for example, a film versus digital camera.

The effects of technology push are not confined to new technology-related products. Changing control devices requires users to adapt to changing technology in familiar products continuously over the life span. For example, a contemporary older adult may be accustomed to an earlier generation of electromechanical controls that accomplished the same purpose as the new, menu-driven controls. Many older adults at the turn of the 21st century may have adapted to several control devices for the telephone—a hand crank for creating a signal of rings, rotary telephones, touch-tone telephones, and now the menu-driven controls combining visual presentation of calling options and a variety of button controls, some of which have multiple functions. Another example is provided by the clothes-washing machine. An older person in the 21st century may have experienced the evolution of controls—called user-interfaces by designers and engineers—ranging from a manually started gas-driven machine to a contemporary electric-powered machine operated by a complex array of digital electronic controls. At this same point in time, a young, first-time user of washing machines might only recognise the contemporary machine as the prototype washing machine. The lessons from these examples are that older adults of any age can expect secular changes in technology both with respect to adapting to new products and novel ways of using familiar products, and that there will always be young adults or children who have never experienced older user-interfaces. The foregoing examples emphasise the importance of changes in user-interfaces as a source of difficulty in using products. These examples do not negate the central importance of good ergonomic principles in the design of interfaces for users of any age or level of experience (Norman 1988).

A central concept of gerontechnology is to include the end user in all phases of the development, distribution and dispersal of technologically based products, environments and services (Bouma 1992; Mollenkopf & Fozard 2004). Significant involvement in the decisions to develop a product or environment in the first place is needed, as well as input into and evaluation of the product under development. The developing and marketing of new products should not be left completely to the imagination of designers or marketers (technology push). Consumer input in distribution means input into and evaluation of consumer education about the product and ease of use of the product. With respect to technology dispersal, consumer input helps define the boundaries or range of application of particular technologies.

Significant consumer input can be useful in many ways. For the manufacturer, it reduces the trial and error approach to developing and marketing products and environments driven primarily by the availability of a particular technology. It improves user-interfaces with products and environments for consumers covering a wide range of ages. It helps older users deal with the problems of adapting to new user-interfaces for products they have used for many years. It serves as a deterrent to unethical marketing practices and product safety and liability issues that might arise in product distribution. It potentially increases the range of uses for products and environments that may be designed for specific uses and users by considering changes in the use of the technology as people age.

In medical technology, physicians and medical scientists provide advocacy as well as knowledge needed to guide technology development and use. In environmental technology, legal experts and engineers serve as the advocates and expert goal-setters for environmental cleaning and greening approaches to environmental quality. In the case of gerontechnology, the roles of advocate and expert must be fulfilled more directly by the ageing user of the technology. The variety of technological advances covers a wide range of products and services, only some of which are of interest to particular subgroups of ageing individuals. Hence, implementing the concept of user involvement in technology in different areas of application takes considerable ingenuity and commitment—significant challenges, especially in areas of application that do not involve assistive technology for specific disabilities.

The emphasis on user involvement in decision making and advocacy is similar to that described in programs of health promotion as related to the environment. As Frankish (2001) notes, health is a product of the interdependence of individuals and sub-systems of the ecosystem. Environments must provide information and resources that enable decisions and behaviours conducive to health.

Activity 11.2

The approaches of gerontechnology—prevention, compensation, enhancement, etc.—are related to public health concepts of primary, secondary and tertiary prevention. Describe and evaluate the usefulness and limitations of this approach for any example of your choice of receptors, structural components or effectors related to ageing and human function.

Age cohorts and secular changes in technology

Model of temporal dynamics of ageing and technology change

The projected changes in the relative distribution of ages across the life span in the 21st century are well described in earlier chapters. Simultaneously, the rapid changes in technology experienced over the past century will continue, probably at a faster rate, particularly in areas of business where technology fulfils functions formerly provided by people (Mollenkopf & Fozard 2004). The interplay between changes in individual ageing and secular changes in the environment are illustrated in Figure 11.1 and may be used in two ways—first as a tool for analysis of specific person–environment situations, and second as a visual aid for describing the changing dynamics of person–environment interactions over time. These uses will be discussed in turn.

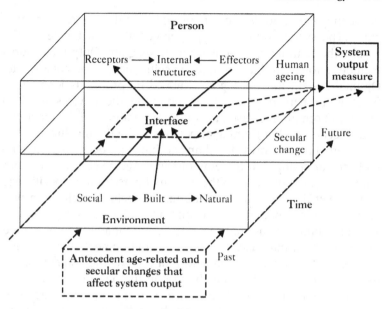

Figure 11.1: Person–environment interface and its changes over time

Information from the environment is received by the person via receptors, for example, visual, auditory, and responded to via effectors, for example, voice, movement of limbs. The environmental information comes from the built or man-made environment, the natural or physical environment, and the social environment. The result of the person–environment interaction is displayed as a system output measure, as shown on the right side of the figure. Over time the quality of the person–environment interface will change, partly because of age-related changes in the physiological and behavioural characteristics of the person and partly because of secular changes in all components of the environment. Antecedent conditions affecting the person–environment interaction are shown at the bottom of the figure. The ageing of a person born in one generation differs from that of person born in a different generation. Adapted from Fozard (2002, Figure 1, vol. 1, no. 3, p. 138).

As a tool for analysis, Figure 11.1 is based on a core concept of ergonomics and engineering according to which people and their environment should be considered as a system. The interface between person and device is represented in the centre of the diagram. The system output is represented in the rectangle on the right of the central person–environment diagram. Output measures include errors, production rate, specific health outcomes, etc. Optimal system functioning is achieved by proper assignment of function to person or machine, adapting the devices used to present information or used to control or manipulate the machine, and selection and/or training of persons using the machine.

Figure 11.1 portrays the changes that may occur with ageing and secular changes in the environment. Ageing can refer to both different age cohorts and to the ageing of persons in a specific age cohort over time. The important changes include declines in perceptual–motor functioning, and internal states including disease. The important secular changes in the environment are not limited to specific user-interfaces in the built environment; they include changes in the social environment that provide the context for the user-interfaces as well as the changes in the natural environment that affect sustainability. Experience with one user-interface can have negative or positive effects on the willingness of a person to use another related or similar one, for example, variations in the displays and controls of different cars or computer software systems. Prior difficulty with a technology-based product may result in avoidance or rejection of a similar product regardless of the ergonomic qualities of the latter.

For purposes of describing the changes in person–environment interactions, Figure 11.1 points to the broad changes in people and the environment that occur over time. Including this feature can improve the descriptive utility of various ecological models inasmuch as it provides a way of describing changes in patterns of interactions between people and their technical environment that may occur as a result of various environmental interventions. This second use of Figure 11.1 will be explored later in the chapter.

To link the shifting age distribution of the human population to the secular changes in technology, social scientists relate the time of introduction of technology to its use by different cohorts of consumers. Sackmann and Waymann (1994) classified successive birth cohorts from the 1930s to the 1970s according to the introduction of various major household technological products, ranging from the radio and telephone to television, automatic clothes-washers and driers, home computers and other advances. They documented how successive cohorts had their first interactions with various technological products at strikingly different ages. More sophisticated analyses of the cohort–technology interaction were reported by Mollenkopf et al (2000).

Structural and individual lag

Sometimes technology develops faster than the needs or abilities of persons to use it (individual lag); at other times technology lags behind human needs and interests (social-structural lag) (Lawton 1998). Lawton's thinking is built on the Rileys' notion of structural lag (Riley & Riley 1994). Age-related illness, cognitive and perceptual-motor declines, and negative attitudes towards old age are the major ingredients of individual lag. The role of gerontechnology in individual lag is compensatory, in other words, the development of products and user-interfaces that facilitate the use of the products by older persons. The core ingredient of social-structural lag results from a social structure that emphasises education for the young, work for middle age and leisure for the old. Current improvements in the longevity and health of older cohorts create demands on the physical and built environment to better support opportunities for leisure, education, creative activities and work for older persons. The role of gerontechnology in social-structural lag is enhancement, the complement of compensation. Lawton goes on to link the complementary gerontechnology functions of compensation and enhancement to feelings of well-being to his domains of well-being, 'health, economics/employment . . . family/friend, sexual relationship, communication' (Lawton 1998, p. 17).

While the dynamics of structural lag have been defined in terms of an interaction between age cohort and secular trends in technology developments, individual lag and social-structural lag are not tied rigidly to members of any specific age group. At any point in time, depending on the specific situation, individual lag may degrade the performance of a 20-year-old person in the same way it affects a 70-year-old. Recognition of this led Mollenkopf (2002) to describe and promote a plan for lifelong learning for gerontechnology that includes job-related and non-job-related learning, and formal and informal learning situations, to reduce problems of structural lag in a changing world. Mollenkopf's plan is specifically aimed at reducing individual lag through education but it may reduce social-structural lag as well.

Life experiences and individual lag

Brauer-Janse et al (1997) vividly described the striking differences in the approaches to learning about and using personal computers exhibited by two groups of first-time users—young children and older people. Research and observational data described by the symposium participants indicated that what was another toy for the youngster was a daunting and delicate machine for the 70-year-old novice. Experienced and novice users profit from different training methods when required to adapt to new production methods (Fozard & Carr 1972; Czaja & Sharit 2002). Age differences and experience are usually confounded in such research inasmuch as the experienced group is usually older and has had previous experience with an earlier device or system.

Docampo et al (2001) examined the implications of individual lag on age differences in the ease of using menu-driven or 'layered-use' interfaces. They observed that many communication devices used electromechanical interfaces before the 1980s and software-style interfaces later (technology generations). Using simulations of these two styles of user-interface they compared the speed and accuracy of their use by young adult participants with early experience (defined as 10–20 years of age) with the user-interface as opposed to three groups of older adults representing cohorts whose early experience was with the electromechanical interface. In addition to the two types of device, levels of difficulty of the task were manipulated so that age-related differences in performance and early experience effects could be distinguished. Age-related performance was lower as task difficulty increased, in keeping with other literature. With task difficulty controlled, the participants whose early experience was with software interfaces performed better on that style of device than any of the cohorts whose early experience was with the electromechanical-style interface. The research results indicate that one source of difficulty in the menu-driven interfaces is related to the requirements to follow a sequence of steps to select the desired outcome. In some devices such as the modern digital camera the difficulty in completing the desired sequence of choices is increased because some controls have multiple functions depending on the way the camera is being operated, for example, creating new images versus editing stored ones.

One major lesson from the research reviewed is that there will continue to be examples of individual lag as successive technology generations interact with different cohorts of ageing people. While the role of early experience is an important contributor to the individual lag, the usefulness of task design and training interventions will be highly specific to particular applications, as suggested by Czaja et al (2001).

Age and motivation to adapt to changing technology

On the basis of anecdotal evidence, one can guess that many basements and garages in homes around the industrialised world contain technological-based appliances and toys that are unused because of the perceived and experienced difficulty of adults and children in using them. For frustrated users of technology, the perceived effort to successfully use the product may not justify the effort to master the techniques for using it. For older users, part of the frustration with the equipment may result from the potential benefits of the technology being unknown to the user because of the technology generation to which that person belongs (Bouwhuis & Melanhorst 2001). As pointed out by Freudenthal (1999), older persons often leave the programming and adjustment of consumer products to their children or technically proficient friends. For this and other reasons, Bouwhuis and Melanhorst point out that older persons may perceive the cognitive effort required to master new technology as considerable, and may choose not to invest the effort to master a technology of uncertain utility to them. Uncertainties about health and time remaining to live contribute to this perception, called 'temporal discounting' by the authors. Temporal discounting may account for the reluctance of many older persons to use the Internet and other communication devices as substitutes for face-to-face communication with family and friends. The role of experience and motivation in adapting to technological change will require continuing research.

Information about gerontechnology

The major sources of existing and new information about gerontechnology are the proceedings of four international conferences on the subject (reported in chronological order by Bouma & Graafmans 1992; Graafmans et al 1998; Pieper et al 2002; Charness et al 2002); the journal *Gerontechnology*, published quarterly since

2001; <http://sts.bwk.tue.nl/gerontech/>; Harrington and Harrington 2000); and <www.gerontechnology.net>, the website of the International Society of Gerontechnology.

In addition, dozens of book chapters and articles in specialty journals have been published since the concept was first developed at the Eindhoven University of Technology in 1988. Two handbook-type volumes related to ergonomics and ageing were recently published (Fisk & Rogers 1997; Steenbekkers & van Beijsterveldt 1998). Other books and articles related to gerontechnology are cited later in the chapter.

Examples of activities and research related to gerontechnology

Because of the rapid developments in gerontechnology, a review of the field would be largely out of date by the time of publication of this book. Therefore, no effort is made to provide a comprehensive review here. Rather a sampling of current activities is described—mostly taken from publications mentioned above with an emphasis on items from the proceedings of the Fourth International Conference on Gerontechnology held in 2002. The summary illustrates some applications of the three major uses of gerontechnology—prevention, compensation and enhancement—to health and functioning, communication, housing, transportation, and work and self-fulfilment activities.

Health and functioning

Gait, stumbles and falls

Compensatory devices to aid personal mobility—rolling walkers, grab bars, hip protectors and other devices—are continually being improved (Charness et al 2002). Interest has grown in the use of technology to prevent problems of poor gait, stumbles and falls. Walking requires muscular strength, known to decline with ageing, but strength is also modifiable by training into very old age. These observations form the basis for proposing a long-term intervention program designed to maintain a physiological reserve of strength required for walking. Unlike cardiovascular training, there are few strength-training guidelines that relate the results of training directly to strength requirements for walking. Studies by Rantanen and Avela (1997) and Kwon et al (2001) have established relationships between gait speed and leg strength that, with some additional refinements, could be used to set goals for strength training, for example, the range of leg strength required for various gait speeds, and sex differences in strength reserve. The next steps involve relating age-dependent strength requirements for optimal gait to the timing and intensity of strength-training programs.

The interventions discussed above address long-term age-related multi-year changes in strength that result in poor gait, stumbles and falls. Muscle strength is not the only factor precipitating stumbles and falls. Gait analyses using motion sensors and dynamic analyses of stride and foot-walking surface contact have yielded important information about age-related differences in gait that are also important factors. Using such technology, Kawai and Hiki (2002) determined that many older persons used greater flexion of hip joints to compensate for relatively weak ankle strength, making them relatively more susceptible to stumbles and falls. The authors describe a simple way to obtain the important information that can be used in clinical settings.

Falls are infrequent and relatively unpredictable in most everyday situations. In an effort to measure walking in the seconds immediately preceding a fall, Tamura et al (2002) and Yoshimura et al (2002) describe a lightweight, unobtrusive, wearable, three-dimensional axial accelerometer that records fall direction, impact acceleration and fall time. The accelerometer is linked to a data logger and microcomputer. While development is still in early stages, the device successfully identified nineteen out of 22 falls amongst a group of older persons with Parkinson's disease. The foregoing examples indicate the wide range of current and potential uses of technology in what would generally be considered primary prevention, in the jargon of public health, but also illustrate the wide range of time intervals between the ascertainment of risk and the event that merit investigation.

Vision and hearing

Exposure to very bright light and loud noise can result in damage to the primary receptors that in some ways resemble those associated with ageing. Examples include members of occupational groups that experience extreme exposure to light, such as professional fishermen, who develop cataracts at an earlier age than workers in noisy environments, for example, airline baggage handlers and rock musicians, who suffer more high-frequency hearing loss than age-matched controls (Fozard & Gordon-Salant 2001). Elevated blood pressure has been shown to be an independent risk factor for elevated intraocular pressure (McLeod et al 1990) and elevated thresholds for frequencies in the speech range (Brant et al 1996). Since circulatory difficulties are secondary to cardiovascular disease risk factors, existing interventions for reducing blood pressure are justified as interventions. There is insufficient evidence for launching a clinical trial of controlling exposure to very bright light. The evidence justifying a noise-reduction intervention is stronger, enough so that the writer has proposed a long-term study of the relationship between noise exposure and age-associated hearing loss. The idea for intervention is to use hearing aid technology to limit exposure, thereby reducing the hearing loss commonly observed with ageing (Fozard 2001).

Early detection of disease

Longitudinal studies of changes in age-associated cardiovascular function and subsequent cardiac disease can be counted amongst the success stories of prevention. The Bogalusa Study of childhood development of risk factors for early onset of heart disease established the importance of early intervention with the conventional risk factors for cardiovascular disease—blood pressure, lipid metabolism, obesity—in children who are clinically free of such disease (Bao et al 1995). In adult males, longitudinal studies of the rate of age-related changes in serum levels of prostate specific antigen (PSA) have been shown by Carter et al (1992) to predict the diagnosis of prostate cancer five to seven years prior to clinical diagnosis. The value of early detection of prostate cancer with respect to its treatment is still controversial. In both these examples the preventive approach has depended on long-term measurements of risk factors in persons who do not have the disease.

Other age-associated changes in function that have the potential for monitoring function and potential risk factors include the relationship between indoor air quality and lung disease, including chronic obstructive lung disease (Snijders et al 2001; Koren et al 2002), and hearing loss and elevated blood pressure (Brant et al 1996). Omenn et al (1997) propose a multiple-component health promotion intervention package related to a half-dozen health problems that have the potential for long-term interventions based on assessments of an accumulation of small traumatic insults over time and the development of interventions targeted toward protection from them.

However, developing the evidence necessary to justify the research and implementation of a prevention program can be expensive and time consuming. Perhaps the best-studied example is the relationship between exposure to tobacco smoke by non-smoking persons ('second-hand smoking') and lung disease. The complexity of the process of establishing relationships between second-hand exposure to smoke and risk for disease and the importance of avoiding second-hand exposure is illustrated in the summary of the research topic described in the United States Public Health Service reports by the US Surgeon General available on the Internet <www.phs.nih.gov> or in the publications listed on the Surgeon General's web page. The number of potential confounders considered in the estimations of risk are formidable—as attested to by the protracted legal battles over the harmful effects of tobacco on health.

Compensation for functional limitations

Devices that compensate for age-associated limitations in functional personal mobility, sensory and perceptual motor function (Fozard 2000) are much more sophisticated than those oriented toward prevention. This is true partly because advances in rehabilitation technology provide products and environments that are potentially useful for older persons with functional limitations. In the general older population, the extent and specificity of the limitations are usually less in 'normal' old age. The quotation marks around 'normal' point out a frequently made distinction between a specific recognised disability that limits function and limitation due to ageing. Older persons often object to using devices designed for persons with specific disabilities because of the perceived stigma associated with the device—'I'm old, not disabled'. This issue is frequently addressed by using universal design principles (Coleman 1998; Coleman & Myerson 2001). Persons with functional limitations related to specific disabilities are, as a group, quite demanding of compensatory products and environments. In contrast, older persons as a group often deny age-associated functional limitations and as a result may not want to use devices that could be useful to them. Miasaki et al (2001) have devised a procedure for a listener to adjust the speech rate of announcers that is adaptable to a wide range of users—an excellent example of a compensatory control device that accommodates a wide range of older users.

The restrictions on coverage by health insurance and the traditional marketing of rehabilitative equipment often magnify the difficulty in accepting the use of compensatory equipment. The legal definition of 20/200 Snellen acuity as the threshold for blindness works against the use by older persons of many low-vision aids, particularly devices that enhance illumination, target size or contrast. The situation is somewhat better for hearing aids and personal broadcast receiving devices such as those available in theatres and concert halls. However, the advertising for such devices is usually uninformative and sometimes misleading to the consumer. For example, the programmable digital hearing aid requires a trained audiologist to adapt it to the needs of the specific user.

Research needed on the natural history of functional decline

Research is needed to improve the use of compensatory devices by older persons (Fozard 2003). While epidemiological information documents an increase in functional limitations in older age groups, information about the ways in which people compensate for them is more limited. Verbrugge and Jette (1994) found that overall, persons with limitations relied on other people for help. Compensatory devices were used relatively more frequently with limitations in lower than in upper extremities. An interview procedure called The Physical Function Inventory (PFI) was developed to identify the ways in which adults compensated for functional limitations. Standard questions in the form of 'Do you have difficulty . . .?' were devised for 23 activities of daily living or instrumental activities and mobility (Whetstone et al 1991). For each activity respondents were asked if they changed how or how frequently the activity was performed. As in other studies, the number of limitations in physical function increased with age. One interesting finding was that a large number of persons denied any difficulty in carrying out the activity because they had already changed how or how frequently they performed the activity. The survey also probed for the specifics of the compensation. An instrument such as the PFI when used in conjunction with a home survey identifying environmental challenges to physical functioning could do much to improve the possibilities for ageing in place by current and future generations of older persons (Pynoos & Regnier 1997).

Communication

Increased communication between people represents the most pervasive manifestation of modern technology. Persons born early in the 20th century have participated in the changes in working and personal life brought about by the evolution of the telephone from its earliest form to the current miniature cell phone which can also be used for playing electronic games and following the ups and downs of the stock market via wireless Internet access. Immediate and easy access to voice communication is now possible throughout much of the world. Technology has brought about reductions in isolation of the homebound, an increase in the availability of safety alarms, remote shopping, telemedicine, business transactions of all kinds and working at home.

The use of advanced communication systems by older persons, such as interactive video, email, Internet access, multimedia and information services, is receiving considerable research and development attention as evidenced in the Fourth International Conference on Gerontechnology (Charness et al 2002). One session, 'Evaluation of computer input devices', contained studies that evaluated the ergonomics of the computer mouse, touch screen devices, etc. Related topics included an evaluation of telephone voice menu systems (Czaja & Sharit 2002). User training and software design were addressed in sessions on 'Navigating the World Wide Web', 'Creativity and socialisation' and 'Domotics and networking'. After reviewing the challenges to users created by rapidly changing technology, Mollenkopf (2002) concluded that clearly focused training in the use of communication technology by older persons will continue to be necessary over future generations, inasmuch as technology changes will almost always render an older person's experience with earlier technology obsolete.

Other sessions and presentations at the Fourth International Conference described the use of advanced communication systems in telemedicine ('Telehealth'), remote monitoring of physiological events related to illnesses and general health, both in the home ('Automation and monitoring') and in long-term care facilities ('Nursing home symposium'), monitoring of mobility of dementia patients ('Technology and dementia'), information and emotional support of caregivers of elderly patients ('Technology, caregiving and training,' 'How does information technology help the family?').

Housing

Consumer pull for increased technology in the home is based on the desire of old persons to remain living independently in their own homes, neighbourhoods and social networks (see Chapter 7). Architects, designers, planners and construction experts argue that the needs of older persons are best served by properly designed new housing—smaller units that can accommodate persons who have or potentially will experience functional limitations and can support smart house technology.

Many plans exist for housing to accommodate the desire to age in place. Homes with flexible interior walls that can be configured to meet the changing needs for space from the time of family rearing to empty nest were available years ago (Fozard & Popkin 1978). Barrier-free housing and height-adjustable work and storage space costs less when included in new construction than when retrofitted into existing housing. The American Association of Retired Persons (Stern & Harootyan 1993) convened a conference to address architecture, technology and retrofit options for senior housing. Later, Goto et al (2001) described current Japanese efforts to develop universal design principles that will accommodate changing needs over the life span.

Enabling environments for ageing in place requires more than barrier-free design. As Levy and Malcolm (1992, p. 88) pointed out, 'problems with home maintenance, mobility and shopping are among those most likely to cause older people to move out of their homes'. A set of twelve design principles to optimise the person–environment fit was provided by Regnier (1993, p. 17): personal privacy, social interaction, personal control and autonomy, orientation and way-finding provisions, safety and security, accessibility to needed services, stimulation and challenge, sensory assistance as needed, familiarity, good aesthetics and appearance, self-expression or personalisation, and adaptable or flexible environments.

The options of new adaptable housing are not possible for most older persons. For economic reasons, adaptation of existing housing is the only option for most (Mutschler 1997). In *Staying Put: Adapting the Places Instead of the People*, Lanspery and Hyde (1997) describe research and programs related to retrofitting existing housing for older persons, including those who are physically frail or have dementia. Several chapters document the variety of economic and policy approaches used to retrofitting (see also Pieper 1994).

Developments in smart home technology cut across all housing options (van Berlo 2002). Smart home developmental research in Europe supported by the European Union is described in Wild and Kirschner (1994). In the Fourth International Conference on Gerontechnology, two sessions, 'Symposium on domotics and networking' and 'General issues in smart home design', described current research on the use of technology for safety and security and environmental control, including lighting, air temperature and quality, accessories such as draperies, and entrances.

Transportation

The automobile will continue to be the preferred or only means of transportation in the daily lives of older persons (Mollenkopf & Fozard 2004). In the United States and Europe, this is due largely to what Barr (2002) calls suburbanisation (increased dispersion) of people's homes. In some European countries and in a few places in the United States, efforts have been made to increase accessibility to public transportation by introducing flexibility into the routes and schedules of buses and vans.

Complex technology helps identify age-associated modifiable perceptual motor skills related to driving. Poor performance on a measure of visual attention, the 'useful field of view', has been identified as a risk factor for automobile accidents (Ball et al 2002). The importance of such interventions for persons with cognitive decline characteristic of early stages of dementia has been recognised in various research activities discussed in a special issue of *Gerontechnology* (2002, vol. 1, no. 4) devoted to driving in relation to age.

Efforts to improve the safety and ease of use of automobiles by older drivers have been documented in an earlier special edition of *Gerontechnology* (2002, vol. 1, no. 2). Hanowski and Dingus (2000) review developments in intelligent transportation systems, such as routing and navigation, safety and collision warning systems.

Highway infrastructure such as signage can be redesigned to be easier to interpret at greater distances, using more illumination, larger characters and more low spatial-frequency elements (Kline 1994; Sagawa 2002). Training and screening older drivers to improve safety has also received considerable attention (Ball & Wahl 2002).

Work and leisure

Physical labour

Age-related losses of physical strength, sensory acuity and behavioural speed are widely believed to decrease the capacity of older workers for work, and to increase their risk for work-related injury. One of the most comprehensive studies of age in relation to capacity for physical work was conducted in Finland by Ilmarinen et al (1992). For some types of heavy labour—repairing electrical utility poles and wires in the case of men, and heavy industrial cleaning in the case of women—it was found that daily performance of the work failed to compensate for losses in muscle strength for workers in their fifties (Nygard et al 1992). It was proposed that additional strength training would partially compensate for the loss. There is an ongoing stream of studies related to job redesign and retraining designed to allow older workers to continue in their jobs. Examples of current activities are described by Scott (2002) and in a session on 'Workplace issues' at the Fourth International Conference of Gerontechnology.

Computer and office work

Czaja et al (2001, 2003) have carried out a number of investigations of age-related difficulties in search and retrieval tasks using simulated computer data bases, and found that training and task redesign are effective interventions. Complex interactions between age and previous experience have been identified.

Leisure and self-expression

The role of technology to enhance the quality of life of older persons in the realms of self-expression and education has received relatively little attention, a situation that should change over time, mostly because of the impact that digital technology is having on the ease of creating and altering visual and auditory images. At present, some of the digital cameras and synthesisers and the associated software used to create and process images and sounds require considerable training to use effectively. Human factors studies are in progress, finding ways to facilitate the use of the Internet by older persons (Ownby & Czaja 2002; Pak et al 2002). Bouma and Harrington (2000) describe a technology-supported system to allow several persons to work simultaneously on painting or creating an image. The technology supporting the application allows the various participants to see their own work as well as that of their fellow artists. The potential of virtual reality for enhancing the endeavours of older persons has not yet received significant research and development efforts.

Relationships between gerontechnology and other approaches to health and ageing

Gerontechnology shares many features with other transactional views of person–environment relationships; while its focus is on the man-made environment, it also considers the social and natural physical environments (Figure 11.1). Marshall (2002) takes another approach to linking a person to the physical environment. As shown in the left panel of Figure 11.2, his model embeds the individual in an ever-broader environmental network that ranges from interpersonal level to public policy. The physical and natural components of environmental influences on behaviour are mediated through the social component of the environment. In contrast, the gerontechnology model includes technology as part of interpersonal relations, as shown in the right side of the figure. The time dimension of Figure 11.2 adds to the comprehensiveness of Marshall's social ecology model.

In the Healthy People 2010 model (Healthy People 2010, 2000), desired health goals and objectives are related to multiple

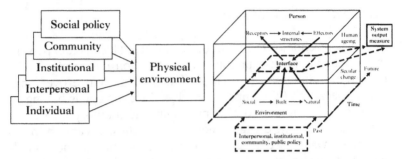

The overlapping rectangles show that a person's behaviour and health is affected by various social interactions, ranging from narrow interpersonal relationships through ever-broader social entities to community and social policy. In this model, the effects of the physical environment are mediated through social interactions. This figure was redrawn from one used by Marshall (2002).

The social determinants of behaviour and health displayed on the left are shown in the box at the base. According to the social ecology model, their contribution to the person–environment interface is through the social component of the environment (no direct arrows from the built or natural components of the environment are shown). Rather, the impact of the physical environment is mediated through the social environment. While the social-ecological model does not specifically discuss the temporal aspects of the social factors, their role in determining behaviour and health are subject to change over time.

Figure 11.2: Marshall's social ecology model of person–environment relationships (left) and its relationship to gerontechnology (right)

determinants of health, as depicted in the left side of Figure 11.3, adapted from Healthy People 2010. In this model, the environment is divided into social and physical components connected to the individual by biological and behavioural pathways. Health-related policies and interventions including those that affect access to quality health care are seen as modifiers of the person–environment interaction that affects measured health status (bottom of figure). Health status is operationally defined by several indices related to public health as well as morbidity and mortality. Changes in such indices measure the progress toward the attainment of the goals and objectives set for the decade. In this model, the interventions and access to health care correspond closely to the prevention, compensation and aid to caregiver uses of gerontechnology.

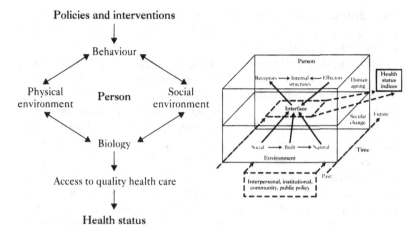

Policies and interventions

Behaviour

Physical environment   **Person**   Social environment

Biology

Access to quality health care

Health status

A person's health status is influenced by the physical and social environment. The interaction is separated into behavioural and biological components, partly reflecting the importance of medical intervention in health status. Public health policies and health interventions as well as assurances of access to medical care are seen as the means to alter health status. Indices of health status (for example, the number of teenage smokers) for each of the many public health goals to be reached by 2010 are described in Healthy People 2010. The figure was adapted from the one presented by Marshall (2002).

The interaction between people and their environments shown in the Healthy People 2010 model is similar to that of the gerontechnology model. The policies and interventions as well as access to health care are shown as specific environmental determiners of the person–environment interface. The impact of the Healthy People interventions as well as all the other components will be reflected in changes in the various health status indices (see the arrow from interface to 'health status' over time), for example, number of persons in different age groups who are hypertensive or overweight.

Figure 11.3: Detail of the Healthy People 2010 model of the factors that influence health status and its relationship to gerontechnology

The right side of Figure 11.3 shows the relationship between the Healthy People 2010 and gerontechnology models. The public health policies and interventions as well as access to medical care are portrayed as environmental determiners of person–environment interactions as shown in the box at the bottom. The health status outcome index (arrow on right) is represented as a measure of the person–environment interface. The time dimension of the gerontechnology scheme captures changes in the health index resulting from the public health interventions.

The gerontechnology version vividly illustrates that many factors in addition to public health policy influence the hoped-for change in the health indices.

Marshall's (2002) model of healthy ageing relates individual well-being at any age to a host of demographic and personal history factors that contribute to health and social integration and along with wealth are considered the necessary proximal conditions for well-being. This model, redrawn slightly from Marshall (2002), is shown in the left side of Figure 11.4. Although the term 'environment' is not shown in the figure, the impact of the physical and social environment on all the factors contributing to well-being is easily discerned. Marshall's model is of particular interest to the present discussion because it identifies a hierarchy of historical factors in a person's life that contribute to well-being. The relationship between Marshall's model and the gerontechnology model is shown on the right side of Figure 11.4. Marshall's antecedent factors are listed as historical environmental factors at the bottom of the figure. The most proximal influences (health, wealth and social integration) are closest to the present in time, while the demographic factors are more in the past. The measure 'well-being' is portrayed as an outcome to the right of measure of the person–environment interface. Marshall's model suggests several environmental interventions across the life span that contribute to well-being in old age. The areas of application named in gerontechnology (communication, housing, work, health) are related to Marshall's factors of social integration—family and household, labour force history, health, respectively. Transportation and mobility cut across all of Marshall's factors.

Other concepts of health related to ageing that extend beyond absence of disease share some of the conceptual elements of gerontechnology. Rowe and Kahn's (1997) definition of successful ageing includes 'maintaining high cognitive and physical function' and 'engagement with life' as well as 'avoiding disease' as the essential components. Baltes and Baltes (1990) use the concepts of compensation and adaptation or accommodation in their eloquent analysis of changing responses to environmental challenges in the face of age-related losses of functional ability. The World Health Organization's definition of health promotion included the notion of the 'enabling environment', which in the gerontechnology model includes prevention, compensation and enhancement

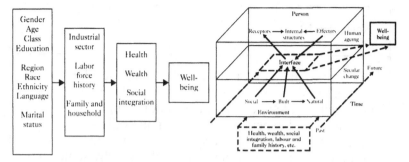

The most proximal influences are current health, wealth and social integration. Less proximal influences (not necessarily less important) include work and family history, and various ethnic and social class factors. Although the factors contributing to well-being are not specifically related to environmental factors, they could be. The left side of Figure 11.4 is slightly redrawn from that presented by Marshall (2002).

In the gerontechnology model (right side), Marshall's (2002) determinants of well-being are seen as environmental factors having their initial influences at various past times in the life of a person. The dynamics of the influences of well-being can change as a result of people ageing as well as changes in the environment in which the person lives.

Figure 11.4: Health promotion model by Marshall (2002) relating well-being at any age to ever more remote factors that impact current well-being and the relationship of determiners of well-being to the person–environment model of gerontechnology

(WHO 1999, as quoted by Williams 2002): 'the process of enabling people to increase control over and to improve, their health . . . and individual or group must be able to identify and to realize aspirations, to satisfy needs, and to change or cope with environment. Health is, therefore, seen as a resource for everyday life, not the objective of living'.

Activity 11.3

The author makes claims that the gerontechnology model in Figure 11.1 provides an improved way of describing other approaches to person–environment interactions illustrated in Figures 11.2, 11.3 and 11.4. Critically evaluate his arguments.

Activity 11.4

The central message of this chapter is that secular changes in the environment over time influence how and how well people in different age cohorts function, live their lives and experience their own and others development and ageing. Using your own experiences and that of family members or friends, identify some examples of technology change that illustrate the concept.

Conclusion

The changes in the technical environment are changing our concepts of distance—what is far and near, how we access people we care about, whether remote or close to us physically and the nature of our social interactions—machines versus people in business and personal interactions (Mollenkopf & Fozard 2004). The way we age and experience the ageing of ourselves and people of other generations living and working alongside us will continue to be shaped by changes in technologies that are becoming more a part of our everyday lives as time goes on. The message of gerontechnology is that ageing and aged people should be actively involved in shaping the technology that affects their lives. Limiting the use of technological products and environments, for whatever reason, may limit their value to both successful and unsuccessful consumers of the technology. Adaptation to the changes in the built environment will be required of us all. How the adaptation is to occur will be a major factor in how and how well we age in the future.

References

ABS. *See* Australian Bureau of Statistics.

ACGP. *See* Australian College of General Practitioners.

Adelman, M 1991, 'Stigma, gay lifestyles and adjustment to aging: A study of later-life gay men and lesbians' in J Lee (ed.) *Gay Midlife and Maturity*, Hawthorn Press, New York, pp. 7–32.

Aged Care Standards and Accreditation Agency 1999, *Accreditation Guide for Residential Aged Care Standards*, Australian Government Publishing Service, Canberra.

AIHW. *See* Australian Institute of Health and Welfare.

Alagiakrishnan, K & Masaki, K 2001, 'Vascular dementia', *eMedicine Journal*, vol. 2, pp. 1–15.

Allan, D & Penning, M 2001, 'Changes in patterns and predictors of physician and hospital utilization among older adults: Regional differences', Presented at the Canadian Association of Gerontologists seminar, Edmonton, Canada.

Allen, T 2000, 'Housing renewal—doesn't it make you sick?' *Housing Studies*, vol. 15, pp. 443–61.

Alzheimer's Association NSW 2002, www.alznsw.asn.au/library/vasclar.htm, *Vascular Dementia HelpNote* (accessed 16 July 2002).

Alzheimer Society of Canada, Toronto, *Statistics* 2002 www.alzheimer.ca/english/disease/stats-people.html

Amar, G & Wilcock, K 1996, 'Fortnightly review: Vascular dementia', *British Medical Journal*, vol. 1, pp. 227–31.

Ambrose, PJ 1997, 'Better housing as preventative medicine', *Housing Review*, vol. 463, pp. 57–9.

American Health Care Association 2003, *Issues of Quality in Home and Community Based Care*, AHCA Health Services Research and Evaluation, http:www.ahca.org (accessed 7 January 2004).

Anderson, J 2002, Ramifications of reminiscence: Dealing with death and personal meaning through reminiscence activity, Unpublished PhD thesis, University of New England, Armidale.

Anderson, R, Hsieh, P & Su, H 1998, 'Resource allocation and resident outcomes in nursing homes: Comparisons between the best and worst', *Research in Nursing and Health*, vol. 21, pp. 297–313.

Andrade, CK & Clifford, P 2001, *Outcome-based Massage*, Lippincott Williams & Wilkins, Baltimore.

Andrews, K 2002, *National Strategy for an Ageing Australia*, Department of Health and Ageing, Canberra.

Antonucci, TC 1985, 'Personal characteristics, social support, and social behavior' in RH Binstock & E Shanas (eds), *Handbook of Aging and the Social Sciences* (2nd edn), Van Nostrand Reinhold, New York.

——1990, 'Social supports and social relationships', in RH Binstock & LK George (eds), *Handbook of Aging and the Social Sciences* (3rd edn), Academic Press, New York.

Anttila, A, Pukkala, E, Soderman, B, Kallio, M, Nieminen, P & Hakama, M 1999, 'Effect of organised screening on cervical cancer incidence and mortality in Finland, 1963–1995: Recent increase in cervical cancer incidence', *International Journal of Cancer*, vol. 83, pp. 59–65.

Arbuckle, NW & de Vries, B 1995, 'Long-term effects of later life spousal and parental bereavement on personal functioning', *Gerontologist*, vol. 35, pp. 637–47.

Arcury, TA, Quandt, SA, Bell, RA, Vitolins, MZ & McDonald, J 2000, 'Complementary and alternative medicine use among rural older adults', *Gerontologist*, vol. 15, p. 141.

Arluke, A, Levin, J & Suchwalko, J 1984, 'Sexuality and romance in advice books for the elderly', *Gerontologist*, vol. 24, pp. 415–8.

Arnold, SB 1991, 'Measurement of quality of life in the frail elderly' in J Birren, J Lubben, J Rowe & D Deutchman (eds), *The Concept and Measurement of Quality of Life in the Frail Elderly*, Academic Press, San Diego.

Astin, JA 1998, 'Why patients use alternative medicine', *Journal of the American Medical Association*, vol. 279, pp. 1548–53.

Astin, JA, Pelletier, KR, Marie, A & Haskell, WL 2000, 'Complementary and alternative medicine use among elderly persons: One year analysis of a Blue Shield Medicare supplement', *Journal of Gerontology*, vol. 55, pp. 4–10.

Astin, L 2003, 'Patterns and predictors of CAM use among older adults' in P Cherniach & N Cherniack (eds), *Alternative Medicine for the Elderly*, Springer, Berlin.

Atchley, RC 1976, *The Sociology of Retirement*, Schenkman Publishing, Cambridge, MA.

Atienza, A, Stephens, MAP & Townsend, AL 2002, 'Dispositional optimism, role-specific stress, and the well-being of adult daughter caregivers', *Research on Aging*, vol. 24, pp. 193–217.

Atkins, S, Adams, M, McKinney, C, McKinney, H, Rose, L, Wentworth, J & Woodworth, J 2003, *Expressive Arts Therapy: Creative Process in Art and Life*, Parkway Publishers Inc, Boone.

Australian Bureau of Statistics 1997, *Retirement and Retirement Intentions, Australia* http://www.abs.gov.au/ausstats/abs%40.nsf/b06660592430724 fca2568b5007b8619/3dc3297faa3cb8abca2568a90013938a!OpenDocument (accessed 23 January 2003).

——1998, *Mental Health and Wellbeing, Profile of Adults*, Australian Bureau of Statistics, Canberra.

——1998, *Survey of Disability, Ageing and Carers*, ACT: Australian Government Publishing Service, Canberra.

——1999a, *Older People, Australia: A Social Report*, http://www.abs.gov.au/ausstats/abs%40.nsf/b06660592430724fca2568b5007b 8619/3be24b1cb70dcae1ca2568a900139 41e!OpenDocument (accessed 23 February 2003).

——1999b, *Disability, Ageing and Carers, Australia*, Australian Bureau of Statistics, Canberra.

——2000, *Population by Age and Sex: Australian States and Territories*, Cat. no. 3201.0, Australian Government Publishing Service, Canberra.

——2000, *Caring in the Community*, http://www.abs.gov.au/Ausstats/abs (accessed 14 October 2003).

——2001, *Census of Population and Housing*, Australian Bureau of Statistics, Canberra.

——2001, *Australian Social Trends, Family Services: Caring in the Community*, http://www.abs.gov.au/aausstats/abs (accessed 14 October 2003).

Australian College of General Practitioners 2002, *Guidelines for Preventive Activities in General Practice*, Australian College of General Practitioners, Melbourne.

Australian Institute of Health and Welfare (AIHW) 1997, *Demand for Disability Support Services in Australia: Size, Cost and Growth*, Australian Institute of Health and Welfare, Canberra.

——2000, *Australia's Health*, Australian Institute of Health and Welfare, Canberra.

——2002, *Older Australia at a Glance*, Cat. no. AGE 25, Australian Institute of Health and Welfare, Canberra.

——2003, Media Release, 6 June.

Australian, The 1995 'Over 65s say sex keeps them active', 26 October, p. 1.

Bachelard, G 1994, *The Poetics of Space*, Beacon Press, Boston.

Baer, HA, Jen, C, Tanassi, LM, Tsia, C & Waahbeh, H 1998, 'The drive for professionalism in acupuncture: A preliminary view from the San Francisco Bay Area', *Social Science and Medicine*, vol. 46, pp. 533–7.

Ball, KK, Wadley, VG & Edwards, JD 2002, 'Advances in technology used to assess and retrain older drivers', *Gerontechnology*, vol. 1, pp. 251–61.

Ball, KK & Wahl, H-W 2002, 'Driving in old age: Use of technology to promote independence', *Gerontechnology*, vol. 1, pp. 217–307.

Ball, MM, Wittington, FJ, Perkins, MM, Patterson, VL, Hollingworth, C & King, SV 2000, 'Quality of life in assisted living facilities: Viewpoints of residents', *Journal of Applied Gerontology*, vol. 19, pp. 304–25.

Ball, RM 1990, 'Public–private solution to protection against the cost of long-term care', *Journal of the American Geriatrics Society*, vol. 382, pp. 156–63.

Baltes, PB & Baltes, MM 1990, *Successful Aging: Perspectives from the Behavioral Sciences*, Cambridge University Press, Cambridge.

Baltes, PB & Smith, J 2003, 'New frontiers in the future of aging: From successful aging of the young old to the dilemmas of the fourth age', *Gerontologist*, vol. 49, pp. 123–35.

Bamford, T 2001, 'Housing and the national health service plan: Reconfiguring the deckchairs?' *Housing, Care and Support*, vol. 42, pp. 4–8.

Bao, W, Strinivasan, SR & Berenson, GS 1995, 'Essential hypertension predicted by tracking of elevated blood pressure from childhood to adulthood: The Bogalusa Heart Study', *American Journal of Hypertension*, vol. 8, pp. 1–8.

Barker, JC 2002, 'Neighbours, friends and other non-kin caregivers of community-living dependent elders', *The Journals of Gerontology*, vol. 57B, pp. S158-S168.

Barr, RA 2002, 'More road to travel by: Implications for mobility and safety in late life', *Gerontechnology*, vol. 2, pp. 50–4.

Barrett, B, Marchand, L, Scheder, J, Appelbaum, D, Chapman, M, Jacobs, C, Westergaard, R & St Clair, N 2000, 'Bridging the gap between conventional and alternative medicine', *Journal of Family Practice*, vol. 49, pp. 234–9.

Barrow, G 1996, *Aging, the Individual and Society*, West Publishing, St Paul, Minneapolis.

Bartlett, H & Burnip, S 1998, 'Quality of care in nursing homes for older people: Providers' perspectives and priorities', *Nursing Research*, vol. 3, pp. 257–68.

Barusch, AS 1988, 'Problems and coping strategies of elderly spouse caregivers', *The Gerontologist*, vol. 28, pp. 677–85.

Bass, DM & Bowman, K 1990, 'Transition from caregiving to bereavement: The relationship of care-related strain and adjustment to death', *The Gerontologist*, vol. 30, pp. 35–42.

Bayer, AH & Harper, L 2000, *Fixing to Stay: A National Survey of Housing and Home Modification Issues*, American Association of Retired Persons, Washington, DC.

Beers, M & Berkow, R 2000, *The Merck Manual of Geriatrics*, Merck Research Laboratories, Whitehouse Station, New Jersey.

Beinfield, H & Korngold, E 1991, *Between Heaven and Earth: A Guide to Chinese Medicine*, Ballantine, New York.

Bell, K & Weinberg, MS 1978, *Homosexualities: A Study of Diversity among Men and Women*, Simon & Schuster, New York.

Bell, PA, Greene, TC, Fisher, JD & Baum, A 2001, *Environmental Psychology* (5th edn), Wadsworth, Belmont CA.

Berger, R 1982, *Gay and Gray*, University of Illinois, Chicago.

Berk, L 2001, *Development Through the Life Span*, Allyn & Bacon, Boston.

Berkman, LF & Syme, SL 1979, 'Social networks, host resistance, and mortality: a nine-year follow-up of Alameda County residents', *American Journal of Epidemiology*, vol. 109, pp. 186–204.

Better Health Commission 1986, *Health for All Australians: Looking Forward to Better Health*, Australian Government Publishing Service, Canberra.

Biegel, DE, Sales, E & Schulz, R 1991, *Family Caregiving in Chronic Illness: Alzheimer's Disease, Cancer, Heart Disease, Mental Illness, and Stroke*, Sage Publications, Newbury Park.

Biggs, S 1993, *Understanding Ageing: Images, Attitudes and Professional Practice*, Open University Press, Buckingham.

Binstock, B & George, L 1990, *Handbook of Aging and the Social Sciences*, Harper & Row, New York.

Binstock, R, Post, S & Whithouse, P 1992, 'The challenges of dementia' in R Binstock, S Post & P Whithouse (eds), *Dementia and Aging: Ethics, Values, Policy Choices*, The Johns Hopkins University Press, London, UK.

Bishop, B 1999a, *The National Strategy for an Ageing Australia: Background Paper*, Department of Health and Aged Care, Publication no. 2517, Canberra.

——1999b, *The National Strategy for an Ageing Australia: Employment for Mature Age Workers: Issues Paper*, Commonwealth of Australia, Canberra.

Bittman, M, Flick, M & Rice, F 2001, 'The recruitment of older Australian workers: A survey of employers in a high growth industry', *SPRC Report*, Social Policy Research Centre, University of New South Wales, Sydney.

Blanks, RG, Moss, SM, McGahan, CE, Quinn, MJ & Babb, PJ 2000, 'Effect of NHS screening program on mortality from breast cancer in England and Wales, 1990–98: Comparison of observed with predicted mortality', *British Medical Journal*, vol. 321, pp. 665–9.

Blondal, S & Scarpetta, S 1998, 'The retirement decisions in OECD countries', *Organisation for Economic Cooperation and Development Working Paper 202*, Paris.

Boaz, RF & Hu, J 1997, 'Determining the amount of help used by disabled elderly persons at home: The role of coping resources', *Journal of Gerontology*, vol. 52, pp. S317–S324.

Bochel, C, Bochel, H & Page, D 1999, 'Housing: The foundation for community care', *Health Society and Community Care*, vol. 76, pp. 492–501.

Boozang, KM 1998, 'Western medicine opens the door to alternative medicine', *American Journal of Law and Medicine*, vol. 24, pp. 185–212.

Bortz II, W, Wallace, D & Wiley, D 1999, 'Sexual function in 1202 aging males: Differentiating aspects', *Journal of Gerontology*, vol. 54, pp. 237–41.

Bouma, H 1992, 'Overview on gerontechnology' in H Bouma & JAM Graafmans (eds), *Gerontechnology*, IOS Press, Amsterdam.

Bouma, H & Graafmans, JAM 1992, *Gerontechnology*, IOS Press, Amsterdam.

Bouma, H & Harrington, TL 2000, 'Information and communication' in TL Harrington & MK Harrington (eds), *Gerontechnology—Why and How*, Shaker Press, Maastricht, NL.

Bourne, C, Minichiello, V & Rohrshiem, R 2002, 'A profile of people over 50 years of age who attend a public sexual health clinic in Sydney, 1991–2001', Paper presented at the Australian College of Sexual Health Physicians Conference, Perth.

Bouwhuis, DG & Melenhorst, AS 2001, 'Perceived cost–benefit ratios of using interactive communication equipment' in K Sagawa & H Bouma (eds), *Proceedings of the International Workshop on Gerontechnology*, National Institute of Bioscience and Human-Technology, Tsukuba, Japan.

Bowling, A 1997, *Measuring Health: A Review of Quality of Life Measurement Scales* (2nd edn), Buckingham, Open University Press.

Braithwaite, V 1998, 'Institutional respite care: Breaking chores or breaking social bonds?' *The Gerontologist*, vol. 38, pp. 610–17.

Braithwaite, VA & Gibson, DM 1987, 'Adjustment to retirement: What we know and what we need to know', *Ageing and Society*, vol. 7, pp. 1–18.

Brant, LJ, Gordon-Salant, S, Pearson, JD, Klein, LL, Morrell, CH, Metter, EJ & Fozard, JL 1996, 'Risk factors related to age-associated hearing loss in the speech frequencies', *Journal of the American Academy of Audiology*, vol. 7, pp. 152–60.

Brauer-Janse, MD, Coleman, R, Fozard, JL, Suri, JF, deVries, G & Yawitz, M 1997, 'User interfaces for young and old', *Interactions*, vol. 4, pp. 34–46.

Brealey, E 2003, *Ten Minute Anti-Ageing*, Cassell Illustrated, London.

Bresher, E & The Editors of Consumer Reports Books 1984, *Love, Sex and Aging: A Consumers Union Report*, Little, Brown & Company, Boston.

Brett, H 2002, *Complementary Therapies in the Care of Older People*, Whurr Publishers, London.

Brice, GC, Gorey, KM, Hall, RM & Angelino, S 1996, 'The STAYWELL program-maximizing elders' capacity for independent living through promotion and disease prevention activities', *Research on Aging*, vol. 18, pp. 2002–218.

Bridge, C & Relf, M 2001, 'An Australian Access Institute: Promoting Research, Education and Information Dissemination', Paper presented at the Inclusion by Design 'Planning the barrier-free world' Congress, Montreal, Canada.

Bridge, C & Simoff, SJ 2000, 'Disability access to the built environment: On-line evaluation and information dissemination' in L Eder (ed.), *Managing Healthcare Information Systems with Web-Enabled Technologies*, Idea Group Publications, Hershey, PA.

Bridge, C, Flatau, P, Whelan, S, Wood, G & Yates, J 2003, *Housing Assistance and Non-Shelter Outcomes*, from http://www.ahuri.edu.au/pubs/finalreports.html

Bridge, C, Kendig, H, Quine, S & Parsons, A 2002, *Housing and Care for Older and Younger Adults with Disabilities*, Final Report, Sydney Research Centre, University of Sydney, Sydney.

Bright, R 1993, *Music in Geriatric Care: A Second Look* (2nd edn), Music Therapy Enterprises, Wahroonga, Australia.

——1995, 'Music therapy as a factor in grief counselling' in T Wigwram, B Saperston & R West (eds), *The Art and Science of Music Therapy: A Handbook*, Harwood Academic Publishers, Switzerland.

——1996, *Grief and Powerlessness: Helping People Regain Control of their Lives*, Jessica Kingsley, London.

——1997, *Wholeness in Later Life*, Jessica Kingsley, London.

Brodaty, H & Hadzi-Pavlovic, D 1990, 'Psychosocial effects on carers of living with persons with dementia', *Australian and New Zealand Journal of Psychiatry*, vol. 24, pp. 351–61.

Brody, EM & Schoonover, CB 1986, 'Patterns of parent-care when adult daughters work and when they do not', *The Gerontologist*, vol. 26, pp. 372–81.

Brody, EM, Hoffman, C, Kleban, MH & Schoonover, CB 1989, 'Caregiving daughters and their local siblings: Perceptions, strains, and interactions', *The Gerontologist*, vol. 29, pp. 529–38.

Brooke, L, Davidson, S, Kendig, H & Reynolds, A 1998, *The Support Needs of Older People in High Rise Public Housing*, Department of Human Services Victoria, Melbourne.

Browning, C & Kendig, H 2003, 'Healthy ageing: A new focus on older people's health and wellbeing' in P Limputtong & I Gardner (eds), *Health, Social Policy and Communities*, Oxford University Press, Melbourne.

Bruce, MF 1986, 'Effects of age-segregated housing on the aging in relation to self-perceived health status, political participation, political cohesiveness and self-esteem', *Dissertation Abstracts International*, vol. 469-A, p. 2779.

Bruce, ML, Leaf, PJ & Rozal, GP 1994, 'Psychiatric status and 9-year mortality data in New Haven Epidemiologic Catchment Area Study', *American Journal of Psychiatry*, vol. 151, pp. 716–21.

Buchner, D, Nicola, R, Martin, M & Patrick, D 1997, 'Physical activity and health promotion in public housing', *American Journal of Preventative Medicine*, vol. 136, pp. 57–62.

Buckle, J 2001, 'The role of aromatherapy in nursing care', *Nursing Clinics of North America*, vol. 36, pp. 57–72.

Bunt, L 1996, *Music Therapy: An Art Beyond Words*, Routledge, New York.

Burbank, PM, Padula, CA & Nigg, CR 2000, 'Changing health behaviors of older adults', *Journal of Gerontological Nursing*, vol. 26, pp. 26–33.

Burridge, R & Ormandy, D 1993, *Unhealthy Housing: Research, Remedies, and Reform*, Spon, London.

Burtless, G & Quinn, JF 2002, *Is Working Longer the Answer for an Aging Workforce? An Issue in Brief*, Centre for Retirement Research, Boston College, Boston, MA.

Butler, R 1963, 'The life review: An interpretation of reminiscence in the aged', *Psychiatry*, vol. 26, pp. 65–76.

——1975, *Why Survive? Being Old in America*, Harper & Row, New York.

——2002, 'The Declaration of Human Rights of Older Persons', United Nations Second World Assembly on Ageing NFO World Forum on Ageing, International Longevity Centre, New York.

Byrne, GJA & Raphael, B 1994, 'Longitudinal study of bereavement phenomena in recently widowed elderly men', *Psychological Medicine*, vol. 24, pp. 411–21.

Byrne, H & MacLean, D 1997, 'Quality of life: Perceptions of residential care', *International Journal of Nursing Practice*, vol. 3, pp. 21–8.

Bytheway, B 1995, *Ageism*, Open University Press, Buckingham.

——1997, *Ageism: Rethinking Ageing*, Open University Press, Buckingham.

Calasanti, TM 1996, 'Gender and life satisfaction in retirement: An assessment of the male model', *Journals of Gerontology*, vol. 51, pp. S18–S29.

Callahan, D 1992, 'Dementia and appropriate care: Allocating scarce resources', in R Binstock, S Post & P Whithouse (eds), *Dementia and Aging*, The Johns Hopkins University Press, Baltimore, MD.

Cameron, P 1970, 'The generation gap: Beliefs about sexuality and self-reported sexuality', *Developmental Psychology*, vol. 3, pp. 272–5.

Campbell, AJ, Robertson, MC, Gardner, MM, Norton, RN, Tilyard, MW & Buchner, DM 1997, 'Randomised controlled trial of a general practice programme of home based exercise to prevent falls in elderly women', *British Medical Journal*, vol. 315, pp. 1065–9.

Campbell, D 1995, *Music Physician for Times to Come* (3rd edn), Quest Books, Wheaton.

Campbell, J & Ikegami, N 2000, 'Long term care insurance comes to Japan', *Health Affairs*, vol. 19, pp. 26–39.

Campbell, LD, Connidis, IA & Davies, L 1999, 'Sibling ties in later life: A social network analysis', *Journal of Family Issues*, vol. 20, pp. 114–48.

Campbell, NC, Thain, J, Deans, HG, Ritchie, LD, Rawles, JM & Squair, JL 1998, 'Secondary prevention clinics for coronary heart disease: Randomised trial of effect on health', *British Medical Journal*, vol. 316, pp. 1434–7.

Canadian Study of Health and Aging Working Group 2002, 'Patterns and health effects of caring for people with dementia: The impact of changing cognitive and residential status', *Gerontologist*, vol. 42, pp. 643–52.

Cannuscio, CC, Jones, C, Kawachi, I, Colditz, GA, Berkman, L & Rimm, E 2002, 'Reverberations of family illness: A longitudinal assessment of informal caregiving and mental health status in the Nurses' Health Study', *American Journal of Public Health*, vol. 92, pp. 1305–11.

Cape, RD & Gibson, SJ 1994, 'The influence of clinical problems, age and social support on outcomes for elderly persons referred to regional aged care assessment teams', *Australian & New Zealand Journal of Medicine*, vol. 244, pp. 378–85.

Carr, A, Samaras, K, Burton, S, Law, M, Freund, J, Chisholm, D & Cooper, D 1998, 'A syndrome of peripheral lipodystrophy, hyperlipidaemia and insulin resistance in patients receiving HIV protease inhibitors', *AIDS*, vol. 12, pp. F51–8.

Carr, D & Utz, RL 2001–2002, 'Late-life widowhood in the United States: New directions in research and theory', *Ageing International*, vol. 27, pp. 65–88.

Carr, D, House, JS, Kessler, RC, Nesse, RM, Sonnega, J & Wortman, C 2000, 'Marital quality and psychological adjustment to widowhood among older adults: A longitudinal analysis', *Journals of Gerontology*, vol. 55, pp. S197–207.

Carrington Reid, M 2003, 'Depressive symptoms as a risk factor for disabling back pain in community-dwelling older persons', *Journal of American Geriatric Society*, vol. 51, pp. 1710–17.

Cartensen, LL 1992, 'Social and emotional patterns in adulthood: Support for socioemotional selectivity theory', *Psychology and Aging*, vol. 7, pp. 331–8.

Carter, HB, Pearson, JD, Metter, EJ, Brant, LJ, Chan, DW, Andres, R, Fozard, JL & Walsh, PC 1992, 'Longitudinal evaluation of prostate-specific antigen levels in men with and without prostate disease', *Journal of the American Medical Association*, vol. 267, pp. 2215–20.

Carter, SE, Campbell, EM, Sanson-Fisher, RW, Redman, S & Gillespie, WJ 1997, 'Environmental hazards in the homes of older people', *Age and Ageing*, vol. 26, pp. 195–202.

Caserta, MS & Lund, DA 1993, 'Intrapersonal resources and the effectiveness of self-help groups for bereaved older adults', *Gerontologist*, vol. 33, pp. 619–29.

Casey, B & Yamada, A 2002, 'Getting older getting poorer: A study of the earning assets, pensions and living arrangements of older people in nine countries', *Organization for Economic Cooperation and Development Occasional Paper no. 60*, OECD, Paris.

Casey, B, Oxley, H, Whitehouse, E, Antolin, P, Duval, R & Leibfritz, W 2003, 'Policies for an ageing society: Recent measures and areas for further reform', *Organization for Economic Cooperation and Development Working Paper 369*, OECD, Paris.

Castle, SC 2000, 'Clinical relevance of age-related immune dysfunction', *Clinical Infectious Diseases*, vol. 31, pp. 578–85.

Center for Health Systems Research and Analysis 2000, *Quality Indicators for Implementation*, http://www.chsra.wisc.edu

Centers for Disease Control 2002a, 'Diagnosis and reporting of HIV and AIDS in states with HIV/AIDS surveillance, United States, 1994–2000', *MMWR*, vol. 51, pp. 595–8.

Centers for Disease Control 2002b, 'Healthy aging: Preventing disease and improving quality of life among older Americans', http://www.cdc.gov/nccdphp/aag-aging.htm (accessed 19 July 2002).

Centers for Medicare and Medicaid Services 2003, *Medicare Information Resource*, http://cms.hhs.gov/medicare/ (accessed 4 February 2004).

Centre for Public Policy 2002, 'The transition from work to retirement', New Social Settlement Project, National Consultation Strategy, Discussion Paper, University of Melbourne, http://www.public-policy.unimelb.edu.au

Chapman, NJ 2001, 'Accessory apartments: Are they a realistic alternative for ageing in place?', *Housing Studies*, vol. 165, p. 637.

Chappell, NL 1989, 'Health and helping among the elderly, gender differences', *Journal of Aging and Health*, vol. 1, pp. 102–20.

——1992, *Social Support and Aging*, Butterworths, Toronto.

——1996, 'Behavioural problems and distress among caregivers of people with dementia', *Aging and Society*, vol. 16, pp. 57–73.

——2001, 'Quality long-term care: Perspectives from the users of home care' in LS Noelker & Z Harel (eds), *Linking Quality of Long-Term Care and Quality of Life*, Springer Publishing, New York.

——2003, 'Correcting cross-cultural stereotypes: Aging in Shanghai and Canada', *Journal of Cross-Cultural Gerontology*, vol. 18, pp. 127–47.

Chappell, NL & Litkenhaus, R 1995, *Informal Caregivers to Adults in British Columbia*, Joint Report by the University of Victoria, Centre on Aging, with the Caregivers Association of British Columbia, Victoria.

Chappell, NL & Penning, MJ 1996, 'Behavioural problems and distress among caregivers to dementia victims', *Ageing and Society*, vol. 16, pp. 57–73.

Chappell, NL, Gee, E, MacDonald, L & Stones, M 2003, *Aging in Contemporary Canada*, Pearson Educational, Toronto.

Chappell, NL, Reid, RC & Dow, E 2001, 'Respite from the caregiver's point of view: A typology of meanings', *Journal of Aging Studies*, vol. 15, pp. 201–16.

Charness, N, Czaja, S, Fisk AD & Rogers, WA 2002. 'Congress issue: Proceedings of the Fourth International Conference on Gerontechnology', *Gerontechnology*, vol. 2, pp. 1–166.

Chauncey, H, Epstein, S, Rose, CL & Hefferren, JJ 1985, *Clinical Geriatric Dentistry*, American Dental Association, Chicago.

Chávez, EM & Ship JA 2000, 'Sensory and motor deficits in the elderly: Impact on oral health', *Journal of Public Health Dentistry*, vol. 60, pp. 297–303.

Chen, J, Ng, E & Wilkins, R 1996, 'The health of Canada's immigrants in 1994–95', *Health Reports*, vol. 7, pp. 33–45.

Chenoweth, L 2003, 'Dedication makes a difference to the elderly', *Nursing Review*, p. 4.

Cherniack, EP, Senzel, RS & Pan, CX 2001, 'Correlates of use of alternative medicine by the elderly in an urban population,' *Journal of Alternative and Complementary Medicine*, vol. 7, pp. 277–80.

Chernoff, R 2001, 'Nutrition and health promotion in older adults', *Journal of Gerontology*, vol. 56, pp. 47–53.

Choi, N & Wodarski, J 1996, 'Relationship between social support and health status of elderly people: Does social support slow down physical and functional deterioration?', *Social Work Research*, vol. 20, pp. 52–63.

Choi, NG 1999, 'Differences in the quality of housing units occupied by elderly men versus elderly women', *Journal of Housing for the Elderly*, vol. 131, pp. 99–113.

Chui, HC, Victoroff, JI, Margolin, D, Jagust, W, Shankle, R & Katzman, R 1992, 'Criteria for the diagnosis of ischemic vascular dementia proposed by State of California Alzheimer's Disease Diagnostic and Treatment Centers', *Neurology*, vol. 42, pp. 473–80.

CHSRA *See* Center for Health Systems Research and Analysis.

Cicero, M 1971 [44BC], *On Old Age*, Penguin, London.

Cicirelli, VG 1982, 'Sibling influence throughout the lifespan', in ME Lamb & B Sutton-Smith (eds), *Sibling Relationships: Their Nature and Significance Across the Lifespan*, Lawrence Erlbaum, Hillside, NJ.

——1985, 'The role of siblings as family caregivers', in WJ Sauer & RT Coward (eds), *Social Support Networks and the Care of the Elderly*, Spring Publishing, Hillside, NJ.

Clair, A 1994, *Music Therapy and Elderly People*, National Association for Music Therapy, Silver Spring.

——1996, *Therapeutic Uses of Music with Older People*, Health Professionals Press, Baltimore, MD.

Clapham, D & Franklin, B 1995, *Housing Management, Community Care and CCT Findings*, Joseph Rowntree Foundation, York, UK.

Clare, R & Tulpulé, A 1994, *Australia's Ageing Society*, Economic Planning Advisory Council Background Paper No 37, Australian Government Publishing Service, Canberra.

Clark, LM & Hartman, M 1996, 'Effects of hardiness and appraisal on the psychological distress and physical health of caregivers to elderly relatives', *Research on Aging*, vol. 18, pp. 379–401.

Clark, PC 2002, 'Effects of individual and family hardiness on caregiver depression and fatigue', *Research in Nursing and Health*, vol. 25, pp. 37–48.

Clark, PJ, Marshall, VW, Ryff, CD & Rosenthal, J 2000, 'Well-being in Canadian seniors: Findings from the Canadian study of health and aging', *Canadian Journal on Aging*, vol. 19, pp. 139–59.

Clemson, L, Cusick, A & Fozard, C 1999, 'Managing risk and exerting control: Determining follow-through with falls prevention', *Disability and Rehabilitation*, vol. 1312, pp. 531–41.

Cobb, S 1976, 'Social support as a moderator of life stress', *Psychosomatic Medicine*, vol. 38, pp. 300–14.

Cohen, CA, Colantonio, A & Vernich, L 2002, 'Positive aspects of caregiving: Rounding out the caregiver experience', *International Journal of Geriatric Psychiatry*, vol. 17, pp. 184–8.

Cohen, CA, Gold, DP, Shulman, KI, Wortley, JT & McDonald, G 1993, 'Factors determining the decision to institutionalize dementing individuals: A prospective study', *Gerontologist*, vol. 33, pp. 714–20.

Cohen, S & Syme, SL 1985, 'Issues in the study and application of social support' in S Cohen & SL Syme (eds), *Social Support and Health*, Academic Press, Orlando, FL.

Coleman, LM, Fowler, LL & Williams, ME 1995, 'Use of unproven therapies by people with Alzheimer's disease', *Journal of the American Geriatrics Society*, vol. 43, pp. 747–50.

Coleman, R 1998, 'Improving the quality of life for older people by design', in JAM Graafmans, V Taipele & N Charness (eds), *Gerontechnology: A Sustainable Investment for the Future*, IOS Press, Amsterdam.

Coleman, R & Myerson, J 2001, 'Improving life quality by countering design exclusion', *Gerontechnology*, vol. 1, pp. 88–102.

Comijs, HC, Pot, AM, Smit, JH, Bouter, LM & Jonker, C 1998, 'Elder abuse in the community: prevalence and consequences', *Journal of the American Geriatric Society*, vol. 46, pp. 885–8.

Commonwealth Department of Community Services and Health 1990, *Mid-Term Review of Aged Care Reform Strategy 1990–1*, Discussion Paper no. 2, Commonwealth Policy and Programs for Dementia Care in Australia, Canberra.

Commonwealth–State Working Party 1987, *Living in a Nursing Home*, Australian Government Publishing Service, Canberra.

Connell, BR & Sanford, JA 2001, 'Difficulty, dependence and housing accessibility for people ageing with a disability', *Journal of Architectural & Planning Research*, vol. 183, pp. 234–42.

Conway, J 1995, 'Housing as an instrument of health care', *Health Society and Community Care*, vol. 33, pp. 141–50.

Cooper, B & Holmes, C 1998, 'Previous psychiatric history as a risk factor for late-life dementia: A population-based case-control study', *Age and Ageing*, vol. 27, pp. 181–8.

Cooper, D & Jenkins, A 1998, *Obtaining Consumer Feedback from Clients of Home Based Care Services: A Review of the Literature*, Welfare Working Paper no. 21, Australian Institute of Health, Canberra.

Cooper, P 1996, *What Happens If: Research into the Housing and Support Needs of Older People with Physical Disabilities*, Paraplegic and Quadriplegic Association of NSW, Sydney.

Cornish, RM 1997, *An Investigation of the Retirement Behaviour of Older Australians*, University of Melbourne, Melbourne.

Costa, PT, McCrae, RR & Zonderman, AB 1987, 'Environmental and dispositional influences on well-being: Longitudinal follow-up of an American national sample', *British Journal of Psychology*, vol. 78, pp. 299–306.

Coulson, I & Ronaldson, S 1997, 'Spiritual care in dementia: Nurturing the human spirit', in S Ronaldson (eds), *Spirituality: The Heart of Nursing*, Ausmed Publications, Melbourne.

Coulson, I, Mariño, R & Minichiello, V 2001, 'Knowledge and practices of older persons in the prevention of vascular dementia', *Archives of Gerontology and Geriatrics*, vol. 33, pp. 273–85.

Coulson, I, Strang, V, Mariño, R & Minichiello, V 2002, *Canadian Lifestyle Perspectives in the Prevention of Vascular Dementia*, Report to the Canadian High Commission, Ottawa.

——2004, 'Knowledge and lifestyle behaviours of healthy older adults related to modifying the onset of vascular dementia', *Archives of Gerontology and Geriatrics*, vol. 39, pp. 43–58.

Courtney, M, Edwards, H, Stephan, J, O'Reilly, M & Duggan, C 2003, 'Quality of life measures for residents of aged care facilities: A literature review', *Australasian Journal of Ageing*, vol. 22, pp. 58–64.

Covey, H 1989, 'Perceptions and attitudes toward sexuality of the elderly', *Gerontologist*, vol. 29, pp. 93–100.

Cram, F & Patton, H 1993, 'Personal possessions and self-identity: Experiences of elderly women in three residential settings', *Australian Journal on Ageing*, vol. 12, pp. 19–24.

Crennshaw, R & Goldberg, J 1996, *Sexual Pharmacology*, WW Norton & Co., New York.

Currie, D 1996, 'Housing issues for women with disabilities', *Shelter NHA*, vol. 11, pp. 20–6.

Czaja, SJ & Lee, CC 2001, 'The Internet and older adults: Design challenges and opportunities' in N Charness, DC Park & BA Sabel (eds), *Ageing and Communication: Opportunities and Challenges of Technology*, Springer, New York.

Czaja, SJ & Lee, CC 2003, 'Designing computer systems for older adults' in J Jacko & A Sears (eds), *The Human–Computer Interaction Handbook: Fundamentals, Evolving Technologies and Emerging Applications*, Lawrence Erlbaum, Mawah, NJ.

Czaja, SJ & Sharit, J 2002, 'The usability of telephone voice menu systems for older Adults', *Gerontechnology*, vol. 2, p. 88.

Czaja, SJ, Sharit, J, Charness, N, Fisk, AD & Rogers, W 2001, 'The Center for Research and Education on Aging and Technology Enhancement (CREATE): A program to enhance technology for older adults', *Gerontechnology*, vol. 1, pp. 50–9.

Dahlin-Ivanoff, S, Klepp, K & Sjorstrand, J 1998, 'Development of a health education program for elderly with age-related macular degeneration: A focus group study', *Patient Education and Counseling*, vol. 34, pp. 63–73.

Daly, MP & Katzel, LI 1997, *Health Promotion and Disease Prevention in the Elderly*, http://cpmcnet.columbia.edu/dept/dental/Dental_Educational_Software/Gerontology_and_Geriatric_Dentistry/prevention/prevention.html

Dartigues, J, Commenges, D, Letenneur, D, Barberger, G, Gilleron, V, Fabrigoule, C, Mazaux, J, Orgogozo, J & Salamon, R 1997, 'Cognitive predictors of dementia in elderly community residents', *Neuroepidemiology*, vol. 16, pp. 29–39.

Davidson, K 2001, 'Late life widowhood, selfishness and new partnership choices: A gendered perspective', *Ageing and Society*, vol. 21, pp. 297–317.

Davis, S 2002, 'Ageism and its implications for the health care of older people', *Northern Health*, 22 April.

Davison, B, Kendig, H, Stephens, F & Merrill, V 1993, *It's My Place: A Report on the Study Options and Preferences: Older People and Their Homes*, Australian Government Publishing Service, Canberra.

de Beauvoir, S 1970, *Old Age*, Penguin, Middlesex.

Deber, R, Narine, L, Baranek, P, Sharpe, N, Masnyk Duvalko, K, Zlotnik-Shaul, R, Coyte, P, Pink, G & Williams, P 1998, 'The public–private mix in health care', *Canada Health Action: Building on the Legacy*, National Forum on Health, Ottawa.

Decker, IM, Sellers, JB, & Stallard, JM, 2002 'Health care for the elderly: A social obligation', *Nursing Forum*, vol. 37, no. 2, pp. 5–11.

Department of Community Services 1987, *Towards a Comprehensive User Rights Mechanism*, Office for the Aged, Australian Government Publishing Service, Canberra.

Department of Education, Science and Training (DEST) 2003, *Australian Aged Care Nursing: A Critical Review of Education, Training, Recruitment and Retention in Residential and Community Settings*, Australian Government Publishing Service, Canberra.

Department of Health (United Kingdom) 2004, *Home Care, Day Care and Meal Provision for Elderly People: By Age 1992 and 1997*, Selected Trends 30, http//:www.statistics.gov.uk

Department of Health (United Kingdom) 2004, *Hospital and Community Health Service Expenditure on the Elderly by Sector 1994–1999*, Social Trends 30, http//:www.statistics.gov.uk

Department of Health and Aged Care 1999, *Aged Care Standards Principles*, Australian Government Publishing Service, Canberra.

Department of Health and Ageing 2002, *Aged Care in Australia*, Australian Government Publishing Service, Canberra.

Department of Health and Family Services 1997a, *Residential Care Guidelines*, Australian Government Publishing Service, Canberra.

——1997b, *Standards for Aged Care Facilities*, Australian Government Publishing Service, Canberra.

——1998, *Resident Classification Scale Training Workbook*, University of Adelaide Press, South Australia.

——2002, *Residential Care Manual*, Aged and Community Care Division, Canberra.

Department of Health, Housing and Community Services 1991, *Report of the Mid-Term Review of the Aged Care Reform Strategy*, Australian Government Publishing Service, Canberra.

DH&FS *See* Department of Health & Family Services.

Diamond, WJ 2001, *The Clinical Practice of Complementary, Alternative and Western Medicine*, CRC Press, Florida.

Diokno, A, Brown, M & Herzog A. 1990, 'Sexual function in the elderly', *Archives of Internal Medicine*, vol. 150, pp. 197–200.

Disley, D & McCormack, T 2002, 'A plea to care', *Sacred Space: The International Journal of Spirituality and Health*, vol. 3, pp. 30–5.

Docampo Rama, M, de Ridder, H & Bouma, H 2001, 'Technology generation and age in using layered interfaces', *Gerontechnology*, vol. 1, pp. 25–40.

Donabedian, A 1966, 'Evaluating the quality of medical care', *Milbank Memorial Fund Quarterly*, vol. 44, pp. 166–206.

Donovan, B, Minichiello, V & Hart, G 1998, 'Australia' in T Brown, R Chan, D Mugrditchian, B Mulhall, D Plummer, R Sarda & W Sittitral (eds), *Sexually Transmitted Diseases in Asia and the Pacific*, Venereology Publishing Inc and East-West Centre, Melbourne.

Doty, P, Benjamin, A, Matthias, R & Franke, T 1998, *In-home Support Services for the Elderly and Disabled: A Comparison of Client-directed and Professional Management Models of Service Delivery*, US Department of Health and Human Services, Washington, DC.

Downer, SM, Cody, MM, McClusky, P, Wilson, PD, Arnott, SJ, Lister, TA & Slevin, ML 1994, 'Pursuit and practice of complementary therapies by cancer patients receiving conventional treatment', *British Medical Journal*, vol. 309, pp. 86–99.

Drossaert, C, Boer, H & Seydel, E 1996, 'Health education to improve repeat participation in the Dutch breast cancer screening programme: Evaluation of a leaflet tailored to previous participants', *Patient Education and Counseling*, vol. 28, pp. 121–31.

Dubé, MP & Sattler, FR 1998, 'Metabolic complications of antiretroviral therapies', *AIDS Clinical Care*, vol. 10, pp. 41–4.

Duncan, R 1998, 'Blueprint for action: The national home modification action coalition', *Technology & Disability*, vol. 8 pp. 85–9.

Dunn, JR 2002, *A Population Health Approach to Housing: A Framework for Research Report*, The National Housing Research Committee & The Canada Mortgage and Housing Corporation, Calgary, Canada.

Dwyer, JW, Barton, AJ & Vogel, BW 1994, 'Area of residence and the risk of institutionalisation', *Journal of Gerontology*, vol. 492, pp. S75–84.

Dwyer, JW, Henretta, JC, Coward, RT & Barton, AJ 1992, 'Changes in the helping behavior of adult children as caregivers', *Research on Aging*, vol. 14, pp. 351–75.

Dychtwald, K 1999, *Age Power: How the 21st Century Will Be Ruled by the New Old*, Tatcher/Putnam, New York.

Edwards, AB, Zarit, SH, Stephens, MAP & Townsend, A 2002, 'Employed family caregivers of cognitively impaired elderly: An examination of role strain and depressive symptoms', *Aging and Mental Health*, vol. 6, pp. 55–61.

Encel, S 1995, 'Retirement and pensions: Social and political context' in V Minichiello, N Chappell, H Kendig & A Walker (eds), *Sociology of Aging: International Perspectives*, ISA, Melbourne.

——1996, 'Retirement ages and pension ages: A complex history', *Social Science Journal*, June, pp. 3–25.

——1998, 'Age discrimination' in M Patrickson & L Hartmann (eds), *Managing an Ageing Workforce*, Woodslane, Sydney.

Engle, JD, Pethtel, L & Zarconi, J 2002, 'Hearing the patient's story', *Sacred Space: The International Journal of Spirituality and Health*, vol. 3, pp. 24–32.

Erickson, L 1997, 'Oral health promotion and prevention for older adults', *Dental Clinics of North America*, vol. 41, pp. 727–50.

Ernst, E 2001a, 'Complementary therapies in palliative cancer care', *Cancer*, vol. 91, pp. 2181–5.

——2001b, 'A primer of complementary and alternative medicine commonly used by cancer patients', *Medical Journal of Australia*, vol. 174, pp. 88–92.

Estes, C 1979, *The Aging Enterprise*, Jossey-Bass, San Francisco.

Estes, CL & Wood, JB 1986, 'The non-profit sector and community-based care for the elderly in the US: A disappearing resource?' *Social Science and Medicine*, vol. 23, pp. 1261–6.

Ettinger, WH, Burns, R, Messier, SP, Applegate, W, Rejeski, WJ, Morgan, T, Shumaker, S, Berry, MJ, O'Toole, M, Monu, J & Craven, T 1997, 'A randomised trial comparing aerobic exercise and resistance exercise with a health education program in older adults with knee osteoarthritis: The Fitness Arthritis and Seniors Trial (FAST)', *Journal of American Medical Association [JAMA]*, vol. 277, pp. 25–31.

Ezzo, J, Berman, B, Hadhazy, VA, Jaded, AR, Lao, L & Singh, BB 2000, 'Is acupuncture effective for the treatment of chronic pain? A systematic review', *Pain*, vol. 86, pp. 217–25.

Fast, J & Da Pont, M 1997, 'Changes in women's work continuity', *Canadian Social Trends*, vol. 46, pp. 2–7.

Faulkner, D & Bennett, K 2002, *Linkages Among Housing Assistance, Residential Relocation, and Use of Community Health and Social Care by Old-Old Adults: Shelter and Non-Shelter Implications for Housing Policy Development*, Final report, The Australian Housing and Urban Research Institute, Southern Research Centre, Melbourne.

Fawcett, M 1995, 'From your secretary', *Journal of the Australian Traditional-Medicine Society*, vol. 1, p. 89.

——2003, 'From your secretary', *Journal of the Australian Traditional-Medicine Society*, vol. 9, p. 5.

Feinberg, LF & Kelly, KA 1995, 'A well-deserved break: Respite programs offered by California's statewide system of caregiver resource centers', *The Gerontologist*, vol. 35, pp. 701–06.

Felce, D 1998, 'The determinants of staff and resident activity in residential services for people with severe intellectual disability: moving beyond size, building design, location and number of staff', *Journal of Intellectual & Developmental Disability*, vol. 232, pp. 103–19.

Feldman, S, Byles, JE & Beaumont, R 2000, 'Is anybody listening? The experiences of widowhood for older Australian women', *Journal of Women and Aging*, vol. 12, pp. 155–76.

Felton, BJ & Berry, CA 1992. 'Do the sources of the urban elderly's social support determine its psychological consequences?', *Psychology and Aging*, vol. 7, pp. 89–97.

Field, TM 1998, 'Massage therapy effects', *American Psychologist*, vol. 53, pp. 1270–81.

Filion, P, Wister, A & Coblentz, E 1992, 'Subjective dimensions of environmental adaptation among the elderly: A challenge to models of housing policy', *Journal of Housing for the Elderly*, vol. 10, pp. 3–32.

Fischer-Rizzi, S 1990, *Complete Aromatherapy Handbook*, Sterling, New York.

Fisk, AD & Rogers, WA 1997, *Handbook of Human Factors and the Older Adults*, Academic Press, San Diego.

Fiske, J, Davis, DM, Frances, C & Gelbier, S 1998, 'The emotional effects of tooth loss in edentulous people', *British Dental Journal*, vol. 184, pp. 90–3.

Fitzgerald, RP, Shiverick, BN & Zimmerman, D 1996, 'Applying performance measures to long term care', *Journal of Quality Improvement*, vol. 22, pp. 505–17.

Fletcher, AE, Dickinson, EJ & Phillip, I 1992, 'Review audit measures: Quality of life instruments for everyday use with elderly patients', *Age and Ageing*, vol. 21, pp. 142–50.

Fogel, BS 1992, 'Psychological aspects of staying at home', *Generations: Quarterly Journal of the American Society on Aging*, vol. XVI, pp. 15–9.

Foster, DF, Phillips, RS & Hamel, MB 2000, 'Alternative medicine use in older Americans', *Journal of the American Geriatrics Society*, vol. 48, pp. 1560–5.

Foucault, M 1973, *The Birth of the Clinic: An Archaeology of Medical Perception*, Vintage Books, New York.

Foucault, M 1975, *Discipline and Punish: The Birth of the Prison* (trans. A. Sheridan), Penguin, London.

Fozard, JL 2000, 'Sensory and cognitive changes with age' in KW Schaie & M Pietrucha (eds), *Mobility and Transportation in the Elderly*, Springer, New York.

——2001, 'Gerontechnology and perceptual-motor-function: New opportunities for prevention, compensation, and enhancement', *Gerontechnology*, vol. 1, pp. 5–24.

——2002, 'Gerontechnology: Beyond ergonomics and universal design', *Gerontechnology*, vol. 1, pp. 137–9.

——2003, 'Enabling environments for physical ageing: A balance of preventive and compensatory interventions' in KW Schaie, H-W Wahl, H Mollenkopf & F Oswald (eds), *Ageing Independently: Living Arrangements and Mobility*, Springer Publishing, New York.

Fozard, JL & Carr Jr, GD 1972, 'Age differences and psychological estimates of abilities and skills', *Industrial Gerontology*, Spring, no. 13, pp. 75–96.

Fozard, JL & Gordon-Salant, S 2001, 'Changes in vision and hearing with ageing', in JE Birren & KW Schaie (eds), *Handbook of the Psychology of Ageing* (5th edn), Academic Press, San Diego, CA.

Fozard, JL & Popkin, SJ 1978, 'Optimizing adult development: Ends and means of an applied psychology of aging', *American Psychologist*, vol. 33, pp. 975–89.

Frain, JP & Carr, PH 1996, 'Is the typical modern house designed for future adaptation for disabled older people?' *Age & Ageing*, vol. 255, pp. 398–401.

Frankental, S 1979, 'Walking the tight-rope: Balancing independence and security in old age', *Social Dynamics*, vol. 52, pp. 18–27.

Frankish, J 2001, 'Health-promoting environments', presented at The Fifth International Conference on Communication, Ageing and Health, Vancouver, Canada.

Free, T & Chambers, L 2001, 'The sweet smell of success', *Journal of Dementia Care*, vol. 9, pp. 9–10.

Freire, P 1970, *Pedagogy of the Oppressed*, Seabury Press, New York.

Freud, S 1961, *Civilization and its Discontents*, WW Norton & Co., New York.

Fries, J 1984, 'The compression of morbidity: Miscellaneous comments about a theme', *Gerontologist*, vol. 24, pp. 354–9.

Fruedenthal, A 1999, *The Design of Home Appliances for Young and Old Consumers*, Delft University of Technology, doctoral dissertation, Delft, NL.

Fry, PS 2001, 'Predictors of health-related quality of life perspectives, self-esteem, and life satisfactions of older adults following spousal loss: An 18-month follow-up study of widows and widowers', *Gerontologist*, vol. 41, pp. 69–81.

Frytak, JR 2000, 'Assessment of quality of life in older adults' in RL Kane & RA Kane (eds), *Assessing Older Persons: Measures, Meaning and Practical Applications*, Oxford University Press, New York.

Gallagher-Thompson, D, O'Hara, R, Simmons, A, Kraemer, HC & Murphy, GMJ 2001. 'Alipoprotein E epsilon4 allele affects the relationship between stress and depression and caregivers of patients with Alzheimer's disease', *Journal of Geriatric Psychiatry and Neurology*, vol. 14, pp. 115–9.

Gardner, I 1994, 'Why people move to retirement villages: Home owners and non-home owners', *Australasian Journal on Ageing*, vol. 131, pp. 36–40.

Garvey, C 1993, 'AIDS care in the elderly: A community-based approach', *AIDS Patient Care*, vol. 8, pp. 118–20.

Gaskins, S & Forte, L 1995, 'The meaning of hope: Implications for nursing practice and research', *Journal of Gerontological Nursing*, vol. 21, pp. 17–23.

Gattuso, S & Shadbolt, A 2002, 'Attitudes toward ageing among Pacific Islander health students in Fiji', *Educational Gerontology*, vol. 26, pp. 99–106.

George, L & Weiler, S 1981, 'Sexuality in middle and late life', *Archives of General Psychiatry*, vol. 38, pp. 919–23.

George, LK & Gwyther, LP 1986, 'Caregiver well-being: A multidimensional examination of family caregivers of demented adults', *The Gerontologist*, vol. 26, pp. 253–9.

Gerasimova, T 1996, 'Elderly women: A challenge to Russia' in A Rotkirch & E Haavio-Mannila (eds), *Women's Voices in Russia Today*, Dartmouth Publishing Group, Aldershot.

Gibson, D 1998, *Aged Care: Old Policies, New Problems*, Cambridge University Press, Cambridge.

Gibson, D & Liu, Z 1995, 'Planning ratios and population growth: Will there be a shortfall in residential aged care by 2021?', *Australian Journal on Ageing*, vol. 14, pp. 57–62.

Gift, HC 1988, 'Issues of aging and oral health promotion', *Gerodontics*, vol. 4, pp. 194–206.

Gilbert, P 1998, 'Evolutionary psychopathology: Why isn't the mind designed better than it is?', *British Journal of Medical Psychology*, vol. 71, pp. 353–73.

Giles, H, Coupland, N, Coupland, J, Williams, A & Nassbaum, J 1992, 'Intergenerational talk and communication with older people', *International Journal of Aging and Human Development*, vol. 34, pp. 271–97.

Gill, TH, Williams, CS, Richardson, ED & Tinetti, ME 1996, 'Impairments in physical performance and cognitive status as predisposing factors for functional dependence among nondisabled older persons', *Journal of Gerontology*, vol. 51, pp. M283–8.

Glass, J & Webb, M 1995, 'Health care educators' knowledge and attitudes regarding sexuality in the aged', *Educational Gerontology*, vol. 21, pp. 713–33.

Glass, N 1998, 'The contested workplace: Reactions to hospital based RNs doing degrees', *Collegian*, vol. 6, pp. 24–31.

Glass, TA, de Leon, CM, Marottoli, RA & Berkman, LF 1999, 'Population based study of social and productive activities as predictors of survival among elderly Americans', *British Medical Journal*, vol. 319, pp. 478–83.

Glickman, L, Stocker, K & Carim, F 1997, 'Self-direction in home care for older people: A consumer's perspective?', *Home Health Care Services Quarterly*, vol. 16, pp. 41–4.

Goffman, E 1969, *The Presentation of Self in Everyday Life*, Penguin, Middlesex.

Gossip, A 1952, 'Exposition on the Gospel according to St. John', *The Interpreter's Bible*, Abingdon Press, New York.

Goto, Y 2001, 'An approach for universal design housing' in K Sagawa & H Bouma (eds), *Proceedings of the International Workshop on Gerontechnology*, National Institute of Bioscience and Human-Technology, Tsukuba, Japan.

Gott, CM 2001, 'Sexual activity and risk-taking in later life', *Health and Social Care in the Community*, vol. 9, pp. 72–8.

Graafmans, J, Fozard, JL, Rietsema, J, van Berlo, A, Bouma, H 1994, 'Gerontechnology: A sustainable development in society' in C Wild & A Kirschner (eds), *Safety-alarm Systems, Technical Aids and Smart Homes*, Akontes Publishing, Knegsel, NL.

Graafmans, JAM, Taipale, V & Charness, N 1998, *Gerontechnology: A Sustainable Investment in the Future*, IOS Press, Amsterdam.

Grainger, R 1990, *Drama and Healing: The Roots of Drama Therapy*, Jessica Kingsley, London.

Grant, C 1996, 'Effects of ageism on individual and health care providers' responses to healthy aging', *Health and Social Work*, vol. 21, pp. 9–15.

Graycar, A 1986, 'Accommodation issues for elderly people', *Australian Journal on Ageing*, vol. 15, p. 8.

Greene, M, Adelman, R & Rizzo, C 1996, 'Problems in communication between physicians and older patients', *Journal of Geriatric Psychiatry*, vol. 29, pp. 13–32.

Gregory, R 1993, *Review of the Structure of Nursing Home Funding Arrangements Stage 1*, Department of Health, Housing, Local Government and Community Services, Australian Government Publishing Service, Canberra.

Gregory, R 1994, *Review of the Structure of Nursing Home Funding Arrangements Stage 2*, Department of Human Services and Health, Australian Government Publishing Service, Canberra.

Gringart, E & Helmes E. 2001, 'Age discrimination in hiring practices against older adults in Western Australia: The case of accounting assistants', *Australasian Journal on Ageing*, vol. 20, pp. 23–8.

Gross, DR & Capuzzi, D 2001, 'Counseling the older adult', in D Capuzzi & DR Gross (eds), *Introduction to the Counseling Profession*, Allyn & Bacon, Boston, MA.

Gross, Z 2000, *Seasons of the Heart*, New World Library, Novato, California.

Grosser, RC & Conley, EK. 1995 'Projections of housing disruption among adults with mental illness who live with aging parents', *Psychiatric Services*, vol. 464, pp. 390–4.

Gui, S 2001, 'Care of the elderly in one-child families in China: Issues and measures', in I Chi, NL Chappell & J Lubben (eds), *Elderly Chinese in Pacific Rim Countries: Social Support and Integration*, Hong Kong University Press, Hong Kong.

Guralnik, JM, Ferrucci, L, Simonsick, EM, Silive, ME & Wallace, RB 1995, 'Lower extremity function in persons over the age of 70 years as predictor of subsequent disability', *New England Journal of Medicine*, vol. 332, pp. 556–61.

Guse, LW & Masesar, MA 1999, 'Quality of life and successful aging in long-term care: Perceptions of residents', *Issues in Mental Health Nursing*, vol. 20, pp. 527–39.

Guzzetta, C 1995, 'Music therapy: Nursing the music of the soul' in D Campbell (eds.), *Music Physician for Times to Come*, Quest Books, Wheaton.

Gyllenhaal, C, Merritt, SL, Peterson, SD, Block, KI & Gochenour, T 2000, 'Efficacy and safety of herbal stimulants and sedatives in sleep disorders', *Sleep Medicine Reviews*, vol. 4, pp 229–51.

Haber, D 1996, 'Strategies to promote the health of older people: An alternative to readiness stages', *Family Community Health*, vol. 19, pp. 1–10.

——1999, *Health Promotion and Aging: Implications for the Health Professions* (2nd edn), Springer Publishing, New York.

Hachinski, V 1992, 'Preventable senility: A call for action against the vascular dementias', *Lancet*, vol. 340, pp. 645–9.

Hagestad, GO 1985, 'Continuity and connectedness' in VL Bengston & JF Roberston (eds), *Grandparenthood*, Sage, Beverly Hills, CA.

Hall, K & Giles-Corti, B 2000, 'Complementary therapies and the general practitioner: A survey of Perth GPs', *Australian Family Physician*, vol. 29, pp. 602–6.

Hamdy, R, Turnbull, J, Edwards, J & Lancaster, M 1998, *Alzheimer's Disease: Handbook for Caregivers*, Mosby, St Louis, MO.

Hanowski, RJ & Dingus, TA 2000, 'Will intelligent transportation systems improve older driver mobility?' in KW Schaie & M Pietrucha (eds), *Mobility and Transportation in the Elderly*, Springer, New York.

Hanser, S 1985, 'Music therapy and stress reduction research', *Music Therapy*, vol. 22, pp. 193–206.

Hardy, MA & Quadagno, J 1995, 'Satisfaction with early retirement: Making choices in the auto industry', *Journals of Gerontology*, vol. 50, pp. S217–28.

Harrington, TL & Harrington, MK 2000, *Gerontechnology: Why and How*, Shaker Press, Maastricht, NL.

Harris, P & Rees, R 2000, 'The prevalence of complementary and alternative medicine use among the general population: A systematic review of the literature', *Complementary Therapies in Medicine*, vol. 8, pp. 88–96.

Harrison, L & Heywood, F 2000, *Health Begins at Home: Planning the*

Health–Housing Interface for Older People, Policy Press, Bristol.

Harvey, A 1995, 'Music in attitudinal medicine', in D Campbell (ed.), *Music Physician for Times to Come*, Quest Books, Wheaton.

Hayes, J, Saunders, W, Flint, E & Blazer, D 1997, 'Social support and depression as risk factors for loss of physical function in late life', *Aging and Mental Health*, vol. 1, pp. 209–20.

Haynes, F 2001, *The Arts: Making Sense, Making Meaning of Ourselves*, http://www.gu.edu.au/centre/atr/opt6/content1i2.html#

Hays, JC, Landerman, LR, George, LK, Flint, EP, Koenig, HG, Land, KC & Blazer, DG 1998, 'Social correlates of the dimensions of depression in the elderly', *Journal of Gerontology*, vol. 53, pp. 31–9.

Hays, T 2002, 'Music in the lives of older people', PhD thesis, The University of New England, Armidale.

Hays, T, Bright, R & Minichiello, V 2002, 'The contribution of music to positive ageing: A review', *Journal of Ageing and Identity*, vol. 7, pp. 165–76.

Hays, T, Fortunato, V & Minichiello, V 1997, 'Insights into the lives of gay older men: A qualitative study with implications for practitioners', *Venereology*, vol. 10, pp. 115–20.

'Healthy People 2010' 2000, *Healthy People in Healthy Communities: A Systematic Approach to Health Improvement*, US Public Health Service, http://www.health.gov/healthypeople/document/htm/uih/uih_bw/uih_1.htm

Hebert, R, Dubois, MF, Wolfson, C, Chambers, L & Cohen C. 2001, 'Factors associated with long-term institutionalization of older people with dementia: Data from the Canadian Study of Health and Aging', *Journals of Gerontology*, vol. 56, pp. M693–9.

Hegge, M & Fischer, C 2000, 'Grief responses of senior and elderly widows: Practice implications', *Journal of Gerontological Nursing*, vol. 26, pp. 35–43.

Hemmings, P 1998, 'Maintaining prosperity in an ageing society', *Ageing Working Papers AWP 6.3*, OECD Study on the Policy Implications of Ageing, OECD, Paris.

Henderson, AS & Jorm, AF 2000, 'Definition and epidemiology of dementia', in M Maj & N Sartorius (eds), *Dementia*, John Wiley & Sons Ltd, Chichester, UK.

Henderson, AS, Korten, AE, Levings, C, Jorm, AF, Christensen, H, Jacomb, PA & Rodgers, B 1998, 'Psychotic symptoms in the elderly: A prospective study in a population sample', *International Journal of Geriatric Psychiatry*, vol. 13, pp. 484–92.

Henrard, JC 1996, 'Cultural problems of ageing especially regarding gender and intergenerational equity', *Social Science and Medicine*, vol. 43, pp. 667–80.

Hess, BB & Soldo, BJ 1985, 'Husband and wife networks', in WJ Sauer & RT Coward (eds), *Social Support Networks and the Care of the Elderly*, Springer, New York.

Hillman, J 2000, *Clinical Perspectives on Elderly Sexuality*, Kluwer Academic/Plenum Publishers, New York.

Hillman, J & Stricker, G 1994, 'A linkage of knowledge and attitudes towards elderly sexuality: Not necessarily a uniform relationship', *Gerontologist*, vol. 34, pp. 256–60.

Hinrichsen, GA, Hernandez, NA & Pollack, S 1992, 'Difficulties and rewards in family care of the depressed older adult', *Gerontologist*, vol. 32, pp. 486–92.

Hite, S 1976, *The Hite Report: A Nationwide Study Of Female Sexuality*, Dell Publishing Co., New York.

Hochschild, A 1973, *The Unexpected Community: Portrait of an Old Age Subculture*, University of California Press, Berkeley.

Hocking, C 1997, 'What possessions say about us: Innovations in promoting occupational performance', Paper presented at the Proceedings of Occupational Therapy Australia's 19th National Conference, Perth, Western Australia.

Hollander, M & Chappell, NL 2002, *Final Report of the National Evaluation of the Cost-Effectiveness of Home Care*, Prepared for the Health Transition Fund, Health Canada, Ottawa.

Hollander, M & Tessaro, A 2001, *Evaluation of the Maintenance and Preventive Function of Home Care (Final Report)*, Home Care/Pharmaceuticals Division, Policy and Communication Branch, Health Canada, Hollander Analytical Services, Victoria, BC.

Holstein, M & Minkler, M 2003, 'Self, society and the new gerontology', *The Gerontologist*, vol. 43, pp. 787–96.

Holt, N, Johnson, A & de Belder, M 2000, 'Patient empowerment in secondary prevention of coronary heart disease', *Lancet*, vol. 356, p. 314.

Home Care NSW 2000, *Helping People Live Independently: Annual Report 1999/2000*, Sydney.

Hooker, K, Monahan, DJ, Bowman, SR, Frazer, LD & Shifren, K 1998, 'Personality counts for a lot: Predictors of mental and physical health of spouse caregivers in two disease groups', *Journals of Gerontology*, vol. 53, pp. P73–P85.

Horowitz, A 1981, 'Sons and daughters as caregivers to older parents: Differences in role performance and consequences', Annual meeting of the Gerontological Society of America, Toronto.

——1985, 'Family caregiving to the frail elderly' in C Eisdorfer (ed.), *Annual Review of Gerontology and Geriatrics*, vol. 5, Guilford Press, New York.

Houben, PP 2001, 'Changing housing for elderly people and co-ordination issues in Europe', *Housing Studies*, vol. 165, p. 651.

House of Representatives Australia 1994, Standing Committee on Community Affairs, *Home But Not Alone: A Report on the Home and Community Care Program*, Australian Government Publishing Service, Canberra.

——2000, Standing Committee on Employment, Education and Workplace Relations, *Age Counts: An Inquiry into Issues Specific to Mature Age Workers*, Australian Government Publishing Service, Canberra.

House, JS & Kahn, RL 1985, 'Measures and concepts of social support' in S Cohen & SL Syme (eds), *Social Support and Health*, Academic Press, Orlando, FL.

House, JS, Robbins, C & Metzner, HL 1982, 'The association of social relationships and activities with mortality: Prospective evidence from the Tecumseh community health study', *American Journal of Epidemiology*, vol. 116, pp. 123–40.

Hraba, J, Lorenz, FO & Pechacova, Z 1997, 'Age and depression in the post-communist Czech republic', *Research on Aging*, vol. 19, pp. 442–61.

http://fehps.une.edu.au/F/d/health/research/rmoralhealthreport.html

http://www.abs.gov.au/aausstats/abs

http://www.detya.gov.au/highered/nursing/pubs/aust_aged_care/3.htm (accessed 12 August 2003).

Hudson, R 2002, 'Welcoming the stranger', *Sacred Space: The International Journal of Spirituality and Health*, vol. 3, pp. 6–12.

Hughes, SL, Giobbie-Hurder, A, Weaver, FM, Kubal, JD & Henderson, W 1999, 'Relationship between caregiver burden and health-related quality of life', *The Gerontologist*, vol. 39, pp. 534–45.

Human Rights and Equal Opportunity Commission 2000, *Age Matters: A Report on Age Discrimination*, Australian Human Rights and Equal Opportunity Commission, Sydney.

Ikels, C 1990, 'The resolution of intergenerational conflict: Perspectives of elders and their family members', *Modern China*, vol. 16, pp. 379–406.

Illmarinin, J, Tuomi, K, Eskelinen, L, Nygard, C-H, Huuhtanen, P & Klockars, M 1992, 'Summary and recommendations of a project involving cross-sectional and follow-up studies on the ageing worker in Finnish municipal occupations (1981–1985)', *Scandinavian Journal of Work, Environment and Health*, vol. 17, Suppl. 1, pp. 135–41.

Imel, S 1996, *Older Workers: Myths and Realities*, ERIC Clearinghouse on Adult, Career and Vocational Education, Columbus, OH.

InterRAL, 2004, http//:www.interrai.org

Ishii-Kuntz, M 1990, 'Social contact and psychological well-being: Comparison across stages of adulthood', *International Journal of Aging and Human Development*, vol. 30, pp. 15–36.

Jacka, J 1989, *Frontiers of Natural Therapies*, Lothian, Melbourne.

Jacobs, JJ, Pham, PTK & Spencer JW 2003, 'Complementary and alternative medicine in the twenty-first century' in JW Spencer & JJ Jacobs (eds), *Complementary and Alternative Medicine: An Evidence Based Approach* (2nd edn), Mosby, St Louis.

Janus, S & Janus, C 1993, *The Janus Report on Sexual Behavior*, John Wiley & Sons, New York.

Jarvik, LF 2000, 'Dementia: Much information, many unanswered questions' in M Maj & N Sartorius (eds), *Dementia*, John Wiley & Sons Ltd, Chichester, UK.

Jarvis, P 2001, *Learning Later Life*, Kogan Page Ltd, London.

Jerrome, D & Wenger, GC 1999, 'Stability and change in late-life friendships', *Ageing and Society*, vol. 19, pp. 661–76.

Johnson, B 1996, 'Older adults and sexuality: A multidimensional perspective', *Journal of Gerontological Nursing*, vol. 22, pp. 6–15.

Johnson, CL & Catalano, DH 1981, 'Childless elderly and their family supports', *The Gerontologist*, vol. 21, pp. 610–8.

Jonas, J 1991, 'Preferences of elderly music listeners residing in nursing homes for arts music, traditional jazz, popular music of the today, and country music', *Music Therapy*, vol. 28, pp. 149–60.

Jones, P 1993, 'The active witness: the acquisition of meaning in dramatherapy' in H Payner (eds), *Handbook of Inquiry in the Arts Therapies: One River, Many Currents*, Jessica Kingsley, London.

Jones, R 2002, ' "That's very rude, I shouldn't be telling you that": Older women talking about sex', *Narrative Inquiry*, vol. 12, pp. 121–43.

Joseph, AE & Chalmers, AI 1996, 'Restructuring long-term care and the geography of ageing: A view from rural New Zealand', *Social Science & Medicine*, vol. 42, pp. 887–96.

Josephek, KJ 2000, 'Alternative medicine's roadmap to the mainstream', *American Journal of Law and Medicine*, vol. 26, pp. 295–310.

Joyce, A 2002, 'Promoting the Social Well-being of Older People', Unpublished PhD thesis, La Trobe University, Melbourne.

Jungmeen, EK & Moen, P 1999, 'Work-retirement transitions and psychological well-being in late midlife', Cornell Employment and Family Careers Institute, Ithaca, NY.

Juslin, P & Sloboda, J 2001, 'Music and emotion: Introduction' in P Juslin & J Sloboda (eds), *Music and Emotion*, Oxford Press, Oxford.

Jutras, S & Veilleux, F 1991, 'Informal caregiving: Correlates of perceived burden', *Canadian Journal on Aging*, vol. 10, pp. 40–55.

Kahana, E & Kahana, B 2001, 'Successful aging among people with HIV/AIDS', *Journal of Clinical Epidemiology*, vol. 54, pp. S53–6.

Kales, HC, Blow, FC, Copeland, LA, Bingham, RC, Kammerer, EE & Mellow, AM 1999, 'Health care utilization by older patients with coexisting dementia and depression', *American Journal of Psychiatry*, vol. 156, pp. 550–6.

Kalisch, DW 2000, *Social Policy Directions Across the OECD Region: Reflections on a Decade of Change*, Policy research paper no. 4, Department of Family and Community Services, Canberra.

Kane, RA 2000, 'Accomplishments, problems, trends and future challenges' in RL Kane & RA Kane (eds), *Assessing Older Persons: Measures, Meaning and Practical Applications*, Oxford University Press, New York.

Kane, RL 1990, 'Introduction' in RL Kane, JG Evans & D MacFadyen (eds), *Improving the Health of Older People: A World View*, Oxford University Press, New York.

Kaplan, GA 1997, 'Behavioural, social and socioenvironmental factors adding years to life and life to years' in T Hickey, M Speers & T Prohaska (eds), *Public Health and Ageing*, The Johns Hopkins University Press, Baltimore, MD.

Kaplan, GA, Salonen, JT, Cohen, RD, Brand, RJ, Syme, SL & Puska, P 1988, 'Social connections and mortality from all causes and from cardiovascular disease: Prospective evidence from eastern Finland', *American Journal of Epidemiology*, vol. 128, pp. 370–80.

Kaplan, GA, Wilson, TW, Cohen, RD, Kauhanen, J, Wu, M & Salonen, JT 1994, 'Social functioning and overall mortality: Prospective evidence from the Kuopio Ischemic Heart Disease Risk Factor Study', *Epidemiology*, vol. 5, pp. 495–500.

Kart, C 1997, *The Realities of Aging: An Introduction to Gerontology*, Allyn & Bacon, Boston, MA.

Karwat, ID 1998, 'Major medical and social needs of disabled rural inhabitants', *Annals of Agriculture and Environmental Medicine*, vol. 52, pp. 117–26.

Katz, J, Chaushu, G & Sharabi, Y 2001, 'On the association between hypercholesterolemia, cardiovascular disease and severe periodontal disease', *Journal of Clinical Periodontology*, vol. 28, pp. 865–8.

Kaufman, S 2000, 'The clash of meanings: Medical narrative and biographical story at life's end', *Generations*, vol. 23, pp.77–82.

Kavanagh, DJ 1990, 'Towards a cognitive-behavioural intervention for adult grief reactions', *British Journal of Psychiatry*, vol. 157, pp. 373–83.

Kawai, H & Hiki, S 2002, 'A system for assessing the walking ability of the elderly', *Gerontechnology*, vol. 2, p. 92.

Kay, E & Locker, D 1998, 'A systematic review of the effectiveness of health promotion aimed at improving oral health', *Community Dental Health*, vol. 15, pp. 132–44.

Kayne, S 1998, 'The sweet smell of health: Medical applications of aromatherapy', *Chemist and Druggist*, vol. 249, pp. 1–3.

Keating, NC, Fast, J, Frederick, J, Cranswick, K & Perrier, C 1999, *Eldercare in Canada: Context, Content and Consequences*, Statistics Canada, Housing, Family and Social Statistics Division, Ottawa.

Keeling, S 2001, 'Relative distance: Ageing in rural New Zealand', *Ageing and Society*, vol. 21, pp. 605–15.

Kellett, J 1991, 'Sexuality of the elderly', *Sexual and Marital Therapy*, vol. 6, pp. 147–55.

——2000, 'Older adult sexuality', in L Szuchman & F Muscarell (eds), *Psychological Perspectives on Human Sexuality*, John Wiley & Sons, Toronto.

Kempen, G, Verbrugge, L, Merrill, S & Ormel, J 1998, 'The impact of multiple impairments on disability in community-dwelling older people', *Age & Ageing*, vol. 27, pp. 595–604.

Kemper, P 1992, 'The use of formal and informal home care by the disabled elderly', *Health Services Research*, vol. 27, pp. 421–51.

Kendig, H 1996a, 'Predictors and consequences of social activity: What matters to older people', *Hong Kong Journal of Gerontology*, vol. 10, pp. 343–6.

——1996b, 'Understanding health promotion for older people' in V Minichiello, N Chappell & H Kendig (eds), *Sociology of Aging: International Perspectives*, International Sociological Association, Research Committee on Aging, Melbourne.

——2000, 'Ageing and the built environment', in P Troy (ed.), *Equity, Environment, Efficiency: Ethics and Economics in Urban Australia*, Melbourne University Press, Melbourne.

Kendig, H & Duckett, S 2001, *Australian Directions in Aged Care: The Generation of Policies for Generations of Older People*, Australian Health Policy Institute, University of Sydney, Sydney.

Kendig, H & Gardner, I 1997, 'Unravelling housing policy for older people' in A Borowski, S Encel & E Ozanne (eds), *Ageing and Social Policy in Australia*, Cambridge University Press, Melbourne.

Kendig, H & McCallum, J 1990, *Grey Policy: Australian Policies for an Ageing Society*, Allen & Unwin, Sydney.

Kendig, H & Neutze, M 1999, *Housing Implications of Population Ageing in Australia*, Paper presented at the Policy Implications of the Ageing of Australia's Population, Canberra.

Kendig, H & Pynoos, J 1996, 'Housing' in J Birren (ed.), *Encyclopaedia of Gerontology*, Academic Press, San Diego, CA.

Kendig, H, Andrews, G, Browning, C, Quine, S & Parsons, A 2000, *A Review of Healthy Ageing Research in Australia*, Publications Production Unit (Public Affairs, Parliamentary and Access Branch), Commonwealth Department of Health and Aged Care, Canberra.

Kendig, H, Helme, R, Teshuva, K, Osborne, D, Flicker, L & Browning, C 1996, *Health Status of Older People Project: Preliminary Findings from a Survey of the Health and Lifestyles of Older Australians*, Victorian Health Promotion Foundation, Melbourne.

Kenyon, J 1987, *Acupressure Techniques*, HarperCollins, London.

Kessler, RC & McLeod, JD 1985, 'Social support and mental health in community samples' in S Cohen & SL Syme (eds), *Social Support and Health*, Academic Press, Orlando, FL.

Khaw, KT 1997, 'Healthy aging', *British Medical Journal*, vol. 315, pp. 1090–6.

Khosh, F 2001, 'Naturopathic approach to Alzheimer's disease', *Townsend Letter for Doctors and Patients*, July, pp. 38–42.

Kicklighter, J 1991, 'Characteristics of older adult learners: A guide for dietetics practitioners', *Journal of the American Dietetic Association*, vol. 91, pp. 1418–25.

Kilander, L, Beglund, L, Boberg, M, Vessby, B & Lithell, H 2001, 'Education, lifestyle factors and mortality from cardiovascular disease and cancer: A 25-year follow-up of Swedish 50-year-old men', *International Journal of Epidemiology*, vol. 30, pp. 1119–26.

Kimmel, DC 1978, 'Adult development and aging: A gay perspective', *Journal of Social Issues*, vol. 34, pp. 113–30.

Kingsberg, S 2002, 'The impact of aging on sexual function in women and their partners', *Archives of Sexual Behavior*, vol. 31, pp. 431–8.

Kinnear, P 2001, *Population Ageing: Crisis or Transition*, Australian Institute of Health and Welfare, Canberra.

Kinsey, AC, Pomeroy, WB & Martin, CE 1948, *Sexual Behavior in the Human Male*, WB Saunders Co., Philadelphia.

Kinsey, AC, Pomeroy, WB, Martin, CE & Gebhard, PH 1953, *Sexual Behavior in the Human Female*, WB Saunders Co., Philadelphia.

Kirkwood, T 2001, *Reith Lecture IV: Making Choices*, BBC Radio4, hhtp:/www.bbc.co.uk/radio4/reith2001/lecture4.shtml

Kitwood, T 1997, 'The concept of personhood and its relevance for a new culture of dementia care' in R Binstock, S Post & P Whithouse (eds), *Dementia and Aging: Ethics, Values, Policy Choices*, The Johns Hopkins University Press, London.

Kline, DW 1994, 'Optimizing the visibility of displays for older observers', *Experimental Ageing Research*, vol. 20, pp. 11–23.

Klinge, I 2000, Paper presented at the *4th European Feminist Research Conference: Body, Gender, Subjectivity*, www.women.it/cyberarchive/files/klinge.htm

Knapman, C 1996, *Older People in Rural Communities: Rethinking the Meaning of Family Based Care* [online], retrieved November 2000. Available: http://www.aifs.org.au/institute/afrcpapers/knapman.htm

Knight, B 1996, *Psychotherapy with Older Adults*, Sage, London.

Kobassa, S 1982, 'The hardy personality: Toward a social psychology of stress and health' in GS Sanders & J Suls (eds), *Social Psychology of Health and Illness*, Erlbaum, Hillsdale, NJ.

Kochera, A 2002, *Falls Among Older Persons and the Role of the Home: An Analysis of Cost, Incidence and Potential Savings from Home Modification*, Issues Brief, AARP Public Policy Institute, Washington, DC.

Koelen, MA, Vaandrager, L & Colomer, C 2001, 'Health promotion research: Dilemmas and challenges', *Journal of Epidemiology Community Health*, vol. 55, pp. 257–62.

Konner, M 1987, *Becoming a Doctor: A Journey of Initiation in Medical School*, Penguin, New York.

Koren, LGH, Pernot, CEE, Snijders, MCL & van Bronswijk, JEMH 2002, 'Supply and demand of indoor air qualities in dwellings', *Gerontechnology*, vol. 2, p. 120.

Kottler, JA 2000, *Nuts and Bolts of Helping*, Allyn & Bacon, Boston, MA.

Kragh-Sorensen, P, Andersen, K, Lolk, A & Nielsen, H 2000, 'Rates and risk factors of dementia: Evidence or controversy?' in M Maj & N Sartorius (eds), *Dementia*, John Wiley & Sons Ltd, Chichester, UK.

Krause, N & Markides, K 1990, 'Measuring social support among older adults', *International Journal of Aging and Human Development*, vol. 30, pp. 37–53.

Kreidler, MC, Campbell, J, Lanik, G, Gray, VR & Conrad, MA 1994, 'A nursing center's use of change theory as a model', *Journal of Gerontological Nursing*, vol. 20, pp. 25–30.

Kristeva, J 1982, *Powers of Horror: An Essay on Abjection* (trans. Leon S. Roudiez), Columbia University Press, New York.

Kuhn, MA 1999, *Complementary Therapies for Health Care Providers*, Lippincott, Williams & Wilkins, Philadelphia.

Kuller, LH 1996, 'Potential prevention of Alzheimer's disease and dementia', *Alzheimer Disorder Association*, vol. 10, pp. 13–16.

Kunzman, U, Little, TD & Smith, J 2000, 'Is age related stability of subjective well-being a paradox? Cross-sectional and longitudinal evidence from the Berlin Aging Study', *Psychology and Aging*, vol. 15, pp. 511–26.

Kwon, I, Oldaker, S, Schrager, MA, Talbot, MA, Fozard, JL & Metter, EJ 2001, 'Relationship between muscle strength and self-paced gait speed: Age and sex effects', *Journal of Gerontology*, vol. 56, pp. B398–B404.

Lachs, MS, Williams, C, O'Brien, S, Hurst, L & Horwitz, R 1997, 'Risk factors for reported elder abuse and neglect: A nine-year observational cohort study', *The Gerontologist*, vol. 37, pp. 469–74.

Lad, V 1985, *Ayurveda: The Science of Self-Healing*, Lotus Press, Wilmot, WI.

Lang, FR & Carstensen, LL 1994, 'Close emotional relationships in late life: Further support for proactive aging in the social domain', *Psychology and Aging*, vol. 9, pp. 315–24.

Lang, FR, Staudinger, UM & Carstensen, LL 1998, 'Perspectives on socio-emotional selectivity in late life: How personality and social context do (and do not) make a difference', *Journal of Gerontology: Psychological Sciences*, vol. 53B, pp. 21–30.

Lanspery, S & Hyde, J 1997, *Staying Put: Adapting the Places Instead of the People*, Baywood Publishing, Amityville, NY.

Larson, R 1978, 'Thirty years of research on the subjective well-being of older Americans', *Journal of Gerontology*, vol. 33, pp. 109–25.

Lassey, WR & Lassey, ML 2001, *Quality of Life for Older People: An International Perspective*, Prentice Hall, New Jersey.

Lawton, MP, Winter, L, Kleban, MH & Ruckdeschel, K 1999, 'Affect and quality of life: Objective and subjective', *Journal of Aging and Health*, vol. 11, pp. 169–98.

Lawton, MP 1998, 'Future society and technology' in JAM Graafmans, V Taipele & N Charness (eds), *Gerontechnology: A Sustainable Investment in the Future*, IOS Press, Amsterdam.

Leake, R & Broderick, JE 1998, 'Treatment efficacy of acupuncture: A review of the research literature', *Integrative Medicine*, vol. 1, pp. 107–15.

Leathers, SJ, Kelley, MA & Richman, JA 1997, 'Postpartum depressive symptomatology in new mothers and fathers: Parenting, work, and support', *The Journal of Nervous and Mental Disease*, vol. 185, pp. 129–39.

Lee, GR 1985, 'Theoretical perspectives on social networks' in WJ Sauer & IRT Coward (eds), *Social Support Networks and the Care of the Elderly*, Springer, New York.

Lee, GR, DeMaris, A, Bavin, S & Sullivan, R 2001, 'Gender differences in the depressive effect of widowhood in later life', *Journals of Gerontology*, vol. 1, pp. S56–S61.

Lee, GR & Ishii-Kuntz, M 1988, 'Social interaction, loneliness, and emotional well-being among the elderly', *Research on Aging*, vol. 9, pp. 459–82.

Lee, JA 1987, 'What can homosexual aging studies contribute to theories of ageing?', *Journal of Homosexuality*, vol. 13, pp. 43–71.

Legge, K 2002, 'Love springs eternal', *The Weekend Australian Magazine*, 31 Aug–1 Sept.

Leibfritz, W 2003, 'Retiring later makes sense', *Organization for Economic Cooperation and Development Observer*, OECD, Paris.

Letvak, S 2002, 'Myths and realities of ageism and nursing', *Association of Operating Room Nurses Journal*, vol. 75, pp. 1101–7.

Leveille, SG, Guralnik, JM, Ferrucci, L & Langlois, JA 1999, 'Aging successfully until death in old age: Opportunities for increasing active life expectancy', *American Journal of Epidemiology*, vol. 149, pp. 654–64.

Levy, D & Malcolm, C 1993, 'Design and problems of ageing' in EJ Stern & RA Harootyan (eds), *Life-span Design of Residential Environments for an Ageing Population*, American Association of Retired Persons, Washington, DC.

Levy, JA, Ory, MG & Crystal, S 2003, 'HIV/AIDS interventions for midlife and older adults: Current status and challenges', *Journal of Acquired Immune Deficiency Syndromes*, vol. 33, pp. 559–67.

Linde, K, Ramirez, G, Mulrow, CD, Pauls, A, Weidenhammer, W & Melchart, D 1996, 'St John's Wort for depression: An overview and meta-analysis of randomised clinical trials', *British Medical Journal*, vol. 313, pp. 253–8.

Lipski, PS 1996, 'Australian nutrition screening initiative', *Australasian Journal on Ageing*, vol. 15, pp. 14–6.

Lis, C & Gaviria, S 1997, 'Vascular dementia, hypertension, and the brain', *Neurological Research*, vol. 9, pp. 471–80.

Little, SJ, Hollis, JF, Stevens, VJ, Mount, K, Mullooly, JP & Johnson, BD 1997, 'Effective group behavioral intervention for older periodontal patients', *Journal of Periodontal Research*, vol. 32, pp. 315–25.

Liu, R 1994, *Baseline Survey Data of Beijing Multidimensional Longitudinal Study of Aging*, Weijin Publishing House, Beijing.

Liu, Z 1998, *The Probability of Nursing Home Use Over a Lifetime*, Working Paper 16, Welfare Division, Australian Institute of Health and Welfare, Canberra.

Loeb, C & Meyer, JS 2000, 'Criteria for diagnosis of vascular dementia', *Archives of Neurology*, vol. 57, pp. 23–35.

Lopata, HZ 1975, 'Support systems of elderly urbanites: Chicago of the 1970s', *The Gerontologist*, vol. 15, pp. 35–41.

Lovestone, S 2000, 'Dementia: Hope for the future', in M Maj & N Sartorius (eds), *Dementia*, John Wiley & Sons Ltd, Chichester, UK.

Luketich, B 1991, 'Sex and the elderly: What do nurses know?', *Educational Gerontology*, vol. 17, pp. 573–639.

Lund, DA, Caserta, MS & Dimond, MF 1986, 'Gender differences through two years of bereavement among the elderly', *Gerontologist*, vol. 26, pp. 314–20.

Luoma, JB & Pearson, JL 2002, 'Suicide and marital status in the United States, 1991–1996: Is widowhood a risk factor?', *American Journal of Public Health*, vol. 92, pp. 1518–22.

Luskin, FM, Dinucci, EM, Newell, KA & Haskell, WL 2003, 'Select populations: Elderly patients' in JW Spencer & JJ Jacobs (eds), *Complementary and Alternative Medicines; An Evidence-based Approach* (2nd edn), Mosby, St Louis.

Lyketsos, CG, Steinberg, M, Tschanz, JT, Norton, MC, Steffens, DC & Breitner, JCS 2000, 'Mental and behavioral disturbances in dementia: Findings from the Cache County Study on memory in aging', *American Journal of Psychiatry*, vol. 157, pp. 708–14.

MacDonald, M, Remus, G & Laing, G 1994, 'Research considerations: The link between housing and health in the elderly', *Journal of Gerontological Nursing*, vol. 207, pp. 5–10.

MacKinnon, ME, Gien, L & Durst, D 2001, 'Silent pain: Social isolation of the elderly Chinese in Canada' in I Chi, NL Chappell & J Lubben (eds), *Elderly Chinese in Pacific Rim Countries: Social Support and Integration*, Hong Kong University Press, Hong Kong.

Maher, S 2001, 'Assessing age-related sleep disorders', *Nursing Older People*, vol. 13, pp. 27–8.

Mahtre, SL & Deber, RB 1992, 'From equal access to health care to equitable access to health: A review of Canadian provincial health commissions and reports', *International Journal of Health Services*, vol. 22, pp. 645–68.

Majerovitz, D 2001, 'Role of family adaptability in the psychological adjustment of spouse caregivers to patients with dementia', *Journal of Mental Health and Aging*, vol. 10, pp. 447–57.

Malmgren, JA, Martin, ML & Nicola, RM 1996, 'Health care access of poverty-level older adults in subsidized public housing', *Public Health Reports*, vol. 1113, pp. 260–3.

Manfredi, R 2002, 'HIV disease and advanced age: An increasing therapeutic challenge', *Drugs & Aging*, vol. 19, pp. 647–69.

Marcantonio, E 2000, 'Dementia' in M Beers & R Berkow (eds), *The Merck Manual of Geriatrics*, Merck Research Laboratories, Division of Merck & Co. Inc, Whitehouse Station, New Jersey.

Marcus, CC 1997, *House as a Mirror of Self: Exploring the Deeper Meaning of Home*, Conari Press, Berkley, CA.

Mariño, R, Wright, FAC, Schofield, M, Minichiello, V & Calache, H 2002, *Oral Health Promotion Program for Older Migrant Adults*, available at: http://fehps.une.edu.au/F/d/health/research/rmoralhealthreport.html

Markham, JP & Gilderbloom, JI 1998, 'Housing quality among the elderly: A decade of changes,' *International Journal of Aging & Human Development*, vol. 461, pp. 71–90.

Marks, NF, Lambert, JD & Choi, H 2002, 'Transitions to caregiving, gender, and psychological well-being: A prospective US national study', *Journal of Marriage and Family*, vol. 64, pp. 657–67.

Marshall, VW 2001, 'Models of health promotion: Towards an integrated vision', paper presented at *The Meeting of the Southern Gerontological Society*, Orlando, FL.

Marsiglio, W & Greer, R 1994, 'A gender analysis of older men's sexuality', in E Thompson (ed.), *Older Men's Lives*, Sage Publications, London.

Martin, C 1981, 'Factors affecting sexual functioning in 60–79-year-old married males', *Archives of Sexual Behaviour*, vol. 10, pp. 399–420.

Martin-Matthews, A 1996, 'Widowhood and widowerhood' in JE Birren (ed.), *Encyclopaedia of Gerontology*, Academic Press, San Diego, CA.

Mason, F, Liu, Z & Braun, P 2001, *The Probability of Using an Aged Care Home over a lifetime 1999–00*, Working Paper no. 36, Australian Institute of Health and Welfare, Canberra.

Masters, WH & Johnson, VE 1966, *Human Sexual Response*, Little, Brown and Company, Boston, MA.

——1970, *Human Sexual Inadequacy*, Little, Brown and Company, Boston, MA.

Mathers, CD, Sadana, R, Salomon, JA, Murray, CJL & Lopez, AD 2001, 'Healthy life expectancy in 191 countries, 1999', *Lancet*, vol. 357, pp. 1685–91.

Matthews, SH 1986, *Friendships Through the Life Course: Oral Biographies in Old Age*, Sage Publications, Newbury Park, CA.

Matthius, R, Lubben, J, Atchison, K & Schweitzer, S 1997, 'Sexual activity and satisfaction among very old adults: Results from a community dwelling medicare population survey', *Gerontologist*, vol. 37, pp. 6–14.

Maule, A, Cliff, D & Taylor, R 1996, 'Early retirement decisions and how they affect later quality of life', *Ageing and Society*, vol. 16, pp. 177–204.

Mayeux, R 1993, 'Neurology of aging: The problem of dementia in the year 2000', in F Lieberman & M Collen (eds), *Aging in Good Health: A Quality Lifestyle for the Later Years*, Plenum Press, New York.

McCallum, J 1986, 'Retirement and widowhood transitions', in HL Kendig (ed.), *Ageing and Families*, Allen & Unwin, Sydney.

——2002, 'The nursing labour force in aged care', *Nursing Review*, September 2002, p. 1.

McColl, M & Friedland, J 1994, 'Social support, aging and disability', *Topics in Geriatric Rehabilitation*, vol. 9, pp. 54–71.

McCracken, A, Fitzwater, E & Lockwood, M 1995. 'Comparison of nursing students' attitudes towards the elderly in Norway and the United States', *Educational Gerontology*, vol. 21, pp. 167–80.

McDaniel, SA & Chappell, NL 1999, 'Health care in regression: Contraindications, tensions and implications for Canadian seniors', *Canadian Public Policy*, vol. 25, pp. 123–32.

McDowell, I & Newell, C 1996, *Measuring Health: A Guide to Rating Scales and Questionnaires*, Oxford University Press, New York.

McLeod, SD, West, SK, Quigley, HA & Fozard, JL 1990, 'A longitudinal study of the relationship between intraocular pressure and blood pressure', *Investigative Ophthalmology and Visual Science*, vol. 31, pp. 2351–66.

McNiff, S 1998, *Trust the Process: An Artist's Guide to Letting Go*, Shambhala, Boston, MA.

Meston, C 1997, 'Aging and sexuality', *The Western Journal of Medicine*, vol. 167, pp. 285–91.

Metz, M & Miner, M 1998, 'Psychosexual and psychosexual aspects of male aging and sexual health', *The Canadian Journal of Human Sexuality*, vol. 7, pp. 245–59.

Miasaki, E, Imai, A, Takagi, T, Imai, T & Ando, A 2001, 'Application trials for the realization of human-friendly broadcasting', *Gerontechnology*, vol. 1, pp. 103–10.

Michael, R, Ganon, J, Laumann, B & Kolate, G 1994, *Sex in America: A Definitive Study*, Little Brown and Company, Boston, MA.

Miller, B & Cafasso, L 1992, 'Gender differences in caregiving: Fact or artifact?', *Gerontologist*, vol. 32, pp. 298–507.

Miller, B, Townsend, A, Carpenter, E, Montgomery, RVJ, Stull, D & Young, RF 2001, 'Social support and caregiver distress: A replication analysis', *Journals of Gerontology*, vol. 56, pp. S249–56.

Mina, J, Nolan, D & Mallal, S 2001, 'Antiretroviral therapy and the lipodystrophy syndrome', *Antiviral Therapy*, vol. 6, pp. 9–20.

Minichiello, V 1995, 'Community care: Economic policy dressed as social concern?', in H Gardner (ed.), *The Politics of Health: The Australian Experience*, Churchill Livingstone, Melbourne.

Minichiello, V, Alexander, L & Jones D 1992, *Gerontology: A Multidisciplinary Approach*, Prentice Hall, Sydney.

Minichiello, V, Browne, J & Kendig, H 2000, 'Perceptions and consequences of ageism: Views of older people', *Ageing and Society*, vol. 20, pp. 253–78.

Minichiello, V, Plummer, D & Loxton, D 2000, 'Knowledge and beliefs of older Australians about sexuality and health', *Australasian Journal on Ageing*, vol. 19, pp. 190–4.

——2004, 'Factors predicting sexual relationships in older people: An Australian study', *Australasian Journal on Ageing*, vol. 23, (in press).

Minichiello, V, Plummer, D & Seal, A 1996, 'The "asexual" older person? Australian evidence', *Venereology: The Interdisciplinary, International Journal of Sexual Health*, vol. 9, pp. 180–8.

Minichiello, V, Plummer, D, Waite, H & Deacon, S 1996, 'Sexuality and older people: Social issues' in V Minichiello, N Chappell, H Kendig & A Walker (eds), *Sociology of Ageing: International Perspectives*, International Sociological Association, Melbourne.

Minister of Public Works and Government Services Canada 1998, Principles of the National Framework on Aging: A Policy Guide, Division of Aging and Seniors, Ottawa.

Minnigerode, F & Adelman, M 1987, 'Elderly homosexual men and women: Report on a pilot study', *Family Co-ordinator*, vol. 27, pp. 451–66.

Mockler, D, Riordan, J & Murphy, M 1998, 'Psychosocial factors associated with the use/nonuse of mental health services by primary carers of individuals with dementia', *International Journal of Geriatric Psychiatry*, vol. 13, pp. 310–4.

Mollenkopf, H 2000, 'Technik im Haurshalt zur Unterstutzung einer selbstbestimmten Lebensfuhrung im Alter. Das Forschungsprojekt "sentha" und erste Ergebnisse des sozialwissenschaftlichen Teilprojekts' (Everyday technologies for senior households: The project 'sentha' and first results of its social science part), *Zeitschrift fur Gerontolgie and Geriatrie*, vol. 33, pp. 155–68.

——2002, 'The significance of lifelong learning in a changing world', *Gerontechnology*, vol. 2, pp. 3–14.

Mollenkopf, H & Fozard, JL 2004, 'Technology and the good life: Challenges for current and future generations of ageing people' in HW Wahl, R Scheidt & P Windley (eds), *Environments, Gerontology and Old Age: Annual Review of Gerontology and Geriatrics*, Springer, New York.

Mooney, G 2000, 'The emperor's quality clothes: For goodness' sake let's take the strain off the word quality!', *Australian and New Zealand Journal of Public Health*, vol. 24, p. 102.

Moore, LB, Goodwin, B, Jones, SA, Wisely, GB, Serabjit-Singh, CJ, Willson, TM, Collins, JL & Kliewer, SA 2000, 'St John's Wort induces hepatic drug metabolism through activation of the pregnane-S receptor', *Proceedings of the National Academy of Science USA*, vol. 97, pp. 7500–2.

Morling, G 2001, 'Massage therapy: The road to professionalism', *Journal of the Australian Traditional-Medicine Society*, vol. 7, p. 131.

Morrow-Howell, N, Sherraden, M, Hinterlong, J & Rozario, P 2001, 'An agenda on productive aging: Research, policy, and practice', George Warren Brown School of Social Work, Washington University, St Louis.

Moss, P 1997, 'Negotiating spaces in home environments: Older women living with arthritis', *Social Science and Medicine*, vol. 451, pp. 23–33.

Moynagh, M & Worsley, R 2001, 'Tomorrow's workplace, fulfilment or stress', Carnegie UK Trust, London.

Mroczek, DK & Kolarz CM. 1998, 'The effect of age on positive and negative affect: A developmental perspective on happiness', *Journal of Personality and Social Psychology*, vol. 75, pp. 1333–49.

Muldoon, MF, Barger, SD, Flory, JD & Manuck, SB 1998, 'What are quality of life measurements measuring?', *British Medical Journal*, vol. 316, pp. 542–5.

Mulligan, T & Moss, C 1991, 'Sexuality and aging in male veterans: A cross sectional study of interest, ability and activity', *Archives of Sexual Behaviour*, vol. 20, pp. 17–25.

Murphy, B, Schofield, H, Nankervis, J, Bloch, S, Herrman, H & Singh, B 1997, 'Women with multiple roles: The emotional impact of caring for ageing parents', *Ageing and Society*, vol. 17, pp. 277–91.

Murray, CJ & Lopez, AD 1997, 'Regional patterns of disability-free life expectancy and disability-adjusted life expectancy: Global Burden of Disease Study', *Lancet*, vol. 349, pp. 1347–52.

Murray, J & Livingston, G 1998, 'A qualitative study of adjustment to caring for an older spouse with psychiatric illness', *Ageing and Society*, vol. 18, pp. 659–71.

Murray, MT & Pizzorno, JE 1990, *Encyclopedia of Natural Medicine*, MacDonald, London.

Mutran, EJ, Reitzes, DJ, Bratton, KA, Fernandez, ME 1997, 'Self-esteem and subjective responses to work among mature workers: Similarities and differences by gender', *Journals of Gerontology*, vol. 52, pp. S89–96.

Mutschler, PH 1997, 'The effects of income on home modification: Can they afford to stay put?' in S Lanspery & J Hyde (eds), *Staying Put: Adapting the Places Instead of the People*, Baywood Publishing, Amityville, NY.

Naleppa, MJ 1996, 'Families and the institutionalised elderly', *Journal of Gerontological Social Work*, vol. 27, pp. 87–111.

National Academy on an Aging Society 1999, The Public Policy and Aging Report, vol. 9, no. 4, The Gerontological Society of America, Washington.

National Center for Health Statistics 1999, *Vital Health and Statistics: Current Estimates from the National Health Interview Survey, 1996*, Series 10, no. 2000, Washington, DC.

National Institute of Aging 1993, *Answers About: The Aging Women and the Aging Man*, US Department of Health and Human Services, Public Health Service and National Institutes of Health, Washington, DC.

National Institute of Health 2003, http://www.nia.nih.gov/health/agepages/aids.htm

Nay, R & Garratt, S 1999, 'Challenging behaviour: The issues of quality of life' in R Nay & S Garrett (eds), *Nursing Older People*, McLennan & Petty, Sydney.

——2002, *Nursing Older People: Issues and Innovations*, McLennan & Petty, Sydney.

Ness, J, Sherman, FT & Pan, CX 1999, 'Alternative medicine: What the data say about common herbal therapies', *Geriatrics*, vol. 54, pp. 33–4.

Nesse, R & Williams, G 1997, 'Are mental disorders diseases?' in S Baron-Cohen (ed.), *The Maladapted Mind: Classic Readings in Evolutionary Psychopathology*, Psychology Press, Hove, East Sussex.

New South Wales (NSW) Health 1992, *Assistants in Nursing Review*, Nursing Branch, Sydney.

New Zealand Ministry of Health 2002, *Health of Older People Strategy: Health Section Action to 2010 to Support Positive Ageing*, Ministry of Health, Wellington.

Neyland, B & Kendig, H 1996, 'Retirement immigration to the coast' in PW Newton & M Bell (eds), *Population Shift, Mobility and Change in Australia*, Australian Government Publishing Service, Canberra.

Nocon, A 1997, 'Until disabled people get consulted: The role of occupational therapy in meeting housing needs', *British Journal of Occupational Therapy*, vol. 603, pp. 115–22.

Nocon, A & Pearson, M 2000, 'The role of friends and neighbors in providing support for older people', *Ageing and Society*, vol. 20, pp. 341–67.

Norman, DA 1988, *The Psychology of Everyday Things*, Basic Books, New York.

Norred, CL 2000, 'Minimising pre-operative anxiety with alternative caring-healing techniques', *Association of Operating Room Nurses (AORN) Journal*, vol. 72, pp. 838–43.

Nygard, C-H, Luopararvi, T & Ilmarinen, J 1992, 'Musculoskeletal capacity and its changes among ageing municipal employees in different work categories', *Scandinavian Journal of Work, Environment, and Health*, vol. 17, Suppl. 1, pp. 110–7.

O'Bryant, SL, Straw, LB & Meddaugh, DI 1990, 'Contributions of the care-giving role to women's development', *Sex Roles*, vol. 23, pp. 645–58.

O'Conner, K 1999, *Estimation of Requirements for and Supply of Registered Nurses in the NSW Nursing Speciality Workforce Groups of: Rehabilitation, Paediatric and Aged Care: Draft Report*, NSW Health Department, Sydney.

Office of Legislative Drafting 1958, *Nursing Home Subsidy Act 1957*, Attorney General's Department, Canberra.

——1970, *States Grants (Home Care) Act 1969*, Attorney General's Department, Canberra.

——1970, *States Grants (Paramedical Services) Act 1969*, Attorney General's Department, Canberra.

——1971, *Delivered Meals Subsidy Act 1970*, Attorney General's Department, Canberra.

——1998, *Aged Care Act 1997*, Attorney General's Department, Canberra.

Office of National Statistics (United Kingdom) 2004a, *Recipients of Selected Benefits for Elderly People 1981/82–1997/98*, Selected Trends 30, http//:www.statistics.gov.uk

——2004b, *Use of Personal Social Services by People Aged 65 and Over Living in Households: By Age 2001/02*, Social Trends 34, http//:www.statistics.gov.uk

OECD *See* Organization for Economic Cooperation and Development.

O'Hanlon, WH & Beadle, S 1999, *Guide to Possibility Land: Fifty-one Methods for Doing Brief, Respectful Therapy*, WW Norton & Co., New York.

O'Loughlin, J, Renaud, L, Richard, L, Sanchez, L & Paradis, G 1998, 'Correlates of the sustainability of community-based health promotion interventions', *Preventive Medicine*, vol. 27, pp. 702–12.

Ommen, GS, Beresford, SAA, Buchner, DA, LaCroix, A, Martin, M, Patrick, DA, Wallace, JI & Wagner, EH 1997, 'Evidence of modifiable risk factors in older adults as a basis for health promotion and disease prevention programs' in T Hickey, MA Speers & TR Prohaska (eds), *Public Health and Ageing*, The Johns Hopkins University Press, Baltimore, MD.

Organization for Economic Cooperation and Development 1996, *Ageing in OECD Countries: A Critical Policy Challenge*, Social Policy Studies no. 20, OECD, Paris.

——2000, *Reforms for an Ageing Society*, OECD, Paris.

——2002, 'Increasing employment: The role of late retirement', *Electronic Outlook*, no. 72, December, OECD, Paris.

Ortiz, J 1997, *The Tao of Music: Using Music to Change Your Life*, Colour Books Ltd, Dublin.

Ott, A, Breteler, MB, van Harskamp, F, Claus, JJ, van der Cammen, TJM, Grobbee, DE & Hofman, A 1995, 'Prevalence of Alzheimer's disease and vascular dementia: Association with education', *British Medical Journal*, vol. 310, pp. 970–4.

Ownby, R & Czaja, S 2002, 'Problems in web page design for the elderly', *Gerontechnology*, vol. 2, p. 101.

Pak, R, Rogers, W & Fisk, AD 2002, 'An investigation of the relationship between spatial abilities and hypertext navigation: It's not as simple as it seems!', *Gerontechnology*, vol. 2, p. 100.

Palmer, J & Molyneux, P 2000, *A Partnership Approach to Health and Housing: A Good Practice Briefing for Primary Care Practitioners*, Health & Housing Network, London.

Parkes, CM 1971, 'Psycho-social transitions: A field for study', *Social Science and Medicine*, vol. 5, pp. 101–15.

——1987, *Bereavement: Studies of Grief in Adult Life*, Penguin, Harmondsworth.

Parks, SH & Pilisuk, M 1991, 'Caregiver burden: Gender and the psychological costs of caregiving', *American Journal of Orthopsychiatry*, vol. 61, pp. 501–9.

Parmenter, G 2003, 'Describing visiting patterns in rural nursing homes', Paper presented at the Australian Association of Gerontology Rural Conference, Coffs Harbour, Australia.

Pearson, A, Nay, R, Koch, S & Ward, C 2002, 'Australian aged care nursing literature reviews' in *National Review of Nursing Education*, Commonwealth of Australia, Canberra.

Pearson, JL & Conwell, Y 1995, 'Suicide in late life: Challenges and opportunities for research', *International Psychogeriatrics*, vol. 7, pp. 131–6.

Peiper, R, Vaarama, M & Fozard, JL 2002, *Gerontechnology: Technology and Ageing—Starting into the Third Millennium*, Shaker Verlag, Aachen.

Penning, M 1998, 'In the middle: Parental caregiving in the context of other roles', *Journal of Gerontology: Social Sciences*, vol. 53, S188–97.

Penning, MJ, Chappell, NL, Stephenson, PH, Rosenblood, L & Tuokko, HA 1998, *Independence Among Older Adults with Disabilities: The Role of Formal Care Services, Informal Caregiving and Self-Care*, Final report submitted to the National Health Research and Development Program (NHRDP), Health Canada, University of Victoria, Centre on Aging, Victoria.

Percival, J 2001, 'Self-esteem and social motivation in age-segregated settings', *Housing Studies*, vol. 166, p. 827.

Perdue, CW & Gurtman, MB 1990, 'Evidence for the automaticity of ageism', *Journal of Experimental Social Psychology*, vol. 26, pp. 199–216.

Perreira, KM & Sloan, FA 2001, 'Life events and alcohol consumption among mature adults: A longitudinal analysis', *Journal of Studies on Alcohol*, vol. 62, pp. 501–8.

Perry, EK, Pickering, AT, Wang, WW, Houghton, PJ & Perry, NS 1999, 'Medicinal plants and Alzheimer's disease: From ethnobotany to phytotherapy', *Journal of Pharmacy and Pharmacology*, vol. 51, pp. 527–34.

Pfeiffer, E & Davis, G 1972, 'Determinants of sexual behavior in middle and old age', *Journal of the American Geriatric Society*, vol. 33, pp. 635–43.

Pfeiffer, E, Verwoerdt, A & Wang, H 1968, 'Sexual behavior in aged men and women: Observations on 254 community volunteers', *Archives of General Psychiatry*, vol. 19, pp. 753–8.

——1969, 'The natural history of sexual behavior in a biologically advantaged group of aged individuals', *Journal of Gerontology*, vol. 24, pp. 193–8.

Pfizer Inc. 2002, *Viagra (sildenafil citrate) tablets*, www.viagra.com (accessed 30 January 2003).

Philips, C, Zimmerman, D, Barnabei, R & Jonsson, R 1997, 'Using the resident assessment instrument for quality enhancement in nursing homes', *Age and Ageing*, vol. 26-S2, pp. 77–81.

Phillips, A 2002, *Equals*, Basic Books, London.

Phillipson, C, Bernard, M, Phillips, J & Ogg, J 2001, *The Family and Community Life of Older People: Social Networks and Social Support in Three Urban Areas*, Routledge, London.

Pieper, R 1994, 'The institutionalization of consultation on home adaptation for the elderly: Some lessons from Munich' in C Wild & A Kirschner (eds), *Safety-alarm Systems, Technical Aids and Smart Homes*, Akontes Publishing, Knegsel, NL.

Pifer, A & Bronte, L 1990, *Our Ageing Society*, WW Norton & Co., London.

Pinkowish, MD 2001, 'Complementary approaches to chronic pain', *Patient Care*, vol. 35, pp. 21–30.

Plassman, BL, Welsch, KA, Helms, BS, Brandt, J, Page, WF & Breitner, JCS 1995, 'Intelligence and education as predictors of cognitive state in late life', *Neurology*, vol. 45, pp. 1446–50.

Poon, L, Clayton, P, Martin, M, Johnson, B, Courtenay, A, Sweaney, S, Merriam, B, Pless, B & Thielman, S 1992, *The Georgia Centerarian Study*, Baywood Publishing, Amityville, NY.

Pot, AM, Deeg, DJH & Knipscheer, CPM 2001, 'Institutionalization of demented elderly: The role of caregiver characteristics', *International Journal of Geriatric Psychiatry*, vol. 16, pp. 273–80.

Potocky, M 1993, 'Effective services for bereaved spouses: A content analysis of the empirical literature', *Health and Social Work*, vol. 18, pp. 288–301.

Pragnell, M, Spence, L & Moore, R 2000, *The Market Potential for Smart Homes*, Joseph Rowntree Foundation, Findings, York, UK.

Prigerson, HG, Maciejewski, PK & Rosenheck, RA 2000, 'Preliminary explorations of the harmful interactive effects of widowhood and marital harmony on health, health service use, and health care costs', *Gerontologist*, vol. 40, pp. 99–108.

Prince, M 1997, 'The need for research on dementia in developing countries', *Tropical Medicine and International Health*, vol. 2, pp. 993–1000.

Proctor, R, Martin, C & Hewison, J 2002, 'When a little knowledge is a dangerous thing . . .: A study of carers' knowledge about dementia, preferred coping style and psychological distress', *International Journal of Geriatric Psychiatry*, vol. 17, pp. 1133–9.

Pruchno, RA 1990, 'Effects of help patterns on the mental health of spouse caregivers', *Research on Aging*, vol. 12, pp. 57–71.

Pynoos, J & Regnier, V 1997, 'Design directives in home adaptation' in S Lanspery & J Hyde (eds), *Staying Put: Adapting the Places Instead of the People*, Baywood Publishing, Amityville, NY.

Pynoos, J, Tabbarah, M, Angelelli, J & Demiere, M 1998, 'Improving the delivery of home modifications', *Technology & Disability*, vol. 8, pp. 3–14.

Queensland Department of Housing 2001, *Universal Housing Design*, Queensland Government, Brisbane.

Quick, HE & Moen, P 1998, 'Gender, employment, and retirement quality: A life course approach to the differential experiences of men and women', *Journal of Occupational Health Psychology*, vol. 3, pp. 44–64.

Quilgars, D 2000, *Low Intensity Support Services: A Systematic Literature Review*, Joseph Rowntree Foundation, Findings, York, UK.

Quinn, JF, Burkhauser, RV & Myers, DA 1990, *Passing the Torch: The Influence of Economic Incentives on Work and Retirement*, WE Upjohn Institute for Employment Research, Kalamazoo, Mich.

Rankin, ED, Haut, MW & Keefover, RW 2001, 'Current marital functioning as a mediating factor in depression among spouse caregivers in dementia', *Clinical Gerontologist*, vol. 23, pp. 27–44.

Rantanen, T & Avela, J 1997, 'Leg extension power and walking speed in very old people living independently', *Journal of Gerontology*, vol. 52A, pp. M325–31.

Ranzijn, E & Luszcz, MA 1994, 'Well-being of elderly Australians: The role of parent–adult child contacts', *Australian Journal on Ageing*, vol. 13, pp. 186–9.

Rauckhorst, L 2001, 'Integration of complementary and conventional health care in Alzheimer's disease and other dementias', *Nurse Practitioner Forum*, vol. 12, pp. 44–5.

Raynor, M 1997, 'Compliance with the DDA: Action planning your way to protection', *The Valuer and Land Economist*, November, pp. 670–3.

Reed, DM, Foley, DJ, White, LR, Heimovitz, H, Burchfeil, CM & Masaki, K 1998, 'Predictors of healthy ageing in men with high life expectancies', *American Journal of Public Health*, vol. 88, pp. 1463–8.

Regnier, V 1993, 'Design principles and research issues in housing for the elderly' in EJ Stern and RA Harootyan (eds), *Life-span Design of Residential Environments for an Ageing Population*, American Association for Retired Persons, Washington, DC.

Reis, MF, Gold, DP, Gauthier, S, Andrew, D & Markiewicz, D 1994, 'Personality traits as determinants of burden and health complaints in caregiving', *International Journal of Aging and Human Development*, vol. 39, pp. 257–71.

Remington, R 2002, 'Hand massage in the agitated elderly' in GJ Rich (ed.), *Massage Therapy: The Evidence for Practice*, Mosby, Edinburgh.

Renzetti, C, Iacono, S, Pinelli, M, Marri, L, Modugno, M & Neri, M 2001, 'Living with dementia: Is distress influenced by carer personality?', *Archives of Gerontology and Geriatrics*, Suppl. 7, pp. 333–40.

Resnick, B 2000, 'Promotion practices of the older adult', *Public Health Nursing*, vol. 17, pp. 160–8.

Ribbe, W, Ljunggren, G, Steel, K, Topinko, E, Hawes, C & Ikegami, N 1997, 'Nursing homes in 10 nations: A comparison between countries and settings', *Age and Ageing*, vol. 26-S2, pp. 3–12.

Richard, F & Richards, E 1912, *Ladies' Handbook of Home Treatment*, Signs Publishing, Melbourne.

Richards, D 2001, 'The remains of the day: Counselling older clients', *Counselling and Psychotherapy Journal*, vol. 12, pp. 10–14.

Riley, MW & Riley, JW 1994, 'Structural lag: Past and future' in MW Riley, RL Kahn & A Foner (eds), *Age and Structural Lag*, Wiley-Interscience, New York.

Riportella-Muller, R 1989, 'Sexuality in the elderly: A review', in K McKinney & S Sprecher (eds), *Human Sexuality: The Societal and Interpersonal Context*, Ablex Publishing Corporation, New Jersey.

Rivara, FP, Grossman, DC & Cummings, P 1997, 'Medical progress: injury prevention', *New England Journal of Medicine*, vol. 337, pp. 613–8.

Rix, S, Rosenman, L & Schulz, J 1999, 'International developments in social security privatization: What risk to women?' *Journal of Cross-Cultural Gerontology*, vol. 14, pp. 25–42.

Roberts, BL, Anthony, MK, Matejczyk, MB & Moore, D 1994, 'Relationship of social support to functional limitations, pain, and well-being among men and women', *Journal of Women and Aging*, vol. 6, pp. 3–19.

Robine, JM, Romieu, I & Cambois, E 1999, 'Health expectancy indicators', *Bulletin of the World Health Organization*, vol. 77, pp. 181–5.

Robinson, BE 1998, 'Depression', *Archives of the American Academy of Orthopaedic Surgeons*, vol. 2, pp. 33–7.

Robinson, P 1983, 'The sociological perspective', in R Weg (ed.) *Sexuality in the Later Years*, Academic Press, San Diego, CA.

Rogers, C 1961, *On Becoming a Person*, Houghton, Mifflin, Boston, MA.

Rogers, J, Grower, R & Supino, P 1992, 'Participant evaluation and cost of a community-based health promotion program for elders', *Public Health Reports*, vol. 107, pp. 417–57.

Rohan, E, Berkman, B, Walker, S & Holmes W. 1994, 'The geriatric oncology patient: Ageism in social work practice', *Journal of Gerontological Social Work*, vol. 23, pp. 201–21.

Rolands, C, Goodwin P & Fiebig, J 1989 *Residents' Rights in Nursing Homes and Hostels: Final Report*, Australian Government Publishing Service, Canberra.

Rook, KS & Pietromonaco, P 1987, 'Close relationships: Ties that heal or ties that bind?', in WH Jones & D Perlman (eds), *Advances in Personal Relationships*, JAI Press, Greenwich, CT.

Roos, NP & Haven, B 1991, 'Predictors of successful aging: A twelve-year study of Manitoba elderly', *American Journal of Public Health*, vol. 81, pp. 63–8.

Rosenkoetter, MM & Garris, JM 1998, 'Psychosocial changes following retirement', *Journal of Advanced Nursing*, vol. 27, pp. 966–76.

Rosenman, L 1996, 'Social security and women's changing patterns of work and retirement', *International Social Security Review*, vol. 4, pp. 5–24.

Rosenman, L & Le Broque, R 1996, 'The price of care: Interpersonal conflict at work and psychological outcomes: Testing a model among young workers' in *Towards a National Agenda for Carers: Workshop Papers*, Australian Government Publishing Service for the Department of Human Services and Health, Canberra.

Rosenman, L & Warburton, J 1997, 'Retirement policy, retirement incomes and women' in A Borowski, S Encel, E Ozanne (eds), *Ageing and Social Policy in Australia*, Cambridge University Press, Melbourne.

Rosenman, L, Warburton, J & Le Brocque, R 1996, 'Early retirement and women', Papers from the Early Retirement Seminar held by the Department of Social Security, Canberra.

Rosenmayr, L & Kockeis, E 1963, 'Propositions for a sociological theory of aging and the family', *International Social Science Journal*, vol. 15, pp. 410–26.

Rosenthal, CJ 1987, 'The comforter: Providing personal advice and emotional support to generations in the family', *Canadian Journal on Aging*, vol. 7, pp. 17–31.

Rosenthal, CJ, Martin-Matthews, A & Matthews, SH 1996, 'Caught in the middle? Occupancy in multiple roles and help to parents in a national probability sample of Canadian adults', *Journals of Gerontology*, vol. 51, S274–83.

Rossi, AS 1994, *Sexuality Across the Life Course*, The University of Chicago Press, Chicago.

Ross, L 1995, 'The spiritual dimension: Its importance to patients' health, well-being and quality of life and its implications for nursing practice', *International Journal of Nursing Studies*, vol. 32, pp. 457–68.

Rowe, JW & Khan, RL 1997, 'Successful aging', *Gerontologist*, vol. 37, pp. 433–40.
——1998, *Successful Aging*, Random House, New York.

Rowland, VT & Shoemake, A 1999, 'How experiences in a nursing home affect nursing students' perceptions of the elderly', *Educational Gerontology*, vol. 21, pp. 735–8.

Rowles, GD 2000, 'Habituation and being in place', *Occupational Therapy Journal of Research*, vol. 20, pp. 52S–67S.

Rubenstein, LZ & Nahas, R 1998, 'Primary and secondary prevention strategies in the older adult', *Geriatric Nursing*, vol. 19, pp. 11–17.

Russell, DW, Cutrona, CE, de la Mora, A & Wallace, RB 1997, 'Loneliness and nursing home admission among rural older adults', *Psychology and Aging*, vol. 12, pp. 574–89.

Ryan, E, Hummert, M & Boich, L 1995, 'Communication predicaments of aging: Patronizing behaviour towards older adults', *Journal of Language and Social Psychology*, vol. 14, pp. 144–66.

Ryff, C 1989, 'Happiness is everything, or is it? Explorations on the meaning of psychological well-being', *Journal of Personality and Social Psychology*, vol. 57, pp. 1069–81.

Ryff, C & Keyes, C 1995, 'The structure of psychological well-being', *Journal of Personality and Social Psychology*, vol. 69, pp. 719–27.

Sacco, RL 2001, 'Newer risk factors for stroke', *Neurology*, vol. 57, pp. S31–4.

Sachdev, PS, Brodaty, H & Looi, JC 1999, 'Vascular dementia: Diagnosis, management and possible prevention', *eMJA*, vol. 170, pp. 81–5.

Sackmann, A & Weymann, A 1994, *Die Technisierung des Alltags: Generationen und technische Innovationen'* (The Technicisation of Everyday Life: Generations and Technical Innovations), Campus, Frankfurt.

Sacks, O 1992, 'Hearing before the Senate Special Committee on aging', *Music Therapy Perspectives*, vol. 10, p. 60.

Sagawa, K 2002, 'Visual functions of older people and visibility of traffic signs', *Gerontechnology*, vol.1, pp. 296–9.

Salkeld, G, Cameron, I, Cumming, R, Seymour, J, Kurrle, S & Quine, S 2000, 'Quality of life related to fear of falling and hip fracture in older women: A time trade-off study', *British Medical Journal*, vol. 320, pp. 341–5.

Sallis, J, Bauman, A & Pratt, M 1998, 'Environmental and policy interventions to promote physical activity', *American Journal of Preventative Medicine*, vol. 154, pp. 379–97.

Sapey, B 1995, 'Disabling homes: A study of the housing needs of disabled people in Cornwall', *Disability and Society*, vol. 101, pp. 71–87.

Sawchuk, K 1995, 'From gloom to boom: Age, identify and target marketing' in M Featherstone & A Wernick (eds), *Images of Ageing: Cultural Representations of Later Life*, Routledge, London.

Schenk, D, Barbour, R, Dunn, W, Gordon, G, Grajeda, H, Guido, T, Hu, K, Huang, J, Johnson-Wood, K, Khan, K, Kholodenko, D, Lee, M, Liao, Z, Lieberberg, I, Motter, R, Mutter, L, Soriano, F, Shopp, G, Vasquez, N, Vandevert, C, Walker, S, Wogulis, M, Yednock, T, Games, D & Seubert, P 1999, 'Immunization with amyloid attenuates Alzheimer-disease-like pathology in the PDAPP mouse', *Nature*, vol. 400, pp. 173–7.

Scherer, P 2002, *Age of Withdrawal from the Labour Force in OECD Countries*, Organisation for Economic Cooperation and Development Occasional Paper No 49, OECD, Paris.

Schiavi, R & Rehman, J 1995, 'Sexuality and aging', *Urological Clinics of North America*, vol. 22, pp. 711–26.

Schiavi, R 1999, *Aging and Male Sexuality*, Cambridge University Press, Cambridge.

Schlossberg, NK 1984, *Counseling Adults in Transition: Linking Practice with Theory*, Springer, New York.

Schmidt, B 2002, *Minnesota Housing Partnership Evaluation of Continuum of Care Support*, http://www.mhponline.org/sidebar/continuumofcare2.htm (accessed June 2004).

Schofield, H, Bloch, S, Herrman, H, Murphy, B, Nankervis, J & Singh, B 1998, *Family Caregivers: Disability, Illness and Ageing*, Allen & Unwin, Sydney.

Schulz, R & Williamson, GM 1991, 'Two-year longitudinal study of depression among Alzheimer's caregivers', *Psychology and Aging*, vol. 6, pp. 569–78.

Schulz, R, Beach, SR, Lind, B, Martire, LM, Zdaniuk, B, Hirsch, C, Jackson, S & Burton, L 2001, 'Involvement in caregiving and adjustment to death of a spouse: Findings from the caregiver health effects study', *Journal of the American Medical Association*, vol. 285, pp. 3123–9.

Schulz, R, O'Brien, A, Czaja, S, Ory, M, Norris, R, Martire, LM, Belle, SH, Burgio, L, Gitlin, L & Coon, D 2002, 'Dementia caregiver intervention research: In search of clinical significance', *Gerontologist*, vol. 42, pp. 589–602.

Schut, HAW, Stroebe, MS & van den Bout, J 1997, 'Intervention for the bereaved: Gender differences in the efficacy of two counselling programmes', *British Journal of Clinical Psychology*, vol. 36, pp. 63–72.

Scott, A 2004, 'Age shall not weary them', *The Daily Examiner*, 13 March, p. 6.

Scott, PA 2002, 'The older worker: Physical and mental attributes essential to retain a viable position in the workplace', *Gerontechnology*, vol. 2, pp. 55–9.

Scott, T, Minichiello, V & Browning, C 1998, 'Secondary school students' knowledge of and attitudes towards older people: Does an education intervention programme make a difference?', *Ageing and Society*, vol. 18, pp. 167–83.

Seccombe, K & Lee, GR 1986, 'Gender differences in retirement satisfaction and its antecedents', *Research on Aging*, vol. 8, pp. 426–40.

Seeman, T, Bruce, M & McAvay, G.1996, 'Social network characteristics and onset of ADL disability: MacArthur studies of successful aging', *Journal of Gerontology*, vol. 51, pp. S191–200.

Shanks-McElroy, HA & Strobino, J 2001, 'Male caregivers of spouses with Alzheimer's disease: Risk factors and health status', *American Journal of Alzheimer's Disease*, vol. 16, pp. 167–75.

Sharpley, CF & Layton, R 1998, 'Effects of age of retirement, reason for retirement, and pre-retirement training on psychological and physical health during retirement', *Australian Psychologist*, vol. 33, pp. 119–24.

Sharps, MJ, Pricesharps, JL & Hanson, L 1998, 'Attitudes of young adults towards older adults', *Educational Gerontology*, vol. 24, pp. 655–60.

Shaw, WS, Patterson, TL, Semple, S & Grant, I 1998, 'Health and well-being in retirement: a summary of theories and their implications' in MHVB Hasselt (ed.), *Handbook of Clinical Geropsychology*, Plenum Press, New York.

Shield, R & Aronson, S 2003, *Aging in Today's World*, Bergmann Books, New York.

Sidoti, C 1997, *Report of Inquiry into Complaints of Discrimination in Employment and Occupation: Redundancy Arrangements and Age Discrimination*, Australian Human Rights and Equal Opportunity Commission, Sydney.

Slade, G 1997, 'Derivation and validation of a short-form oral health impact profile', *Community Dentistry and Oral Epidemiology*, vol. 25, pp. 284–90.

Slater, R 1995, *The Psychology of Growing Old: Looking Forward*, Open University Press, Buckingham.

Smith, A, Rissel, C, Richters, J, Grulich, A & deVisser, R 2003, 'Sex in Australia: Reflections and recommendations', *Australian and New Zealand Journal of Public Health*, vol. 27, pp. 251–6.

Smola, S, Justice, AC, Wagner, J, Rabeneck, L, Weissman, S & Rodriguez-Barradas, M 2001, 'The VACS 3 Project Team: Veterans aging cohort three-site study (VACS 3)', *Journal of Clinical Epidemiology*, vol. 54, pp. S61–76.

Snijders, MCL, Koren, LGH, Kort, HSM & van Bronswijk, JEMH 2001, 'Clean outdoor air increases physical independence: A pilot study', *Gerontechnology*, vol. 1, pp. 124–7.

Snowdon, D 2001, *Aging with Grace*, Bantom Dell Publishing Group, Random House Inc., New York.

Snyder, E & Spreitzer, E 1976, 'Attitudes of the aged towards non-traditional sexual behaviour', *Archives of Sexual Behavior*, vol. 5, pp. 249–54.

Solem, PE 1987, 'Mortality during the first five years after reaching retirement age' in L Levi (ed.), *Society, Stress, and Disease*, Oxford University Press, New York.

Solomon, LJ, Mickey, RM, Rairikar, CJ, Worden, J & Flynn, BS 1998, 'Three-year prospective adherence to three breast cancer screening modalities', *Preventive Medicine*, vol. 27, pp. 781–6.

Somerville, M 2002, 'Learning potentials and limitations under globalisation in aged care workplaces', *International Journal of Workplace Learning*, vol. 14, pp. 68–76.

SoRelle, R 1998, 'Vascular and lipid syndromes in selected HIV-infected patients', *Circulation*, vol. 98, pp. 829–30.

Sorensen, S, Pinquart, M & Duberstein, P 2002, 'How effective are interventions with caregivers? An updated meta-analysis', *American Journal of Geriatric Psychiatry*, vol. 10, pp. 407–16.

Sprenkle, DG 1999, 'Therapeutic issues and strategies in group therapy with older men' in M Duffy (ed.), *Handbook of Counselling and Psychotherapy with Adults*, John Wiley & Sons Inc, Rochester.

Standards and Accreditation Agency 2001, *The Standard*, vol. 3, p. 1.

Standards Australia and Standards New Zealand 1994, *Quality Systems—Model for Quality Assurance in Production, Installation and Servicing*, AS/NZS ISO 9002, Homebush, Australia.

Statistics Canada 2002, *Profile of the Canadian Population by Aged and Sex: Canada Ages*, Report Number 96F0030XIE2001002, Government of Canada, Ottawa.

Stead, A, Winbush, E, Eadie, D & Teer, P 1997, 'A qualitative study of older people's perceptions of ageing exercise: The implications for health promotion', *Health Education Journal*, vol. 56, pp. 3–16.

Steenbekkers, LPA & van Beijsterveldt, CEM 1998, *Design-relevant Characteristics of Ageing Users*, Delft University Press, Delft, NL.

Stegner, W 1976, *The Spectator Bird*, Doubleday, New York.

Steinbach, U 1992, 'Social networks, institutionalization and mortality among elderly people in the United States', *Journal of Gerontology*, vol. 47, pp. S183–90.

Steinke, E 1994, 'Knowledge and attitudes of older adults about sexuality in aging: A comparison of two studies', *Journal of Advanced Nursing*, vol. 19, pp. 477–85.

Steptoe, A, Wardle, J, Fuller, R, Holte, A, Justo, J, Sanderman, R & Wichstrom, L 1997, 'Leisure-time physical exercise: Prevalence, attitudinal correlates, and behavioural correlates among young Europeans from 21 countries', *Preventative Medicine*, vol. 26, pp. 845–54.

Stevens, J 2003, 'The ennursement of old age in NSW: A history of nursing and the care of older people between white settlement and federation', *Collegian*, vol. 10, pp. 19–24.

Stewart, AL, Shelbourne, CD & Brod, M 1996, 'Measuring health related quality of life in older and demented populations' in B Spiker (ed.), *Quality of Life and Pharmacoeconomics in Clinical Trials*, Lippincott-Raven, Philadelphia.

Stewart, J, Harris, J & Sapey, B 1999, 'Disability and dependency: Origins and futures of "special needs" housing for disabled people', *Disability & Society*, vol. 141, pp. 5–20.

Strain, LA & Chappell, NL 1982, 'Confidants—do they make a difference in quality of life', *Research on Aging*, vol. 4, pp. 479–502.

——1985, 'Measuring choice of care: When is an interview technique adequate?' *Canadian Association on Gerontology*, Hamilton, Ontario.

Prime Minister's Science, Engineering and Innovations Council 2003, *Promoting Healthy Ageing in Australia*, retrieved July 2003, from http://www.dest.gov.au/science/pmseic/documents/promoting healthy ageing report.doc

Strawbridge, WJ, Cohen, RD, Shema, S & Kaplan, GA 1996, 'Successful aging: Predictors and associated activities', *American Journal of Epidemiology*, vol. 144, pp. 135–41.

Streib, GF 1987, 'Old age in sociocultural context: China and the United States', *Journal of Aging Studies*, vol. 1, pp. 95–112.

Strombeck, R 2003, 'Finding sex partners on-line: A new high-risk practice among older adults', *Journal of Acquired Immune Deficiency Syndrome*, vol. 33, pp. 5225–8.

Struyk, RJ & Katsura, HM 1988, *Ageing at Home: How the Elderly Adjust Their Housing Without Moving*, Haworth Press, New York.

Stull, DE, Kosloski, K & Kercher, K 1994, 'Caregiver burden and generic well-being: Opposite sides of the same coin?', *Gerontologist*, vol. 34, pp. 88–94.

Sun Herald, The 2003, 'Sex no problem after all', 19 January, p. 27.

Tame, D 1984, *The Secret Power of Music: The Transformation of Self and Society Through Musical Energy*, Destiny Books, Rochester, NY.

Tamura, T, Yoshimura, T, Nagaya, M & Chihara, K 2002, 'A fall analysis system', *Gerontechnology*, vol. 2, p. 149.

Taylor, RJ, Morrell, SL, Mamoon, HA & Wain, GV 2001, 'Effects of screening on cervical cancer incidence and mortality in New South Wales implied by influences of period of diagnosis and birth cohort', *Journal of Epidemiology and Community Health*, vol. 55, pp. 782–8.

Tebb, SS 1995, 'Aid to empowerment: A caregiver well-being scale', *Health and Social Work*, vol. 20, pp. 87–92.

Tennstedt, SL, McKinlay, JB & Sullivan, LM 1989, 'Informal care for frail elders: The role of secondary caregivers', *The Geronotologist*, vol. 29, pp. 677–83.

Thomson, N 2003, *The Health of Indigenous Australians*, Oxford University Press, Melbourne.

Tilley, J & Wiener, J 2001, *Consumer Directed Home and Community Services: Policy Issues*, The Urban Institute, Occasional Paper no. 44, Washington, DC.

Tinnion, J & Rothman, G 1999, 'Retirement income adequacy and the emerging super system: New estimates', *The Seventh Colloquium of Superannuation Researchers*, University of Melbourne, Melbourne.

Tirrito, T 2003, *Aging in the New Millennium: A Global View*, University of South Carolina, Columbia, SC.

Townsend, P 1957, *The Family Life of Old People: An Enquiry in East London*, Penguin, Harmondsworth.

Trepanier, L, Baillargeon, J & Bouffard, L 2001, 'Tenacity and flexibility in the pursuit of personal goals: Impact of retirement and well-being', *Canadian Journal on Aging*, vol. 20, pp. 557–76.

Tucak, L 2002, 'New love drug easy on the heart', *The Australian*, 22 April.

Turkoski, B, Pierce, LL, Schreck, S, Salter, J, Radziewicz, R, Guhde, J & Brady, R 1997, 'Clinical nursing judgement related to reducing the incidence of falls by elderly patients', *Rehabilitation Nursing*, vol. 22, pp. 124–30.

Turner, B & Adams, C 1988, 'Reported change in preferred sexual activity over the adult years', *Journal of Sex Research*, vol. 25, pp. 289–303.

UK Department for Work and Pensions 2002, 'Simplicity and choice: Work and savings for retirement', *Green Paper*, UK Government, London.

Umberson, D, Wortman, CB & Kessler, RC 1992, 'Widowhood and depression: Explaining long-term gender differences in vulnerability', *Journal of Health and Social Behavior*, vol. 33, pp. 10–24.

United Kingdom 2001, *Our Healthy Nation*, http:www.ohn.gov.uk/ohn (accessed 19 February 2004).

US National Academy on an Aging Society 1999, 'Public Policy and Aging Report', vol. 9, no. 4, The Gerontological Society of America, Washington.

US Preventive Service Taskforce (USPSTF) 2002, 'Screening for breast cancer: Recommendations and rationale', *American Family Physician*, vol. 65, pp. 2537–44.

Utz, RL, Carr, D, Nesse, R & Wortman, CB 2002, 'Effect of widowhood on older adults' social participation: An evaluation of activity, disengagement, and continuity theories', *Gerontologist*, vol. 42, pp. 522–33.

Vacha, K 1985, *Quiet Fire: Memoirs of Older Gay Men*, The Vrossing Press, Trumansburg, NY.

Vaillant, G 2002, *Aging Well*, Little, Brown & Company, Boston, MA.

van Berlo, A 2002, 'Smart home technology: Have older people paved the way?', *Gerontechnology*, vol. 2, pp. 77–87.

van Bronswijk, JEMH, Bouma, H & Fozard, JL 2003, 'Linking the impacts of technology to its areas of application that most affect quality of life', *Gerontechnology*, vol. 2, pp. 169–72.

Van der Rit, P 1993, 'Effects of therapeutic massage on pre-operative anxiety in a rural hospital: Part 1', *The Australian Journal of Rural Health*, vol. 9, pp. 11–16.

Ventura, MR, Young, DE, Feldman, MJ, Pastore, P, Pikula, S & Yates, MA 1984, 'Effectiveness of health promotion interventions', *Nursing Research*, vol. 33, pp. 162–97.

Verbrugge, LM 1979, 'Marital status and health', *Journal of Marriage and the Family*, vol. 41, pp. 267–85.

Verbrugge, LM & Jette, AM 1994, 'The disablement process', *Social Science and Medicine*, vol. 38, pp. 1–14.

Vickers, A 2000, 'Complementary medicine', *British Medical Journal*, vol. 321, pp. 683–9.

Vickers, A & Zollman, C 1999, 'Herbal medicine', *British Medical Journal*, vol. 319, pp. 1050–3.

Vikstrom, A 2003, *Towards an Access Standard for Housing Within the Building Code of Australia*, Discussion paper, Australian Network for Universal Housing Design, Sydney.

Vincent, C & Furnham, A 1996, 'Why do patients turn to complementary medicine? An empirical study', *British Journal of Clinical Psychology*, vol. 35, pp. 37–48.

Vitaliano, PP, Russo, J, Young, HM, Teri, L & Maiuro, RD 1991, 'Predictors of burden in spouse caregivers of individuals with Alzheimer's disease', *Psychology and Aging*, vol. 6, pp. 392–402.

von Faber, M, Wiel, ABD, Exel, E, Gussekloo, J, Lagaay, AM, Dongen, EV, Knook, DL, Geest, SVDG & Westendorp, RGJ 2001, 'Successful aging in the oldest old: Who can be characterized as successfully aged?', *Archives of Internal Medicine*, vol. 161, pp. 2694–700.

Walker, N 1997, 'Wellness for elders' in B Spradley & J Allender (eds), *Readings in Community Health Nursing*, MacLennan & Petty, Sydney, pp. 459–67.

Walker, A & Maltby, T 1997, *Ageing Europe*, Open University Press, Buckingham.

Walker, A & Minichiello, V 1996, 'Emerging issues in sociological thinking, research and teaching' in V Minichiello, N Chappell, H Kendig & A Walker (eds), *Sociology of Aging: International Perspectives*, ISA, Melbourne.

Walker, M, Orrell, M, Manela, M, Livingston, G & Katona, C 1998, 'Do health and use of services differ in residents of sheltered accommodation? A pilot study', *International Journal of Geriatric Psychiatry*, vol. 139, pp. 617–24.

Walker, A, Walker, C & Ryan, T 1996, 'Older people with learning difficulties leaving institutional care: A case of double jeopardy', *Ageing and Society*, vol. 16, pp. 125–50.

Walker-Bone, K, Jaraid, K, Arden, N & Cooper, C 2000, 'Medical management of osteoarthritis', *British Medical Journal*, vol. 321, pp. 936–40.

Ware, J, Kosinski, M & Keller, S 1995, *SF-12: How to Score the SF-12 Physical and Mental Health Summary Scales*, The Health Institute, New England Medical Center, Boston, MA.

——1996, 'A 12-item Short Form Survey: Construction of scales and preliminary test of reliability and validity', *Medical Care*, vol. 34, pp. 220–33.

Watson, E & Mears, J 1996, 'Stretched lives: Working in paid employment and caring for elderly relatives', *Australian Institute of Family Studies: Family Matters*, vol. 45, pp. 5–9.

Watson, P 1990, 'The Americans with Disabilities Act: More rights for people with disabilities', *Rehabilitation Nursing*, vol. 156, pp. 325–8.

Wells, Y 1996, 'Older people as care-providers: Costs and benefits', Paper presented at the International Association of Gerontology, Adelaide, Australia.

Wells, YD & Kendig, HL 1997, 'Health and well-being of spouse caregivers and the widowed', *Gerontologist*, vol. 37, pp. 666–74.

——1999, 'Psychological resources and successful retirement', *Australian Psychologist*, vol. 34, pp. 111–5.

Wenger, GC, Davies, R, Shahtahmasebi, S & Scott, A 1996, 'Social isolation and loneliness in old age: Review and model refinement', *Ageing and Society*, vol. 16, pp. 333–58.

Wenger, GC, Scott, A & Patterson, N 2000, 'How important is parenthood? Childlessness and support in old age in England', *Ageing and Society*, vol. 20, pp. 161–82.

Wetzel, MS, Eisenberg, DM & Kaptchuk, TJ 1998, 'Courses involving complementary and alternative medicine at US medical schools', *Journal of the American Medical Association*, vol. 280, pp. 784–7.

Whetstone, LM, Fozard, JL, Metter, EJ, Hiscock, BS, Burke, R, Gittings, NE & Fried, LP 2001, 'The Physical Functioning Inventory: A procedure for assessing physical function in adults', *Journal of Ageing and Health*, vol. 13, pp. 467–93.

White, C 1982, 'Sexual interest, attitudes, knowledge and sexual history in relation to sexual behavior in the institutionalized aged', *Archives of Sexual Behavior*, vol. 11, pp. 11–21.

White, C & Catania, J 1982, 'Psychoeducational intervention for sexuality with the aged, family members of the aged, and people who work with the aged', *International Journal of Aging and Human Development*, vol. 15, pp. 121–38.

Whitlock, G, MacMahon, S, Anderson, C, Neal, B, Rodgers, A & Chalmers, J 1997, 'Blood pressure for the prevention of cognitive decline with cognitive disease', *Clinical Hypertension*, vol. 19, pp. 843–55.

WHO. *See* World Health Organization.

Wild, C & Kirschner, A 1994, *Safety-alarm Systems, Technical Aids and Smart Homes*, Akontes Publishing, Knegsel, NL.

Williamson, GM & Shaffer, DR 2001, 'Relationship quality and potentially harmful behaviors by spousal caregivers: How we were then, how we are now', *Psychology and Aging*, vol. 16, pp. 217–26.

Wilson, DR 1998, 'Evolutionary epidemiology and manic depression', *British Journal of Medical Psychology*, vol. 71, pp. 375–95.

Wister, AV 1989, 'Environmental adaptation by persons in their later life', *Research on Aging*, vol. 113, pp. 267–91.

Withers, G 1994, *Australia's Ageing Society*, Economic Planning Advisory Council, Background Paper no. 37, Foreword, Australian Government Publishing Service, Canberra.

Woelk, H 2000, 'Comparison of St John's Wort and imipramine for treating depression: randomised controlled trial', *British Medical Journal*, vol. 321, pp. 536–9.

Wolcott, I 1998, *Families in Later Life: Dimensions of Retirement*, Australian Institute of Family Studies, Melbourne.

Wolcott, I & Glezer, H 1999, 'Older workers, families and public policies', *Family Matters*, vol. 53, pp. 77–81.

Wolf, SL, Sattin, RW, O'Grady, M, Freret, N, Ricci, L, Greenspan, AI, Xu, T & Kutner, M 2001, 'A study design to investigate the effect of intense Tai Chi in reducing falls among older adults transitioning to frailty', *Controlled Clinical Trials*, vol. 22, pp. 689–704.

Woolf, L 2003, *Gay and Lesbian Aging*, www.webster.edu/~woolfim/oldergay.html

Woolfe, R & Briggs, S 1997, 'Counselling older adults: Issues and awareness', *Counselling Psychology Quarterly*, vol. 10, pp. 1989–94.

World Health Organization 1988, *Global Medium-Term Programme, Programme 9.5, Health of the Elderly*, WHO HEE/MTP/88, WHO, Geneva.

——1997, *Jakarta Declaration on Leading Health Promotion into the 21st Century*, from http://www.who.int/hpr/NPH/docs/JakartaDeclarationEnglish.pdf

——1998a, *Statement Developed by WHO Quality of Life Working Group*, WHO Health Promotion Glossary 1998, WHO/HPR/HEP/98.1, WHO, Geneva.

——1998b, *Growing Older—Staying Well: Ageing and Physical Activity in Everyday Life*, WHO/HPR/AHE/98.1, WHO, Geneva.

——1999, *A life Course Perspective of Maintaining Independence in Older Age*, WHO/HSC/99.2, WHO, Geneva.

——2000, *The World Health Report 2000: Health Systems: Improving Performance*, WHO, Geneva.

——2001, *Men, Ageing and Health: Achieving Health across the Lifespan*, Pub. no. 01WHO/NHM/NPH/01.2, WHO, Geneva.

——2002, *Active Ageing: A Policy Framework*, WHO, Geneva.

——2002, *Policy Response Contained in Active Ageing: A Policy Framework*, www.who.int/hpr/ageing (accessed, 9 April, 2002).

World Health Organization/International Network for the Prevention of Elder Abuse [INPEA] 2002, *Missing Voices of Older Persons on Elder Abuse*, WHO, Geneva.

Worthington, D 1998, *A Research Report on a National Strategy for an Aging Australia and the 1999 International Year of Older Persons (Quantitative Second Stage)*, Prepared for the Office for the Aged, Department of Health and Family Services, Canberra.

Wortman, CB & Conway, TL 1985, 'The role of social support in adaptation and recovery from physical illness' in S Cohen & SL Syme (eds), *Social Support and Health*, Academic Press, Orlando, FL.

Wortman, CB & Silver, RC 1990, 'Successful mastery of bereavement and widowhood: A life-course perspective', in P Baltes & M Baltes (eds), *Successful Aging: Perspectives from the Behavioral Sciences*, Cambridge University Press, Cambridge, England.

Wright, LK 1991, 'The impact of Alzheimer's disease on the marital relationship', *Gerontologist*, vol. 31, pp. 224–37.

Wright, PR 2002, 'Playing "betwixt" and "between" learning and healing: Playback theatre for a troubled world' in B Rasmussen & A Ostern (eds), *The IDEA Dialogues 2001*, International Drama Education Association, Bergen.

Wylde, M 1998, 'Consumer knowledge of home modifications', *Technology and Disability*, vol. 8, pp. 51–68.

Xia, C & Ma, F 1995, 'The impact of the number of children on family support for the elderly', *Population Research*, vol. 19, pp. 10–16.

Yamamoto, K 1994, 'Revision of nursing curricula in Japan to meet the needs of an ageing society', *Educational Gerontology*, vol. 20, pp. 495–502.

Yamamoto, N & Wallhagen, MI 1998, 'Service use by family caregivers in Japan', *Social Science and Medicine*, vol. 47, pp. 677–91.

Yates, PM, Beadle, G, Clavarino, A, Najman, JM, Thompson, D, Williams, G, Kenny, L, Roberts, S, Mason, B & Schlect, D 1993, 'Patients with terminal cancer who use alternative therapies: Their beliefs and practices', *Sociology of Health and Illness*, vol. 15, pp. 198–216.

Yoshimura T, Nakajima, K & Tamura, T 2002, 'An ambulatory fall monitoring system for the elderly' in R Pieper, M Vaarama & JL Fozard (eds), *Gerontechnology: Technology and Ageing Starting into the Third Millennium*, Shaker Verlag, Aachen.

Young, K 1996, 'Health, health promotion and the elderly', *Journal of Clinical Nursing*, vol. 5, pp. 241–8.

Young, MG 2000, 'Chronic pain management in the elderly', *Patient Care*, vol. 34, pp. 31–40.

Zarit, SH & Zarit, JM 1983, *The Burden Interview*, Ethel Percy Andrus Gerontology Center, Los Angeles.

Zashin, SJ 2000, 'Complementary and alternative therapies for arthritis: Science or fiction?', *The Journal of Musculoskeletal Medicine*, vol. 17, pp. 330–45.

Zeiss, M & Kasel-Godley, J 2001, 'Sexuality in older adults' relationships', *Generations*, vol. 25, pp. 128–5.

Zhao, L, Tatara, K, Kuroda, K & Takayama, Y 1993, 'Mortality of frail elderly people living at home in relation to housing conditions', *Journal of Epidemiology & Community Health*, vol. 474, pp. 298–302.

Zhu, X, Kitano, H, Chi, I, Lubben, JE, Berkanovic, E & Zhang, C 1994, 'Living arrangements and family support of the elderly in Beijing', in GH Stopp (ed.), *International Perspectives on Healthcare for the Elderly*, Peter Lang, New York.

Zimmerman, DR, Karon, SL, Arling, G, Clark, RN, Sanforth, F & Ross, R 1995, 'Developing and testing of nursing home quality indicators', *Health Care Financial Review*, vol. 16, pp. 107–27.

Zollman, C & Vickers, A 1999, 'What is complementary medicine?', *British Medical Journal*, vol. 319, pp. 693–6.

Index

Printed in the United States
by Baker & Taylor Publisher Services

Printed in the United States
by Baker & Taylor Publisher Services